DISTRICT NURSING
Second Edition

DISTRICT NURSING

SECOND EDITION

Monica E. Baly

PhD, BA(Hons), SRN, SCM, HVCert, FRCN
Researcher in the History of the Queen's Nursing Institute

Barbara M. Robottom

MSc, BA, SRN, RSCN, QN, RNT, CHNTCert
Professional Adviser (District Nursing), English National Board for Nursing, Midwifery and Health Visiting, London

June M. Clark

PhD, RGN, RHV, FRCN
Director of Nursing (Community), West Lambeth Health Authority, London

HEINEMANN NURSING

Heinemann Nursing
An imprint of Heinemann Professional Publishing Ltd
Halley Court, Jordan Hill, Oxford OX2 8EJ

OXFORD   LONDON   SINGAPORE
NAIROBI   IBADAN   KINGSTON

First published as *A New Approach to District Nursing* 1981
Reprinted 1983, 1984, 1986
Second edition 1987
Reprinted 1988

British Library Cataloguing in Publication Data
Baly, Monica E.
    District nursing.—2nd ed.
    1. Community health nursing—Great Britain
    I. Title   II. Robottom, Barbara M.
    III. Clark, June   IV. A New approach to
    district nursing
    610.73'43'0941   RT98

ISBN 0 433 01163 7

Typeset D.P. Media Limited, Hitchin, Herts
Printed and bound in Great Britain by
Biddles Limited, Guildford and King's Lynn

Contents

Acknowledgements   vii
Foreword   viii
Preface   ix

Section I: Background to care

1. Patients are people   3
2. The world we live in   8
3. People as individuals   34
4. People in groups   56
5. The primary care setting   77

Section II: Approaches to care

6. The nature of district nursing   101
7. Assessment of need   112
8. Planning care   133
9. Implementation   146
10. Evaluating care   170

Section III: Special needs

11. Sick children   189
12. Handicap and disability   196
13. Mental illness   209
14. Acute and chronic illness   218
15. Elderly people   228
16. Terminal care   243

Section IV: Policies for care

17. Financing the health and social services   259
18. The development of the National Health Service   273

19. The social services   291
20. Policies for nursing   ·311

Section V: The professional district nurse

21. The development of district nursing   333
22. Ethical and legal considerations   346

Appendices

1. UKCC code of professional practice   371
2. Guide to health and social services   373
3. Guide to voluntary organisations   388
4. Guide to social security and other financial benefits   395
5. A synoptic history of district nursing   396
6. Curriculum in district nursing   400
7. Selected relevant official reports and related legislation   407

Index   409

District Nursing is essentially the work of a team; each contributor has learnt from and borrowed from the others. At times material has changed its section regardless of authorship. However, responsibility is primarily as follows:

Chapters 1, 2, 3, 4, 5, 12 and Appendices 3 and 4   June Clark

Chapters 6, 7, 8, 9, 10, 11, 14, 15 and 16   Barabara Robottom

Chapters 13, 17, 18, 19, 20, 21, 22
    and Appendices 5 and 7   Monica Baly

Acknowledgements

The authors of *District Nursing* would like to acknowledge the help given by many people in the preparation of the first edition, and to thank the many district nurse tutors, and district nurses themselves, who responded to the questionnaire which was sent out by William Heinemann Medical Books and organised by Miss Cathy Watson, whom we thank for her help and advice.

Our thanks are also due to Miss Alison Bramley, the librarian of the Royal College of Nursing, for help with updating material and suggestions for further reading. Miss Robottom wishes to thank Mrs Dorothy Jones OBE, formerly Nursing Officer at the Department of Health and Social Security, for her continued help and interest. Dr Baly thanks Miss Val Cowie, Director of the Labour Relations and Legal Department of the Royal College of Nursing, for reading Chapter 22 and for her helpful suggestions, and members of the Primary Health Care Society for their help and interest. Our gratitude is also due to the Office of Health Economics for supplying information, for updating our statistics and for producing new charts.

Finally, our thanks go to William Heinemann Medical Books for their help and encouragement in what has been an over-long gestation period, during which events relating to district nursing changed as we wrote.

MEB, JMC, BMR, 1987

Foreword

The first edition of this work has proved to be a useful resource for students and practitioners of district nursing. Since its publication in 1981, there have been significant changes in the managerial context in which district nursing contributes to the National Health Service, in the statutory regulation of district nursing through the National Boards, the UKCC and the epidemiological and social trends to which district nursing has responded. Further changes are envisaged with the recommendations of the Cumberlege report and Project 2000 (UKCC). This second edition has taken all these factors into account and there has been considerable up-dating of the text and reference material.

The importance of primary health care has been emphasised by the WHO declaration of Alma Ata. In achieving the aims of 'health for all', the district nursing service plays a crucial role. Unless the district nurse is adequately prepared and her function supported by knowledge, her vital contribution may be eroded.

This popular and authoritative book is a compendium of much of the knowledge needed for practice by district nurses. It sets district nursing in the context of social policies for care, surveys various approaches and examines the needs of special groups for whom the district nurse is responsible. It stresses the importance of the individual within the group, and the authors illustrate examples of everyday problems with reference to representative patients and their families. This serves to give flesh and blood to the bones of knowledge.

Monica Baly, Barbara Robottom and June Clark are all leaders in the profession, and the high standards they set will ensure that this book remains a classic.

McFarlane of Llandaff, 1987

Preface

Never has the aphorism 'half that which you teach your students today will be out of date in five years; the trouble is you do not know which half' been more clearly demonstrated. In the five years since the first edition of this book, ideas about the nursing process have changed. What was a pioneer concept is now accepted practice, and there have been many modifications. This is as it should be: advances are made by research and experimentation.

Aware of the many developments in the practice of district nursing and new proposals for the education of district nurses, and warned by the dangers of today's *avant garde* being tomorrow's out of date, we have tried to keep principles and avoid the minutiae of the latest concept; district nurses will read these for themselves in their professional journals.

Before preparing this second edition of *District Nursing* the authors sought the advice of the main users of the book through a questionnaire. Our thanks are due to the many tutors and district nurses who have helped us in the preparation of this second edition; that we could not include all the suggestions is not due to wilfulness but to the fact that it is not possible to encompass everything a district nurse might want to know within one medium-sized text book.

MEB, BMR, JMC, 1987

Background to Care

'Unless the nurse can appreciate the psychological, emotional, spiritual and social needs of her patients and their families, in addition to the physical needs, her assessment of the nursing aspects could be suspect'.

Panel of Assessors: *Report on the Education and Training of the District Nurse* (1976)

District nursing is concerned with people in their normal social setting, in their own homes, with their families. The social circumstances are as varied as the individuals themselves, but these circumstances have considerable significance for their health and nursing needs, the way in which they are managed, and the way in which the nurse can respond. The five chapters in Section I describe the context in which district nursing is practised—the physical and social environments in which both nurse and patient live and the organisational setting which provides the framework for the delivery of care.

Chapter 1

Patients are People

Mr Adams

Mr Adams, who is 85 years old, had a cerebrovascular accident 2 years ago. He now has a right-sided hemiplegia, is incontinent of urine and faeces, his speech is slurred, and he is very confused. He is cared for by his elderly wife, whose mobility is becoming increasingly limited by arthritis.

The couple's only son was killed in France in 1944; a rather faded photo of a handsome young soldier standing between his smiling parents still has pride of place on the mantlepiece. Mr Adams was the youngest of four brothers, all of whom are now dead, and apart from a nephew and niece with whom he lost contact many years ago, he has no other relatives. Mrs Adams has a younger sister, but she lives more than a hundred miles away and so they rarely see each other.

They live in a terraced cottage in a small village. The house has not been modernised, so the only heating is by open fires, supplemented when necessary with a paraffin heater. There is no bathroom, and only an outside toilet.

Mr Adams is cared for in a living room, which, in addition to the large double bed contains a comfortable clutter of rather old-fashioned furniture. Mrs Adams rarely goes further afield than the village post office where she does most of her shopping, especially since the bus service to the nearest town was stopped some months ago.

Mrs Baker

Mrs Baker, who is 48, lives with her three children (girls of 17 and 12, and a boy of 14), her marriage having broken up about 6 years ago. Her husband has since remarried, and never visits now. The eldest girl, Sarah, is staying at home from work to care for her mother, who has carcinoma of the liver and is now in the terminal stages of her illness.

They live in a modern semidetached house on a suburban housing estate. The neighbours are kind and willing to help, but most of them are at work all day.

Mrs Baker obviously used to take a pride in her house but it is now showing signs of neglect, Sarah does her best, but without much help from her younger brother and sister; Paul spends very little time at home and Angela seems continually immersed in her school work.

Mrs Baker is aware of her prognosis, but she has not shared the knowledge with her children, although she suspects that Sarah guesses the truth. Each morning Mrs Baker dresses herself carefully and comes downstairs. She spends most of the day 'resting' on the settee in the living room. At present her pain is well-controlled and this has helped her to avoid showing the seriousness of her condition to the two younger children and to visitors.

Mrs Cray

Mrs Cray is a 68-year-old widow who lives alone in a flat on the fourth floor of a high-rise block of flats in a big city. She is obese and has varicose ulcers of both legs. She also has mild diabetes which is controlled by diet and drugs. She is not very mobile and is inclined to sit by an electric fire most of the day. She has not been out of the flat for a long time—saying that if the lift broke down (which happens frequently) she could not climb the stairs to get back home.

She has a home help who brings the shopping when she comes on Wednesday mornings to do the housework. A lady came once and offered her 'meals on wheels', but she refused. Mrs Cray's married daughter lives in one of the new neighbourhoods which have sprung up around the outskirts of the city. She works full-time now that both her children are at secondary school, but she manages to get over to see her mother about once a fortnight.

Mrs Cray's constant companion is a large white cat called Snowie, whom she has had for 7 years ever since he was a kitten. Snowie is just as fat as his owner and, like her, he spends most of the day curled up in front of the fire; his sleek white coat is Mrs Cray's pride and joy.

John Davis

John Davis, who is 22 years old, became tetraplegic following an accident on his motorbike 2 years ago. He is the youngest child of the family; his older sisters are married and living away from home. Before his accident his main interests were motorbikes and discos and he was engaged to be married but his fiancée now only visits occasionally.

John lives at home with his parents. To enable him to be transferred home from the regional spinal injuries unit where he spent the months following his accident, the family were rehoused into a bungalow which has been converted to accommodate the equipment he requires. He has a POSSUM apparatus, a pneumatic bed, lifting hoist and many other aids for his care.

He is incontinent and has a condom drainage fitted. Two nurses visit daily in the mornings, his parents managing his care for the rest of the day. John's father works for an insurance company; they have been very understanding about his rather poor work performance since John came home from hospital, but this is, of course, reflected in his commission. John's mother has devoted all her time to his care since giving up her part-time job when John came home.

Mr Evans

Mr Evans has just been discharged home from the local district hospital following the repair of an inguinal hernia; there is some infection of the wound, so the district nurse has been asked to visit to dress it.

Mr Evans is 38 years old and works as a bricklayer. He was very relieved to get his operation done relatively quickly because he had to have a lot of time off work, and he is anxious to get back to work as soon as possible, before the winter weather starts. Mrs Evans works part-time in a greengrocer's shop now that the youngest of their two children has just started school. The primary school which the children attend and the shop where she works are part of the 'precinct' which is the centre of the big council estate where the Evans family live.

Mr Fisher

Mr Fisher, who is now in his mid-forties, was first diagnosed as having multiple sclerosis about 10 years ago. At first he was able to continue his work as an accountant with a finance house in the City by doing most of the work at home instead of commuting daily as he had done before, but he was forced to give up about three years ago; he continues to work from home, however, as an accountant and tax adviser. Mrs Fisher teaches history in the local high school for girls and has recently been appointed deputy headmistress. The couple have no children.

The Fishers live in a detached house in a small private cul-de-sac quite near the station. They chose the house, and indeed the town, because of its easy access to London, although Mr Fisher came originally from the north of England and Mrs Fisher from the west country.

Rose Johnson

Rose Johnson, who is 7 years old, has sickle-cell anaemia. She is the middle of three children; her older sister and baby brother are not affected by the disease. The Johnsons live in a Victorian terraced house in a run-down part of one of Britain's large cities. Some parts of the city not far away have been redeveloped but the development programme has now stopped. The waiting list for council housing is long because no new houses are being built. Mrs Johnson came to England from the West Indies as a child in the early 1950s and has lived in this area ever since; her mother lives in the next street, and her sister, who also has three children, lives two streets away. Mr Johnson, who is also West Indian, works for the council in the Parks Department. Rose has been in and out of the children's hospital many times, but now that it is closing she will go, if necessary, to the main district general hospital. She attends a new school which opened last year in the part of the city which has been redeveloped; the head teacher and the school nurse are well aware of the problem of the neighbourhood and of Rose's disease.

District nurses are concerned with patients who have widely different nursing needs and who are supported by families or other carers who have markedly different abilities and capabilities. Moreover, patients come from the whole social spectrum and live in conditions ranging from the impoverished to the affluent. All these variations must be noted by the nurse when she makes her assessment and be considered when the plan of care is being made. For these reasons we refer to the histories of these seven patients in all parts of the book in order to illustrate the complexity of the factors that the nurse must take into account when carrying out her responsibilities.

Chapter 2

The World We Live In

Compare the seven patients in Chapter 1 with the following account by a district nurse of her 'typical working day', written in 1893.[1]

'For instance, a few days ago, starting at 8 a.m., I go first to see the patient who is more dangerously sick than any of the others—a little girl with bronchial pneumonia and whooping-cough. I find her mother has kept the room warm and well-aired, and carefully carried out the directions given about her medicine, stimulant, and nourishment. As her temperature is high, I give her a sponge bath, I then rub her chest with camphorated oil, and put on a cotton jacket I had made for her.

Then I go to see a little boy just recovering from pneumonia, who is weak and very stiff. I give him a good rubbing, and show his mother how to make a custard and beef-tea for him.

Then to see our oldest case, who says she is a hundred. She has had a grippe, has been quite sick, but is now improving. She is not in pain so I wash her face and hands, rub her back with alcohol, make an eggnog, and leave her calling down numberless blessings on me.

The next case is a two-year-old girl who has bronchitis. I have been at this house before, and am glad to find the sick child in bed with a hot flannel on her chest. I give her medicine and milk, which she refused to take from her grandmother.

I notice the four-weeks-old baby is being fed from a cup of tea, as there is no milk in the house. I promise to ask the doctor for a diet order, and show the grandmother how to prepare the baby's food properly.

I next see a woman who has erysipelas. I show her daughter how to make and apply the wash ordered by the doctor, and how to make some beef-tea.

Then I go to the dispensary to get some supplies, and to the loan closet to get some sheets and pillow-cases for a needy patient. I meet the physician at 12 o'clock and report the cases I have seen this morning and the preceding afternoon; ask for the diet order, get the new orders, and go with the doctor to see a man who has an abscess which needs to be lanced. When this is done I wash the arm, make a poultice, and put on a sling.

After my luncheon I begin the afternoon round by going to see a woman who has a bruised and crushed ankle. This patient ought to be in hospital, but does not want to leave her young baby and five children. I dress the wound, put on a splint, and caution her to use it as little as possible.

Then to see two chronic cases—one a woman with an ulcer on her leg. I show her how to dress this. As she cannot leave her room and is fond of reading. I lend her some of the books given by one of the managers for this purpose. The other patient is a young girl with phthisis, whose mother is glad of any suggestions for Maggie's pleasure or comfort.

The next call is to a family where the seven children have a painful skin disease. I showed their mother how to wash them and to apply the ordered ointment. Any amount of old linen is needed here. One of the children had brought home a stray dog that was afterward found to be covered with sores. The children had all played with the dog, and this was the result—truly a case of mistaken kindness.

The next house I visit is one of the most dismal in the district. Sounds of quarrelling come from every room. The halls and stairs are dark and dirty. The patient's room is up three flights, and contains only a stove, table and old sofa-bed. He is a boy with acute rheumatism. They have not yet sent for the medicine which the doctor ordered the day before. I get the mother to go for this while I do up the patient's knees in cotton-wool and bandage. This boy's sister was also a patient; her neck and face were burned. As I dressed this for her she explained that in a friendly scuffle she fell across the stove. She neglected doing anything for it until afraid that her neck was growing crooked. I have twice since found this young woman so intoxicated that she could not be roused sufficiently to have her neck dressed; so I fear this is one of the few hopeless cases.

The next visit is to a German woman, who is in bed, with her face and head, particularly about her eyes, badly burned. She had been heating a can of milk with the stopper in, and it exploded in her face. One of her neighbours told her to put ink on it. She did so, and the result was startling, to say the least. It takes much time and patience to get this properly dressed, as the woman is weak and nervous and understands very little English. She has five small children, and her husband is doing the best he can for her. I stay and show him how to make some gruel for the patient and to prepare the milk for the baby.

Then I go to the little girl I saw first in the morning, take her temperature and pulse, and make her comfortable for the night.

The last visit is to a woman who has gastritis. She cannot retain nourishment, and has much pain. A neighbour who had been a patient some time before came in, made the bed, put the room in order, and offered to make a poultice. She did this very nicely while I peptonized some milk which the patient was able to take.

Almost every day I find some former patient carrying out many of the simple directions that have been given during some former sickness. While this may be taken as a fair day's work, there are many cases requiring hours of care, as, for example, where a child is very sick and the mother is also sick, or in emergencies—as haemorrhages, confinements, or operations.

How, and for what reasons, does this nurse's account differ from district nursing today?

The first difference to be observed is in the age structure of the nurse's clientele: of the thirteen patients described, four are small children and only one patient is described as elderly. One family has six children, a second has seven children and a third five children. The clientele of today's district nurse would include relatively few children, and a much higher proportion of elderly people, and most of the families she meets will contain only one or two children. These differences illustrate the effect of demographic changes on the work of today's district nurse.

A second difference is in the kind of illnesses from which her patients are suffering. The terms 'grippe' and 'phthisis' do not even appear in a modern dictionary although the conditions themselves still exist under the modern diagnostic labels of influenza and tuberculosis. In 1855 one in six of all deaths was caused by tuberculosis. Today, diseases such as tuberculosis, erysipelas, acute rheumatism, skin infections and even pneumonia would only rarely figure in a district nurse's caseload.

A third difference is shown by what the nurse does for her patients. Today's district nurse is unlikely to spend much time rubbing children's chests with camphorated oil or patients' backs with alcohol, applying poultices, or making gruel and beef-tea. The fact that she does not illustrates the tremendous recent advances in scientific and medical knowledge, especially in the development of new drugs and in modern technology. Yet this difference is perhaps rather superficial—a difference in the technique rather than in the underlying task—because the basic activities described such as monitoring the patient's condition, attending to the patient's toilet needs, dressing wounds, teaching relatives how to care for the sick member of the family, teaching the principles of sound nutrition and healthy living, and mobilising resources, are aspects of the 'unique function' of the nurse[2] wherever and whenever nursing is practised.

Demographic changes

The size and structure of a population over a period of time is determined by the relationships between the number of births and the number of deaths. A population's size will increase rapidly if the birth rate is constant or increasing while the death rate is falling, as in the underdeveloped countries at present; and less rapidly if the death rate falls while the birth rate is constant or falling less than the death rate, as in Britain and other developed countries during the present century.

The growth of the population of Britain can be described in four stages:

Stage 1 (up to about 1750), characterised by high birth rates and high death rates; the population increased very slowly and by 1750 reached approximately 8 million.

Stage 2 (1750–1880), characterised by a high birth rate and a fall in the death rate from about 30–40 per thousand in the mid-eighteenth century to about 20 per thousand by 1850; the result was a rapid increase in population to 38 million by the end of the nineteenth century.

Stage 3 (1880–1950), characterised by falling birth rates and even more rapidly falling death rates, the population reached 50 million by 1951.

Stage 4 (1951 to present day), characterised by a low birth rate and a low death rate; the population is still increasing but very slowly with slight decreases in some years; it reached 56 million by 1981 and is expected to reach about 58 million by the end of the century.

The birth rate (the number of babies born per year per thousand of the population) is determined not only by the number of babies which each woman has, which is in turn affected by a variety of factors, but also by the number of woman of childbearing age in the population. In Britain the birth rate has fallen significantly during the past century, mainly because of the reduction in family size. Two-thirds of the women who married about the year 1860 gave birth to six or more children; women who married a century later rarely gave birth to more than four, and the average number of children per family was fewer than 2.5. Many factors have contributed to this change—among them the advent of reliable contraception and changes in the role and status of women—but the net result is that families are much smaller than they used to be.

The death rate has fallen even more dramatically: from 22.7 per thousand in 1851 to 11.6 (males) and 11.1 (females) in 1984, mainly as a result of the different pattern of health and disease which is discussed below. The crude death rate figures, however, do not by themselves show the aspect of the change which is even more significant—the change in the age distribution of deaths. A century ago about 30% of the population died before reaching adulthood, and women who survived until maturity faced a high risk of death in childbirth. Now more than 90% of the population can expect to see their 50th birthday and about two-thirds their 70th. The significant change is thus not the reduction in the death rate as such, but the increase in life expectancy from 41 years in 1841, to 71 years for men and 77 years for women at present.

This complex interaction between birth rates, death rates, causes of death and life expectancy determines the age structure of the population which can be shown in the form of a 'population pyramid'. Figure 2.1 shows how the shape of Britain's population pyramid changed between 1871 and 1985. The most obvious and significant change is the number and proportion of elderly people in the population. Since 1961 the total population has increased by about 7% but the over-65 population has increased by more than 25% and the trend is continuing. There are now more than 8 million people aged 65 years or over in the United Kingdom, and they constitute nearly 15% of the total population.

Figure 2.1 also shows an even more significant change in the age structure *within* the elderly population—the increase in the number and the proportion of the over-75s and the over-85s.

The significance of these changes is not simply the weight of numbers. The elderly, and especially the very elderly, are also the greatest users of health services. More than half of all the hospital

Fig. 2.1. Population profiles 1871 and 1985. Shaded areas indicate dependent population (children and elderly population).

beds are occupied by patients over the age of 65 years, and more than 80% of district nurses' visits in 1985 were to patients aged over 65 years. Figure 2.2 shows the demands on primary health care services made by the very elderly.

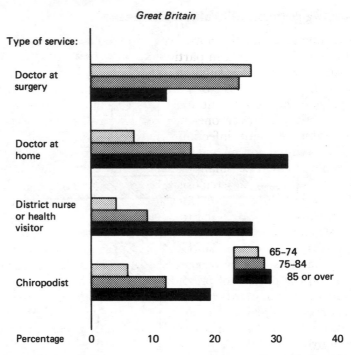

Great Britain

Type of service:

Doctor at
surgery

Doctor at
home

District nurse
or health
visitor

Chiropodist

65–74
75–84
85 or over

Percentage   0   10   20   30   40

Fig. 2.2. Use of health services by the elderly (from *Social Trends 1986*, with permission).

Other demographic factors increase the difficulties. Smaller families mean fewer children to care for elderly parents—the burden of care falling entirely on the one or two instead of being shared among perhaps six or eight. As life expectancy increases, the sons and daughters caring for their elderly parents are often themselves elderly. Moreover the effects of these demographic changes are exacerbated by social changes: For example, working wives have less time to devote to ageing parents than wives who stay at home; greater mobility means that children have often moved away from their parents' neighbourhood; small houses on modern estates do not provide room to accommodate elderly relatives. The 1983 General Household Survey found that more than a quarter of the over-65s and almost half (46.6%) of the over-75s live alone.

Changing patterns of health and disease

The dramatic decline in mortality is due to changing patterns in health and disease, and in particular to the decline in infectious disease. McKeown[3] has suggested that 86% of the total reduction of the death rate from the beginning of the eighteenth century to the present day is attributable to the decline of the infectious diseases. In 1850 over one-third of all deaths recorded were attributable to eight infectious diseases—tuberculosis (which alone accounted for one-sixth of the total mortality), typhus, scarlet fever, cholera, smallpox, whooping-cough, measles, and diphtheria. By 1978 tuberculosis accounted for 0.1% of all deaths and other infectious diseases for a further 0.2%. In that year half of all deaths were attributed to circulatory disease (of these half were attributed to ischaemic heart disease and a quarter to cerebrovascular disease), and one-fifth to cancer.

Why has this change occurred, and what is the effect of the change on the pattern of present-day health care?

Contrary to popular belief the change was not due to the rapid advance in medical knowledge, nor even to the discovery of immunisation, nor to the advent of the National Health Service, although all of these things have played some part. As McKeown has shown, the decline in the death rate and the change in the pattern of mortality was due primarily to improvements in nutrition, hygiene and sanitation, and in general standards of living. An understanding of this change offers many clues to coping with today's health problems, and for this reason three examples are considered in more detail:

    tuberculosis
    cholera
    maternal mortality

Tuberculosis

Three hundred years ago John Bunyan described tuberculosis as 'this captain of the men of death', and in 1850 this disease accounted for one-sixth of all deaths. Figure 2.3 shows the decline in the mortality rate from tuberculosis between 1838 and 1960. Since 1960 the mortality rate has continued to fall. Events which

Fig. 2.3. Respiratory tuberculosis: mean annual death rates (standardised to 1901 population) for England and Wales (from McKeown T. (1979) *The Role of Medicine*. Oxford: Blackwell Scientific).

might have been thought to be significant in the decline are shown, but it is clear that these factors alone cannot explain the change although they may have contributed to it. One clue is given by the fact that even before 1900, tuberculosis was far more prevalent in the towns and cities than in rural districts. Another clue is the short-term increase in mortality during both world wars. Yet another is the fact that in Britain today tuberculosis is most common among recent immigrants from developing countries. McKeown has analysed the decline in tuberculosis in detail and has shown convincingly that the major factors in the 'success story' were the improvements in the conditions which allowed tuberculosis to flourish, namely low resistance as a result of malnutrition and heavy exposure due to overcrowding.[3]

Cholera

It was the great cholera epidemics of the nineteenth century which, in the words of the historian Trevelyan, 'scared society into the tardy beginnings of sanitary self-defence'. Chadwick's great *Report on the Sanitary Conditions of the Labouring Population of Great Britain*, published in 1842, showed that insanitary conditions, defective drainage and inadequate water supply were invariably associated with infectious disease and high mortality; but the great breakthrough in the defeat of cholera is attributed to a London doctor, John Snow, whose detailed records of patients who contracted the disease revealed one factor common to them all: all had drunk water or eaten food prepared with water from the Broad Street pump. When, on his advice, the handle of the pump was removed the outbreak abated, and Snow rightly concluded that the disease was caused by an organism which contaminated the water, although the cholera vibrio was not actually identified until 1883, some 30 years later. Cholera is now confined largely to the tropics—but it is important to recognise that it occurs in certain countries not because they are 'tropical' but because their water supplies are contaminated.

The story of the conquest of cholera illustrates three principles which are as relevant today as they were a century ago in the prevention of disease: first, the value of epidemiology in identifying causes and pointing to possible solutions, secondly, the importance of environmental control and thirdly, the fact that preventive action can be effective even in the absence of complete knowledge.

Maternal mortality

At the beginning of this century and before, childbirth was recognised and feared as a life-threatening as well as a life-giving process; upwards of 2500 mothers died in childbirth each year. The novels of the nineteenth century, notably those of Dickens, are rich in accounts of death in childbirth. In 1983 there were only 50 maternal deaths, a reduction of 98%.

The decline in the maternal mortality rate, shown in Table 2.1, shows quite a different pattern from that of tuberculosis and cholera. It can be seen that the decline began much later, during the 1930s.

A departmental committee to consider maternal mortality, set up by the Ministry of Health in 1927, suggested that 48% of maternal deaths were avoidable and recommended investment in antenatal care and provision of more maternity homes and hospital beds. The work of the original committee continues in the

Table 2.1. The decline in the maternal mortality rate 1900–1985

Year	Maternal deaths per thousand live births (United Kingdom)
1900–1902	4.71
1910–1912	3.95
1920–1922	4.37
1930–1932	4.54
1940–1942	3.29
1950–1952	0.88
1960–1962	0.36
1970–1972	0.17
1978	0.08
1980	0.11
1982	0.10
1984	0.09
1985	0.07

Source: CSO Annual Abstract of Statistics 1987. London: HMSO.

Reports on Confidential Enquiries into Maternal Deaths, which were instituted in 1950.

Analysis of the causes of maternal mortality gives some clues to the reasons for the different patterns and provides some lessons which are different from those of the two previous examples. The principal causes between 1950 and 1978 are shown in Table 2.2, and they highlight the importance of the contributions made by the control of infection. The prevention of infection was achieved through understanding of the principles of asepsis, and cure through chemotherapy and antibiotics; by the provision of health services, in particular the development of antenatal services during the 1930s and birth control and abortion services in the late 1960s; by developments in medical technology such as anaesthesia and blood transfusions; and by other social provisions such as protective employment legislation and financial benefits, as well as by the general improvement in living standards, especially nutrition. Moreover, it shows more clearly than in any other field (except perhaps for the example of cholera) the importance of a political commitment to take the action necessary to tackle a recognised problem.

Table 2.2. Principal causes of maternal mortality 1950–1983

Cause	Number of deaths				
	1950	*1960*	*1970*	*1978*	*1983*
Abortion	103	62	32	5	1
Puerperal sepsis	26	8	9	1	1
Thrombosis and embolism	62	27	10	11	7
Haemorrhage	82	44	12	4	2
Toxaemia	185	63	24	23	6
All other causes	162	106	59	24	34
ALL CAUSES	620	310	146	68	51

Source: OPCS (1978). *Birth statistics.* London: HMSO (updated).

Mortality today

The victims of infectious disease were young; today three-quarters of all deaths occur after the age of 65 years. The change is reflected in the major causes of death: more than half of all deaths nowadays are due to circulatory disease—heart disease and stroke—and a further fifth to cancer. The leading causes of death at different ages are shown in Fig. 2.4. Although this chart was published in 1972 there has been little change since. Apart from old age, the most vulnerable period is the first week of life, when the main causes are prematurity and congenital malformation. During childhood and early adulthood accidents stand out as the leading cause. During the middle years the pattern is very different for men compared with women: for men the greatest killer by far is ischaemic heart disease, although cancer, especially lung cancer, is also important. For women the cancers are the major cause of death with breast cancer the most important type.

The present pattern of mortality offers new challenges. There is still some scope for advances in curative medicine, the investment in the search for a cure for cancer is massive and there is considerable scope for preventive action against accidents and coronary heart disease; but the greatest challenge is that 'the wheel has gone full circle; what can be prevented has been prevented, what can be cured is largely cured, what is left is care'.[4]

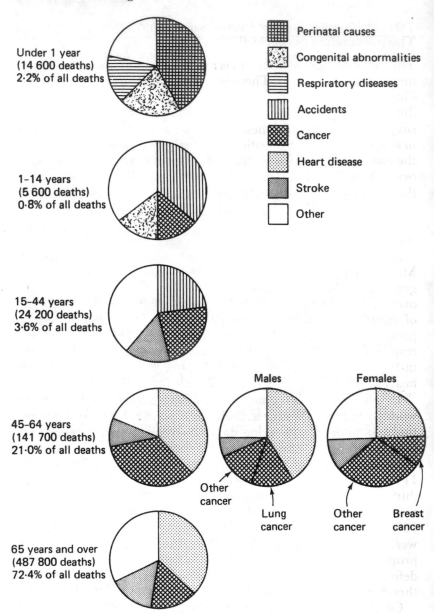

Fig. 2.4. Deaths in age groups indicating the main causes: United Kingdom 1972 (from *Prevention and Health: Everybody's Business*. London: HMSO).

The prevalence of morbidity

The measurement of ill-health is a far more complex task than the measurement of death. There is no clear line beween health and illness as there is between life and death, and the definition of illness, which is discussed in more detail in Chapter 3, is a subjective assessment. These difficulties are increased by changes in diagnostic labels as medical knowledge increases (for example the grippe and phthisis of 1893) and it is difficult to trace changes over a long period of time. Several different kinds of yardstick for the measurement of ill-health are currently in use and techniques are still being refined and developed.

The number of people admitted to hospital rises each year, but this may be a truer reflection of demand and of people's expectations about health care than of the prevalence of sickness. More than half of all hospital beds in psychiatric hospitals, and in general hospitals more than half of all beds are occupied by people over the age of 65 years, so the stereotype of the hospital as a place of curative technology is not particularly accurate. Excluding psychiatric and maternity patients, diseases of the digestive and respiratory systems account for a quarter of all admissions, while in terms of the length of time spent in hospital, diseases of the heart and circulation including strokes take first place.

In any given month about one million workers are absent from work by reason of sickness. Sickness accounts for more than ten times as many lost working days as strikes. The incidence and prevalence of ill-health among the non-working population is difficult to estimate, but in the *General Household Survey of 1983* 11% of men and 14% of women reported 'restricted activity' during the 14 days prior to interview and 31% of men and 33% of women reported a long-standing illness. About 12% of men and 16% of women had consulted a general practitioner in the 2 weeks prior to the interview. The discrepancy between the proportions indicates something of the subjectivity of the definition of 'being ill' and also the extent of unreported (and therefore untreated) illness.

Of particular interest to the district nurse, however, who receives her patients by referral from the general practitioner, is the distribution of sickness patterns in a general practice population. A national survey of general practitioner consultation patterns showed that in 1970–71 about a quarter of the population saw their general practitioner about a respiratory complaint, a further 11% for a disease of the nervous system, and the same proportions for skin diseases and mental disorders.

When all the statistics are put together it can be seen that the spectrum of today's health problems contains three main elements:

1 The diseases and disabilities of old age
2 Diseases caused by individual behaviour
3 Hazards relating to our changing environment

Diseases and disabilities of old age

An increasing number of old people inevitably means more cases of disability and chronic degenerative disease. The common chronic degenerative diseases include arteriosclerosis, cerebro-vascular disease, cardiovascular disease, multiple sclerosis, osteoarthritis, rheumatoid arthritis, Parkinson's disease, and chronic chest disease. Defects of sight, hearing and disability increase with advancing years. Troubles rarely come singly: multiple pathology is one of the characteristics of disease in the elderly. Health problems, both physical and mental, are exacerbated by social factors such as social isolation resulting from problems such as bereavement, deafness and immobility, poor nutrition, unsuitable housing conditions and inadequate income. The complexity of the disease and disability in the elderly is well illustrated by our descriptions of Mr Adams and Mrs Cray and this subject is further discussed in Chapter 15.

Diseases caused by individual behaviour

The review of present-day mortality and morbidity showed that the most common causes of premature death were heart disease, cancer (especially lung cancer) and accidents, and the most common reasons for consulting a doctor were respiratory diseases, nervous disorders and mental disorders. All these diseases are directly affected, and in some cases actually caused, by aspects of our behaviour—in particular our eating and drinking habits, smoking, sexual behaviour, and our use of leisure. As a nation we eat too much food and food of the wrong kind, drink too much alcohol, smoke too many cigarettes, are sexually promiscuous and take too little physical exercise.

Diet

The malnutrition associated with poverty and the diseases which flourished as a result (e.g. tuberculosis, rickets) have been replaced by a malnutrition associated with affluence in which general over-eating leads to obesity which increases the risk of diabetes and heart disease and exacerbates other conditions such as respiratory disease and arthritis. Specific dietary habits lead to problems such as dental caries (sugar), coronary heart disease (saturated fats and sugar), bowel cancer and diverticular disease (inadequate roughage) and allergy (food additives). Men who are more than 25% heavier than average for their age and height have a death rate twice as high as those within 5% of the average.

Alcohol

Excessive drinking is the direct cause of disorders such as cirrhosis of the liver and alcoholism, and the indirect cause of a large proportion of road traffic and other accidents. Alcoholism causes serious social problems not only for the victim but also for his family. This problem is discussed in Chapter 13.

Drugs

The rise in drug addiction, especially addiction to heroin, has given much concern in recent years. The numbers of new addicts notified by doctors to the Home Office increased from 307 in 1973 to 5415 in 1984; in 1983 more than 3700 people were admitted to psychiatric wards with a drug-related diagnosis. The number of drug misusers, however, is much greater than the number of notifications or admissions to hospital. Of special concern to the district nurse is the number of people who would never call themselves drug addicts but who are dependent on antidepressants, tranquillisers and sedatives.

Smoking

Smoking is known to be associated with lung cancer, chronic bronchitis, coronary heart disease and increased perinatal mortality. The proportion of adults who smoke has fallen in recent years but is still too high—36% of men and 32% of women in 1984 smoked cigarettes. The most dramatic decline in smoking in recent years has, significantly, occurred among doctors, whose death rate has declined correspondingly. The increase in the number of women who smoke is now beginning to be reflected in a reduction of the gap between the sexes in mortality rates. There is particular concern also over the prevalence of smoking among schoolchildren; according to the OPCS survey in 1982, 19% of schoolchildren between the ages of 11 and 16 smoke cigarettes, and other smaller-scale surveys since have suggested that the numbers have increased.

Sexual behaviour

One change in sexual behaviour—namely the widespread use of contraception—has led to health benefits in the reduction of maternal mortality. However, the increase in sexual activity outside marriage has also contributed to the dramatic increase of more than four-fold between 1959 and 1984 in venereal disease, which is now the most common of all the infectious diseases. The number of sexual partners and the age at which sexual activity was commenced have also been shown to be associated with cervical cancer.

Most recently concern has focused on the spread of the virus HIV and acquired immune deficiency syndrome (AIDS). This will have an impact on the work of the district nurse as many of these people will die, possibly alone, at home. New literature and information on this condition appears almost daily and district nurses are reminded of their responsibilities within the UKCC Code of Professional Conduct (see Appendix 1) for keeping their own professional knowledge updated. Further discussion regarding the needs of such patients and the role of the district nurse takes place in Chapter 22.

Other behavioural health problems

Reduction in the length of the working week and the increased availability of domestic aids such as washing machines has increased the amount of leisure time available for most people, but not much leisure time is spent on health-inducing activities. The 1983 General Household Survey found that the average weekly time spent watching television was about 29 hours during January and only 10 hours less in August; only 19% of men and 17% of women had been for a walk longer than 2 miles in the 4 weeks prior to interview. More people than ever before work in sedentary jobs and travel by car instead of walking. The result is inadequate physical activity which exacerbates the problems of obesity but in addition is directly associated with an increased risk of coronary heart disease.

Other leisure pursuits carry their own specific hazards. The hazards of hang-gliding may be obvious, but less obvious are the hearing loss and migraines associated with discos, the paraplegia and head injuries associated with motorbikes, and the injuries caused by violence on the football terraces.

These patterns of illness are well represented among our seven patients. The health problems of Mrs Adams and Mrs Cray are typical of those of the elderly; Mr Fisher, although comparatively young at present, is the victim of a chronic disease for which there is no known cure and no means of prevention; Mrs Baker will die prematurely from one form of the disease which is the most common cause of premature death among women; and John Davis is a casualty of his life style.

The physical environment

The importance of environmental factors in the causation of disease has been clearly demonstrated by epidemiological studies in the tradition of pioneers such as Chadwick and Rowntree, but environmental factors are also important in the treatment and care of patients.

The importance of environmental factors is clearly exemplified by chronic bronchitis. The death rate from this disease differs widely in different parts of the country and increases with each step down the social class scale. Other factors which have been shown to be significant include climate, levels of air pollution, occupation and smoking habits. Measures such as smokeless zones, the protection of workers from dust and a reduction in cigarette smoking would considerably reduce the prevalence of the disease. For patients suffering from chronic bronchitis the extent of their recovery and their chances of becoming ill again depend less on the effectiveness of the treatment by antibiotics and bronchodilators than on whether or not they give up smoking, go home to a damp house in an inner city area, or return to work in the same dusty conditions as before.

The following environmental factors have a particularly significant influence upon health:

Nutrition
Environmental pollution
Occupational environment
Housing conditions

Consider the effect of these environmental influences on the health problems of the seven families in Chapter 1.

Nutrition

Adequate nutrition is little mentioned; there is no evidence that any of the patients are malnourished in the sense of not having enough to eat. However, the effect of misguided eating habits on Mrs Cray's condition can be seen, as well as how much worse the situation might be without the home help to buy the food.

Because of the system of protective legislation established over the last century in recognition of the fact that contaminated food is a source of disease, all the families can reasonably assume that their milk will be free from tubercle and other organisms and that their meat will be free from parasites and will have been inspected at the port of entry if it is imported from abroad. One can expect that food will be unadulterated by harmful additives (except for those additives which are specified and controlled), and will be prepared and sold on premises whose standards of hygiene are required to meet a certain standard, and that the nutritional content of staple foods such as bread, margarine and flour meets certain minimum requirements.

1989 - Listeria   salmonella   (cook chill foods, paté)

Environmental services

These are not mentioned in any of the pen portraits. The reason is not that they are unimportant, but that facilities such as sewage and refuse disposal and a pure water supply are taken for granted in Britain today. One has to read the history of the nineteenth century to appreciate the difference that these facilities have made to health.

Occupation

None of the patients is suffering from an illness which can be directly attributed to their occupation. Prescribed industrial diseases and industrial accidents account for over a tenth of working days lost through sickness. However, it is likely that Mr Evans' occupation has contributed to his health problem and the effect of employment on the management of patient care can be seen in the cases of Mr Evans and Mr Fisher.

Housing

Probably the most influential environmental factor from the district nurse's point of view is housing conditions, and the effects of housing, particularly on the way in which the district nurse can provide care, is seen in the stories of several of our families. The Adams' housing conditions—a small unmodernised cottage with no central heating, no bathroom, and only an outside toilet—lie at one extreme of the continuum. The bungalow which has been specially converted for John Davis lies at the other. Housing conditions affect a patient's susceptibility to certain illnesses and to accidents, and the course of his illness, as well as being an important factor to be considered in the management of illness.

The Johnson family are lucky in that at least they occupy the whole house, but in the area where they live many larger houses are likely to be occupied by several families. Several families may have to share a single lavatory, water may have to be carried by families living at the top of the house from a tap on the floor below, and cooking facilities may consist of a single gas ring on a small landing. It is not difficult to imagine the risks to health which life in such conditions involves. Overcrowding leads to the rapid spread of airborne infections such as tuberculosis. Damp conditions, caused by defective roofs or gutters, or the lack of a damp course, lead to exacerbation of rheumatic and respiratory disorders. Poor sanitation and inadequate facilities for food preparation lead to gastroenteritis. There is no space for the children to play, and the inadequate cooking and heating arrangements predispose to accidents, especially burns and scalds. Altogether the stress produced by trying to cope with life in these surroundings causes a great deal of mental ill-health.

The implications of housing conditions for the management of care are considerable. For example, a patient suffering from a chronic cardiac condition must avoid stairs. In a modern house it may be possible to turn a downstairs room into a bedroom; but the poorly housed may not only have to climb stairs, but have to carry water up and down them as well. Similarly the management of a colostomy may be extremely difficult if the lavatory is at the bottom of the garden and there is no bathroom. Moreover, so far only the physical aspects of housing conditions have been considered. The social aspects, which include location, the type of ownership and the type of neighbourhood, are also important.

New environmental hazards

In many respects our environment today is healthier than it has ever been. We enjoy pure water, clean food, clean air, safe sanitation, drainage and refuse disposal services, and a relatively safe working environment. However, as one environmental hazard is conquered another emerges, and each innovation brings unintended disadvantages as well as its intended benefits. The use of the motor car produces an annual toll of 8000 deaths and almost 100 000 serious injuries; new chemicals are constantly being developed for use in industry and the home; chemical and radioactive pollution of the atmosphere is increasingly causing concern. Knowledge is increasing about the effects, particularly on mental health, of less tangible environmental factors such as noise.

Environmental control and personal freedom

Discussion of environmental factors, particularly in relation to the prevention of illness, raises the dilemma of environmental control versus individual freedom. It is a fact that most of the improvements in today's environment compared with that of the last century, and the improvement in health which this has produced, are due to environmental controls imposed by legislation. Some of today's environmental hazards could be controlled in the same way. Legislation to enforce the wearing of seat belts in cars reduced the number of deaths and serious injuries to front-seat occupants of cars by a third; many people are in favour of similar legislation to add fluoride to all drinking water, which has been conclusively shown to reduce the prevalence of dental caries, and to reduce the availability of alcohol and cigarettes. Opponents of such measures argue that they are an unwarrantable intrusion on personal freedom, exactly as did the very many and powerful opponents of the environmental legislation of the last century. The debate is well summarised in the *Report of the Royal Commission on the NHS* (1979).[5] Meanwhile the dilemma confirms the overwhelming need for health education as an integral part of the role of the district nurse into the 1990s as it was in the 1890s.

The social environment

The social environment is as important to patterns of illness and to the management of care as is the physical environment, and the changes which have taken place during this century have been just as dramatic and their effects no less profound. Demographic changes have already been discussed, but other significant social changes include changes in family structure and patterns of family life, changes in the role of women, in education, in working and in patterns of income and spending. All these factors are closely inter-related; for example, the reduction in family size is both a cause and a result of changes in the role of women and the pattern of women's work outside the home.

Perhaps the most striking changes are those in family structure and patterns of family life, particularly since the 1930s. The family is discussed in more detail in Chapter 4, but must be considered here also as an aspect of social change. Compared with 1900, more people marry and they marry younger; there is a corresponding decrease in the number and proportion of single women; women have, on average, fewer children, and their childbearing period is completed earlier than previously, releasing them for paid work outside the home. In 1921 fewer than one in ten married women worked outside the home compared with one in two now; very high proportions of women return to work after having their children and women are also increasingly returning to work between births. Divorce is much more common and there is a corresponding increase in the number of one-parent families (13% of all families with dependent children in 1983).

To social statisticians the terms 'families' and 'households' mean different things; households are groups of people who live and eat together, while families consist of a married couple with or without children, or a lone parent with children. A household may consist of a single family or more than one family living together, or occupants who are unrelated. The change in the number and proportion of the different types of household is another indicator of change in family life. The increased number of households reflects a fall in household size, which is due not only to a reduction in family size but a reduction in the number of households containing two or more families and to an increase in the number of elderly people living alone.

Changes in the pattern of family life have been exacerbated by changes in housing patterns and town planning. In city areas the old back-to-back slums have been cleared and replaced by tower blocks of flats; in rural areas the lack of work opportunities for young people and problems of public transport have forced young people to move nearer to towns; the modern semidetached house on a surburban estate is too small to accommodate elderly grandparents and unsuitable for an elderly person living alone.

Some of the implications of these changes in the social environment can be seen in the stories of our seven patients, but they are no doubt particularly problematic for Mr Adams, Mrs Baker, Mrs Cray and Mrs Fisher. Who will care for Mr and Mrs Adams as they become older and more frail? Who will care for Mrs Baker's children when their mother is dead? How will Mrs

Cray's daughter cope with the conflicting needs of her mother and her children? How will Mrs Fisher resolve the conflict between a promising career and an increasingly disabled husband? How will Mr Fisher avoid adding the problems of social isolation to the problems of his physical disability? All these questions must be asked by the district nurse—and answered—in assessing each patient's needs and planning and implementing her programme of care.

Unemployment

The link between unemployment and health has been much debated. For a few people—those whose occupations expose them to health hazards—unemployment has brought an improvement in health. For many victims, however, the frustration and anxieties associated with redundancy have led to stress-related illnesses (including mental illness) and even to suicide, and the poverty associated with long-term unemployment can seriously affect health at all ages, and especially the health of children.

The effect of techology

The kind of nursing action which was open to our district nurse in 1893 seems extremely limited when compared with the resources which would be available to her today. Such resources include not only increased medical knowledge, but powerful drugs, sophisticated diagnostic techniques, and equipment such as ripple beds and electric wheelchairs, pre-sterilised dressings, and disposable syringes and needles. District nurses no longer depend on 'old linen' or dressings sterilised in a biscuit tin in the family's oven. While such modern devices make district nursing much easier in some ways, in others they make it more difficult; the modern district nurse needs greater knowledge and more varied skills than ever before if she is to get the best from the resources available.

One aspect of technological development which has revolutionised the lives of all of us is the development of communication media, especially the telephone and television. Television brings the remote and esoteric into the family living-room, increasing people's knowledge and influencing their expectations about health care as about other things; its potential as a medium for health education has scarcely begun to be exploited. Computers and the microchip have already revolutionised the storage, manipulation, and retrieval of information in industry and commerce, and their implications for health care are tremendous. Technological advance also brings problems in the pace of life and the rate of change which make considerable demands on human adaptability, and produces stresses which may lead to individual and social breakdown.

Social conditions and the role of the nurse

A constant problem for all those who work in the health and social services is the knowledge that social conditions are affecting a patient's health or recovery from illness, without the ability to change those conditions. It is easy to advise a patient suffering from bronchitis that a change of job is essential and to move out of the damp inner-city basement. In practice, however, it may be quite impossible for this advice to be followed. It is important in planning an individual patient's care to make a realistic assessment of the social circumstances, including the possibilities for change, and to plan care accordingly. It is equally important to recognise the nurse's role as the patient's advocate in attempting to improve the situation. Caring for a patient must include measures to improve, whatever way is possible, the social conditions which are affecting health, and also the support which may be necessary to help maintain health at the optimum level in whatever conditions the patient may live.

References

1 Somerville C. E. M. (1893). District Nursing. In: Hampton I.A. *et al.* (1949). *Nursing of the Sick 1893: papers and discussions from the International Congress of Charities Correction and Philanthropy, Chicago 1893*. New York: McGraw Hill.
2 Henderson V. (1960). *Basic Principles of Nursing Care*. Geneva: International Council of Nurses.
3 McKeown T. (1979). *The Role of Medicine*. Oxford: Blackwell Scientific.
4 Baly M. (1973). *Nursing and Social Change*, 1st edn. London: Heinemann Medical.
5 *Report of the Royal Commission on the National Health Service* (1979). Cmnd. 7615. London: HMSO.

Further Reading

Baly M. (1980). *Nursing and Social Change*, 2nd edn. London: Heinemann Medical.

Black N., ed. (1984). *Health and Disease: A Reader*. Milton Keynes: Open University Press.

Central Statistical Office (1986). *Social Trends*. London: HMSO.

Department of Health and Social Security (1976). *Prevention and Health: Everybody's Business*. London: HMSO.

Doyal L. (1980). *The Political Economy of Health*. London: Pluto Press.

Halsey A. H., ed. (1972). *Trends in British Society Since 1900*. London: Macmillan.

Health Education Council (1981). *The Great Divide*. London: HEC.

McKeown R., Lowe C. R. (1974). *An Introduction to Social Medicine*, 2nd edn. Oxford: Blackwell Scientific.

Pratt R. J. (1986). *AIDS: A Strategy for Nursing Care*. London: Edward Arnold.

Royal College of Nursing (1986). *Nursing guidelines on the management of patients in hospital and the community suffering from AIDS*. London: RCN Publications.

Townsend P., Davidson N., eds. (1982). *Inequalities in Health: The Black Report*. Harmondsworth: Penguin.

Watkin B. (1975). *Documents on Health and Social Services 1831 to the Present Day*. London: Methuen.

Chapter 3

People as Individuals

The idea that each patient is a unique individual is basic to the philosophy of nursing care. But what do we mean by the term 'unique individual'? Clearly human beings have many shared characteristics and one can detect and describe patterns of bodily function and of behaviour which are common to all mankind. Moreover in accepting Alexander Pope's belief that 'the proper study of mankind is man', one must recognise that man can be studied from a number of perspectives; the disciplines of chemistry, anatomy, physiology, psychology, anthropology and sociology all make a contribution to our understanding of man both as a species and as a unique individual. It is important that nurses recognise and use the contribution which the theories, concepts and discoveries of other disciplines can make to their own unique function of giving nursing care.

This chapter and the following one draw heavily upon the resources of psychology and sociology. They should not, however, be regarded as a 'potted textbook' of those disciplines, nor is the line between the two disciplines distinct, although this chapter draws more heavily on psychology and the following chapter on sociology.

The uniqueness of the human individual

The complexity of the human individual arises not so much from the number and complexity of the elements from which he or she is made, as from the infinite variety of ways in which they interrelate. Of particular importance is the inter-relationship between heredity and environment. Heredity includes all the characteristics with which a person is endowed from the moment of conception as a result of the particular combination of genes carried by the chromosomes contained within the nucleus of each body cell. It is important to recognise that genetic factors determine not only physical characteristics such as sex or eye

colour, but also some mental characteristics such as temperament. Except in the case of uniovular twins, each individual's
genetic endowment is unique. The term 'environment' includes
all the external physical, mental and social experiences which
happen to an individual from the moment of conception onwards.
In practice each individual's environment is also unique. Studies
of twins which have attempted to estimate the relative influence of
heredity and environmental factors on many different characteristics have confirmed the complexity and the uniqueness of the
human individual. Uniovular twins differ from each other
because of the differences in their environments, while even if a
completely uniform environment could be provided people would
experience it differently.

Moreover, a human being is more than simply the sum of
certain genetic and environmentally determined elements. As the
biologist H. J. Muller has remarked:

> Although parts and processes may be isolated for analytical purposes,
> they cannot be understood without reference to the dynamic unified
> whole that is more than their sum. To say for example that man is
> made up of certain elements is a satisfactory description only for those
> who intend to use him as fertiliser.[1]

Individual personality

One aspect of the uniqueness of the individual is the phenomenon
which we call 'personality'. Personality is the complex of
psychological and emotional attributes, of feelings, attitudes,
thought patterns, emotions and drives, that characterises a
person. Like other attributes, personality is the product of
hereditary and environmental factors. Different schools of
psychological thought lay different emphasis on the various
factors which contribute to personality and offer different
explanations of how personality develops and why a particular
person's personality is the way it is.

Personality is an important, although not the only, determinant
of behaviour. Some people are more consistent in their reactions
and behaviour than others because personality is more organised
in some people than in others. We apply the terms 'stable' and
'unstable' to the personality as an explanation of the consistency

or inconsistency of a person's behaviour, and by using the terms 'mature' and 'immature' we also imply that the acquisition of personality is a developmental process; experience is an important aspect of environment, and childhood experience in particular is an important determinant of adult personality.

Personality is usually described in one of three ways—by attributes referred to as personality traits, by temperament, or by personality type. *Personality traits* are attributes such as patience, tolerance, assertiveness, which indicate a tendency to behave in a consistent manner in particular situations; psychologists such as Eysenck and Cattell have devised techniques for testing the strength of various personality traits and have tried to relate them to specific behaviours. *Temperament* refers to a person's emotional state, particularly to the way in which emotions are expressed over a long period of time, for example placidness, irritability. *Mood* describes the emotion prevailing for a short period.

Psychologists such as Kretchmer and Sheldon have associated different temperaments with different body types, and even at an everyday level reference is often made to the 'fat and happy' type of person. The link between temperament and physical factors, especially endocrine factors, has important implications for the nursing care of individual patients. Temperament may change with age and may be seriously distorted by endocrine imbalance whether associated with age (e.g. the menopause) or therapy (e.g. steroids). Classifications based on temperament overlap with those based on *personality type*, the most common of which is Jung's distinction between *introverts* and *extroverts*. *Introverts* are defined as people who 'turn inwards' in their behaviour, i.e. are quiet, shy, and reserved with other people, while *extroverts* 'turn outwards' and use their relationship to other people as the main guide to their behaviour.

It is important to recognise, however, that personality is by definition unique to the individual, and no individual exactly conforms to an ideal type.

Individual experience

One definition of psychology is 'the scientific study of behaviour and experience'.[2] Some psychologists believe that behaviour alone is a legitimate subject for study, because only behaviour can be objectively observed; the behaviourist school of psychology, originated by the psychologist Watson, is based on this view. The conception of experience is, however, at least as relevant to the practice of nursing because it explains and justifies the need to adapt nursing care to the individual patient.

When a nurse sticks an injection needle into a patient's buttock, this stimulus produces a behavioural response such as crying (if the patient is a baby) or a grimace (if the patient is a more controlled adult), which can be observed. The nurse will probably assume that the patient is experiencing pain, inferring this both from the observed behavioural response and from expectations based upon her own experience of receiving injections, but she cannot feel his pain in exactly the way that he feels it, however close her relationship or however great her empathy. This view forms the basis of the work of psychologists and psychiatrists such as R. D. Laing, philosophers such as Husserl and Sartre, and of the sociological approach known as phenomenology. It is particularly important for the nurse because it shows the danger of responding to patients on the basis of what the nurse thinks the patient 'ought' to feel rather than on what he does feel. The nurse must recognise and take account of the limitations imposed by the fact that her only entry to a patient's experience, which is unique and peculiar to him, is by what the patient tells her either verbally or by other behaviour; for example, if a patient says he is in pain, there is no justification for the nurse to say that he is not. When taking into account environmental factors, such as those described in the previous chapter, it is important to recognise that every individual's environment is different and unique because he experiences it differently from other people. Similarly, his experience of his illness and the way in which he responds to it is individual and unique, and his behaviour will vary accordingly.

Individual behaviour

Why do people behave in the way they do? What are the determinants of human behaviour?

Behaviour can be defined as the activity of an organism in response to the situation in which it finds itself. At its simplest level, for example at the level of the amoeba, behaviour is merely the response to a stimulus; the particular response produced by a particular stimulus occurs automatically and is always the same. In more complex organisms, including man, this type of behaviour persists in the form of *reflex behaviour* whose main function is to ensure physical survival, for example protective responses such as blinking or coughing and the maintenace of essential processes such as heartbeat and digestion. In complex animals, however, most behaviour is controlled through a *central nervous system*, in which sensory nerves carry information from the receptors to the brain, where the information is sorted, interpreted and translated into instructions which are transmitted by motor nerves to appropriate effectors. The processes which take place within the brain are extremely complex and little understood, but it is these activities or *mental processes* which direct human behaviour and which are the subject of study of the discipline called psychology.

It would be impossible in this book to describe, even briefly, all the mental processes involved in individual behaviour, this section merely outlines some of the main concepts and factors which the study of psychology has shown to affect human behaviour, and which are particularly relevant to the task of the district nurse; readers are strongly advised to pursue the suggestions for further reading.

Factors which have been the subject of intensive investigation and which have been found to be particularly important include:

Perception
Motivation
Attitudes and value
Memory
Learning

Perception

Perception is the interpretation in the brain of the sensory stimuli received by the sense organs. It is a learnt activity which involves remembering previous stimuli, comparing the new stimulus with them, and recognising it as similar or different. Since the amount of information bombarding the sense organs at any one time is greater than the mind can cope with, material is selected through the mechanism of *attention*. No two individuals will make exactly the same selection, and because people's previous knowledge, expectations and standards of comparison differ, no two people will perceive the same thing or event in exactly the same way; perception, like experience is unqiue.

Because the process is so complicated and affected by so many factors, misinterpretation of the information received is common, and this is important because it may lead to inappropriate behaviour. Misinterpretation may result from inadequacies in the information gathered by the sense organs, deficiencies in attention, the 'wrong kind' of previous knowledge, or conflict between the new perception and previous perceptions or expectations.

Motivation

Motivation can refer either to the goal of an action or to the energising force which initiates action, and it is variously analysed in terms of drives, antecedents or purpose. A *drive* is a state of arousal to remedy a felt need, e.g. hunger drive, sex drive; needs may be physiological, psychological, or social. Explanations based on *antecedents* try to link cause and effect; for example a child's response to admission to hospital may be determined by any previous experience of separation from the mother. The third approach to motivation sees behaviour as *goal-oriented*; for example a child may respond to the birth of a baby brother by reverting to babyish behaviour in order to obtain more of the mother's attention. It is important to realise that motivation is often unconscious; few people can recognise their own motivation when asked to account for their behaviour although they may recognise that their behaviour was not rational.

Attitudes and values

An *attitude* is a persistent predisposition to think, feel and act in a certain way, favourably or unfavourably, in relation to something. *Values* are collections of interrelated attitudes. Attitudes and values certainly influence behaviour, but the exact relationship between them is much debated. Attitudes are learned, mainly during the process of socialisation (Chapter 4), and those which are acquired early are usually strongly held and very resistant to change. Attitude change is one of the most important and one of the most difficult tasks of education.

Memory

Memory is the mental process concerned with the storage and recall of information; it is therefore an important component of the processes of perception and learning. The process of remembering events just perceived is referred to as short-term memory; the storage capacity of short-term memory is small, so any overflow of information is either forgotten or transferred to the long-term memory. Retrieving information from the long-term memory is often difficult and incomplete and considerable attention has been applied to investigating what factors improve the ability to recall. The inability to recall unpleasant or worrying events acts as a protective mechanism; material which is hidden in the memory in this way is said to be *repressed*. The activity of remembering depends on a healthy and intact brain; brain damage, whether caused by disorders such as epilepsy or by the process of ageing, produces memory impairment.

Learning

Learning is the acquisition of a new and better adapted pattern of behaviour; it is the process by which changes are brought about in an individual's response to the environment. Learning is an important topic in psychology which has wide application for nursing and is discussed in more detail in Chapter 9. Not all learning is conscious and this has important implications for behaviour. Experimental work has led to a number of theories to explain learning, but basically two broad types can be distinguished: stimulus-response learning or conditioning, and cognitive learning or learning by insight. Conditioning was first described by Pavlov who conditioned a dog to salivate in response to a bell by ringing the bell every time the dog was given food until the dog would salivate in response to the bell alone. Pavlov's discoveries were developed by Watson and later by Skinner who showed that a response to a stimulus could be strengthened by consistently following it with a reward (a *reinforcer*); this process of 'operant' conditioning forms the basis of the behaviour therapy used in psychiatric nursing to help patients overcome phobias or unacceptable behaviour (however defined), but the concept of *reinforcement* has a much wider application.

Insight or cognitive learning involves solving problems by thinking about the relationships between different ideas and actions and relating general principles to specific problems. An important aspect of learning is the learning of skills, and Argyle has shown that the process of learning a motor skill such as riding a bicycle applies equally to the learning of social skills.

Anxiety and stress

Stress is an important concept in nursing for two reasons: first because it has been shown to be an important causative factor in illness and secondly because illness itself is a stress-producing event. At a common-sense level most people would define stress as a 'feeling' which is provoked by any situation which is 'too much to cope with'. Writers such as Selye and Antonovsky have analysed stress from a more scientific perspective. From the physiological perspective stress is a physiological adaptation, manifested by physiological events such as increased heart rate, to physiological threat; from the psychological perspective—which must be included because even physiological stressors depend on the individual's perception of the threat—stress is consciously experienced through the emotions of fear or anxiety as well as through the assessment of the situation made by the rational or cognitive aspect of the mind. We do not know why some people are able to tolerate stress better than others, but we do know that when stress exceeds the level which an individual is able to tolerate—whatever the level may be for the particular indi-vidual—it becomes manifest in their behaviour, sometimes to the extent of mental or psychosomatic illness.

Stress mobilises mechanisms which help an individual to cope, and part of the task of the nurse is to enhance these coping mechanisms, for example by listening empathetically and by counselling, as well as to try to reduce the stress wherever possible by removing the cause. Some coping mechanisms, however, operate below the level of consciousness; the form which these *mental defence mechanisms* take depends on the particular individual and the particular circumstances. James[3] has distinguished six types:

1   Mechanisms involving substitution—
     e.g. *compensation*: when energy is redirected from the problem area into a different and less threatening channel; *sublimation*: when energy is redirected towards a similar but more attainable goal.

2   Mechanisms for improving the chances of coping with the problematic environment—
     e.g. *regression*: returning to earlier patterns of behaviour which were previously successful; *identification*: adopting the attitudes and behaviour of other people who seem to cope more successfully.

3   Mechanisms for converting mental anxieties into physical terms which are thought to be more acceptable—
     e.g. *psychosomatic illness*: where an individual develops a physical illness such as asthma or gastric ulcer; *conversion hysteria*: where an individual develops a physical incapacity which enables him to withdraw without loss of face.

4   Mechanisms for ignoring the existence of the problem—
     e.g. *repression*: when the unpleasant experience is stored away so far into unconsciousness that it cannot be recalled; *rationalisation*: when information about the problem is reinterpreted so that it is made tolerable.

5   Mechanism for redirecting the conflict—
     e.g. *projection*: when the blame for one's own unsatisfactory responses is transferred to other people.

6   Mechanisms for avoiding the problem by retreating from it—
     e.g. *withdrawal*: when the person withdraws from normal social interaction 'into his own shell'; *hyperactivity*: when the person busies himself with so many other activities that he has no time to think about the real problem.

These mental defence mechanisms are used by everyone to some extent, and they are a valuable means of relieving anxiety and coping with stress, but when pursued to extremes can interfere with normal behaviour even to the extent of mental illness.

Psychological concepts and nursing

All these concepts and theories, which are the specific concern of psychologists and which have been demonstrated and tested in mainly 'artificial' (i.e. experimental) settings, are nevertheless directly relevant to the district nurse's everyday task of caring for patients. An understanding of the patient's personality, mental processes and behaviour, and of her own, is fundamental to the nurse's ability to assess and to meet an individual patient's needs. Effective teaching, which is an important part of her role, requires an understanding of how people learn, including the processes of perception, memory and motivation. Effective communication, which is a prerequisite for the use of all other nursing skills, is itself a learnt skill which also incorporates these processes. For this reason, many of the concepts introduced in this chapter reappear in later chapters as practical factors in patient care.

The individual definition of illness

Illness is not merely a physiological phenomenon. People differ in their experience of particular symptoms, in their readiness to accept a particular symptom as a symptom of illness, and in what they decide to do about it. Nor is *illness* the same thing as *disease*; it is possible to feel ill when no disease exists. *Disease* is a medical concept based on the presence of certain observable pathological abnormalities of body function which are indicated by a set of signs or symptoms. *Illness* on the other hand is a subjective experience indicated by the person's feelings of pain or discomfort. The difference was well described by an American woman (note that Americans use the word 'sick' where English people use the word 'ill') as follows:

> 'I wish I knew what you mean by being sick. Sometimes I felt so bad I could curl up and die but I had to go on because of the kids who have to be taken care of, and besides we didn't have the money to spend for the doctor. How could I be sick? Some people can be sick anytime with everything, but most of us can't be sick, even when we need to be'.[4]

PERSON'S PERCEPTION

- Person with chronic condition–lives within limits
  Sick role rejected

O Neurotic or malingerer–sick role desired

■ Shared definition–sick role legitimatized

Fig. 3.1. Perceptions of illness (from Chapman C. (1977) *Sociology for Nurses.*
London: Ballière Tindall).

Because the 'disease theory' approach to illness, which is the
basis of most medical training and practice, is outside the
experience of most patients, it is perhaps not surprising that
doctors, nurses and patients may have different perceptions, as
shown in Fig. 3.1. Illness is defined by individuals in terms of their
own experience, feelings and values and the nurse must recognise
that just as she is entitled to her own experience, feelings and
values, so that patient is entitled to his.

The term *illness behaviour* is used to describe 'the way in which
symptoms may be differently perceived, evaluated, and acted (or
not acted) upon by different kinds of persons',[5] and both the
concept and the way it is manifested in people's behaviour has
been extensively studied by medical sociologists such as Robinson, Mechanic and others.

Individual responses to illness

Balint has pointed out that 'With the starting of an illness a
number of secondary processes are also set in motion. One may
say that illness creates a new-life situation to which the patient
must adapt himself'.[6]

The response of different individuals depends on their
definition of illness, their experience of it, and what it means to
them; it will also be coloured by their personality. Illness is a
psychological as well as a physiological stressor and therefore

provokes various coping mechanisms including all the *mental defence mechanisms* previously described. One of the mechanisms most commonly adopted by people who are ill is regression—that is they revert to previous patterns of behaviour, especially to those of childhood. They may be unreasonably demanding, seeking constant attention from those around them rather like a toddler constantly demanding the attention of its mother, and they may become more dependent on other people, physically and emotionally, than their physical condition warrants. Some people will repress and deny the seriousness of their situation because they cannot consciously face it; this mechanism must always be considered in dealing with patients for whom the prognosis is poor or who are dying (Chapter 16).

Emotional responses are very varied. Almost everybody who becomes ill experiences anxiety not only because of fears about the illness itself but also about consequential events such as having an operation or being admitted to hospital. Relieving anxiety is an important nursing function about which much has been written which is considered in more detail in later chapters. The question 'Why did this happen to me?' often provokes anger, which may be expressed directly in angry behaviour, channelled inwards as guilt, or towards other people in the mental mechanism of projection. Some patients feel guilty because they look upon the illness as a punishment for something they have done or not done; this is especially common among children. Guilty feelings are also experienced by anxious relatives and are sometimes the reason for trying to take on too much responsibility for their loved one's care. For some people the worst part of illness is the damage which it does to their self-esteem. It is difficult for people to think well of themselves when they are helpless, robbed of their privacy and their independence; yet self-esteem is a basic human need (Chapter 7).

Some illnesses and treatments cause disturbances in the *body image* which individuals develop in early childhood and which includes not only awareness and perception of their physical shape but also the values and emotional attitudes which they attach to it. The way in which people respond to and come to terms with disfigurement depends on many factors, including their age, the speed at which the change occurred and how visible the disfigurement is.

Social responses to illness

Although each individual's experience of illness is unique, his behaviour also takes account of other people's views about it, and their behaviour towards the sick person depends on their views about illness and their expectations about how sick people behave. This pattern of expectations and the behaviour which occurs in response to it is an application of the concept of *role* which is discussed in more detail in the next chapter. The pattern of expected behaviour associated with being ill, which the sociologist Parsons called 'the sick role',[7] has four aspects:

1   The sick person is exempted from normal social responsibilities. This is accepted as the 'right' of the sick person, but only when it has been 'recognised' or *legitimised* by others, i.e. when *other people* define the sick person as sick.

2   The sick person cannot be expected to make himself well by an act of decision or will. It is recognised that he 'cannot help' his illness. This also depends on *other people's* definition of the sick person's sickness.

These two 'rights' carry associated responsibilities:

3   The sick person should want to get well, and as speedily as possible. Everybody assumes that illness is temporary, and 'makes allowances' for it on that basis.

4   The sick person should seek expert (medical) help and should cooperate with it in order to get well.

While these expectations do govern the behaviour of people who are ill to a considerable extent, and a good deal of our health care system assumes that this behaviour will occur, there are many cases which do not fit the pattern. For example, some conditions require the person to be exempted from normal responsibilities, but there is no possibility that he will 'get well': should one treat as 'sick' a patient who is paralysed after an accident, like John Davis? Similarly some people who have been defined—rightly or wrongly—by other people as 'sick' refuse to behave in the way expected. These discrepancies in behaviour cause problems for the patient, his family, and the nurse, but they confirm the uniqueness of the individual and of his experience.

Another way in which other people's perceptions of the illness affect both their behaviour and that of the sick person is based on the concept of 'stigma'. The word stigma means mark or blemish, but is used as a technical term in sociology to mean any characteristic which marks out an individual as being inferior in some way; in other words it is an expression of people's moral judgements, and is closely related to the idea that illness is a punishment and the sufferer is 'to blame'. Some illnesses—especially mental illness, mental handicap, epilepsy, and venereal disease—carry a stigma which results in the sufferer being treated by other people as an 'outcast'. This has serious effects not only on the individual patient but also on his family, for frequently the stigma is attached to the whole family.

Individual behaviour

People's behaviour and personality are moulded by their life's experiences and must therefore be considered in relation to their age and stage of development. Although the term 'life cycle' conjures up an image of a smoothly rounded circle, the process of individual development is more like a series of steps as shown in Fig. 3.2. The horizontal lines in the diagram represent the relatively stable stages of childhood, adulthood and old age. The diagonal lines represent the jump from one relatively stable stage to the next; the stages of infancy, adolescence, and middle age are 'critical periods' in development, periods of imbalance before stability returns. During these 'critical periods' the individual is especially vulnerable to stressors in the external environment which are indicated by arrows on the diagram; physical and mental changes coincide with changes in roles and responsibilities, some of which are listed alongside each diagonal line or 'critical period'. The term 'critical period' is also used in another sense, to imply that for each step forward or upward there is a 'right' time; the step cannot be taken before the individual is 'ready' and although some indication of the typical chronological ages at which these changes occur is given in the diagram, the age at which each step forward occurs varies from person to person. Like physical development, psychosocial development follows a

BIRTH

INFANCY

maternal rejection →

broken home →

establishment of relationship with mother

establishment of relationship with other people

acquisition of basic skills

acquisition of language

urge for independence

starting school

5 yrs

CHILDHOOD

disturbed parent-child relationships →

drug abuse →

sexual experimentation →

12 yrs

puberty

rapid growth and body changes

role confusion and rebellion

establishment of self identity

awakening of sexuality

establishment of a career

ADOLESCENCE

20 yrs

marriage

starting a family

ADULTHOOD

50 yrs

MIDDLE AGE

children leave home

woman: menopause

man: no further progress in career

retirement

progressive physical deterioration

marital breakdown →

bereavement →

65 yrs   OLD AGE

Fig. 3.2. Steps in psychosocial development.

characteristic sequence which is the same for everyone although the rate of development, and therefore the timing of a particular step, varies. Like physical and intellectual development, psychosocial development may be arrested—an individual may be unable to achieve the leap from one level to the next.

Different psychologists use different theories of development and concentrate on different stages or aspects of behaviour or personality. However, all agree on two basic principles: first, that what happens at one stage of development affects what happens at later stages, and secondly the earliest stages, especially early childhood, are especially important.

The exact number of stages identified varies but they can be broadly grouped into six:

Infancy
Childhood
Adolescence
Adulthood
Middle age
Old age

Infancy

There are many ways of approaching the study of infant development. For example, paediatricians such as Sheridan and Illingworth have concentrated on establishing norms of physical development; Freud and his followers have concentrated on emotional development; Piaget on intellectual development; Erikson on psychosocial adjustment to developmental 'tasks'. Clearly physical, mental and social development are closely interrelated, but the age at which children reach particular developmental milestones varies considerably.

From many points of view the first year of life is the most important. During this time the baby develops from the helpless, completely dependent newborn whose range of behaviour is very limited, to the one-year-old who has achieved considerable, although not complete, control over his body movements; has learnt that he exists as an independent being which is separate from the rest of the world; has learnt to use his sense organs as a means of collecting information about the world; and has established social relationships with other people, including a special social relationship with his mother or mother-substitute, and a sophisticated means of communicating with them.

During the second year his ability to walk enables him to explore a far larger segment of the world around him, but his confidence to do so depends very much on the security of a safe and constant base to which he can return at will; the absence of this base, usually his mother, causes considerable distress, and the consequences of long-term absence or complete loss of this base-person may be far reaching. Around the age of two he is beginning to discover the extent of his independence and to use the power which this gives him, in manipulative or negativistic behaviour; he is beginning to use language as the main means of communicating his needs and feelings to other people. By the age of four or five he is relatively independent in terms of basic self-care skills, completely mobile, manually dextrous, fluent in language, and able to establish and maintain social relationships with relative strangers. By the age of five the foundations of his personality, self-concept, and basic patterns of behaviour are well and truly laid, and the experiences of this early period will have a profound effect on his future development.

Childhood

The rate of change is much slower between the age of about five years and puberty. Starting school, however, is an important step because it provides opportunities for learning far more than facts and skills; the social learning which takes place during the primary school years includes responses to authority and discipline, the establishment of peer-group relationships especially friendships, and the rights and obligations involved in being a member of a group. Social learning is accompanied by moral learning—not only an awareness of right and wrong but of the ability to choose between them—and rapid intellectual development.

Adolescence

Adolescence is a period of transition from childhood to adulthood. The physical changes associated with the development of sexual maturity are reflected in the coming to terms with one's sexuality and in the awakening of sexual feelings. Endocrine instability causes instability of mood which is reflected in instability of behaviour. Socially the transition is from the dependence of childhood to the independence of adulthood. Erikson[8] describes the adolescent mind as 'essentially a mind of the moratorium . . . between the morality learned by the child and the ethics to be developed by the adult . . . an ideological mind' in search of 'identity'; the achievement of 'identity' represents the achievement of maturity.

Adulthood

Although adulthood is associated with the achievement of 'maturity', maturity is an elusive concept. In terms of physical development it carries the connotation of completion, or even of an optimal stage which is followed by a decline. Emotional maturity, however, implies integration and self-control, the ability to give love as well as to receive it, and the ability to accept responsibility for other people as well as for oneself. Maturity is expressed in attitudes to work, in social responsibility and in the creation—socially as well as physically—of the new generation. Some adults, however, continue to be motivated in their behaviour by emotions which properly belong to childhood, and to persist in behaviour patterns which were appropriate to an earlier stage of development; an adult who behaves in this way could be described as physically mature but emotionally immature. This kind of immaturity is frequently brought to light when the individual has to face a particular stress such as illness.

Middle age

It has been said that middle age is a modern invention which can be attributed to improved standards of living; life has been stretched out in the middle so that what used to be old age is now middle age. Defining the stage in chronological terms is not easy; 'middle age' is usually considered to cover the years from the middle or late forties to retirement, but chronological age may not be exactly reflected in physiological or psychological age. Point of view alters the definition—while the child or the adolescent may consider the 45-year-old to be quite ancient, the 45-year-old may consider himself young.

In terms of psychosocial development, however, middle age represents a critical developmental period analogous to adolescence in that it is a stage of 'becoming'—shown in Fig. 3.2 as a diagonal line. As in adolescence, the physiological changes associated with the climacteric, and especially in women with the menopause, have psychological and social as well as physical effects. In the field of family relationships instability may result from the fact that the children are no longer dependent but have left the parental home to establish their own homes and families. This changes the marital relationship at the same time as the menopause may be causing changes in ideas about sexual activity and changing body image. At work a man must accept that he has 'reached his peak' whether this point is at or short of his aspirations or capabilities; for a woman this period may mark a new career. The death of elderly parents may be the first real experience of bereavement. The early stages of degenerative disorders such as arthritis may be beginning to make their presence felt.

This period offers an important challenge for health education because intervention at this stage can considerably mitigate some of the problems of old age; in particular preparation for retirement can make the adjustment to retirement, for both men and women, considerably easier.

Old age

Ageing, like adolescence, is a process that is social and psychological as well as physical, and as in adolescence, physical changes affect personality and behaviour. Unlike adolescence, however, the onset of old age is not marked by an identifiable event; the onset is insidious and its definition, like that of illness, is very subjective.

Deterioration of the special senses such as vision and hearing have important mental and social consequences. The organic degeneration of the brain which is termed dementia disrupts the personality and affects intelligence, memory, emotional state, and learning—that is, the ability to adapt to a changing environment. One manifestation of these changes is that personality becomes more rigid; old people tend to be set in their ways. Conservatism and apprehension about change increase, although how far this is due to mental changes and how far to social changes is uncertain. The older people get the more dependent they become on the stabilising effect of their own home and their own possessions; familiar ornaments and old photographs are not only treasured mementoes but an important prop to maintaining identity. Short-term memory becomes poor while long-term memory is retained—even appearing, relative to the short-term memory loss, to improve. Old people like to reminisce, and it is possible that this is a means of 'reworking' previous experiences in such a way as to come to terms with them. Erikson sees 'coming to terms' with oneself as the mark of the successful achievement of the last stage of development:

> Only in him who in some way has taken care of things and people and has adapted himself to the triumphs and disappointments adherent to being—only in him may gradually ripen the fruit of these seven stages. I know no better word for it than ego integrity. . . . It is the acceptance of one's one and only life cycle as something that had to be and that, by necessity, permitted of no substitution. . . . The lack of this accrued ego integration is signified by fear of death: the one and only life cycle is not accepted as the ultimate of life.[8]

Other writers have described the elderly person's method of adjustment as *disengagement*. Disengagement involves reducing the extent of social interaction, reducing the number of social roles played, reducing life space and social activity. Emotional disengagement involves a flattening of emotion which may be manifested as a certain 'mellowness' or equanimity of temperament. The prospect of death is no longer terrifying and may be looked forward to peacefully.

Conclusion

Each individual experiences illness differently and copes with it differently; this chapter has described some of the factors which explain individual differences. The nurse must consider all these factors in relation to each patient, but one might apply them to just one of the seven patients as follows:

John Davis is 22 years old, and is tetraplegic as the result of a motorbike accident 2 years ago. At the time of his accident he was at the threshold of healthy adulthood, recently 'flown' from the family 'nest', launched upon a promising career, about to marry. All his hopes and expectations of a wonderful future—and those of his parents—were shattered. Imagine the immediate psychological effects of the accident. John's immediate reactions might have been masked by the intensive care required for his survival, but his parents' response might have been first numbed shock, then anger, then despair. Does John's father blame himself for allowing John to have a motorbike, and is that why he feels he must contribute to John's care even at the risk of his job? During the months in hospital the realities of his situation will gradually have dawned upon John, but the environment of the hospital, where he could identify with and derive support from other patients in similar situations, may have protected him for a time. Now that he is living at home and his condition is stable is he still 'sick'? Do other people treat him as 'sick', and does he want them to do so? How has he adjusted his body image to take account of his paralysis? How does he cope with the fact that his sexual drives, which are strongest at this age, are unimpaired although the means by which they would normally have been expressed are no longer available? What mental mechanisms does he use to cope with his situation—does he compensate for his physical loss by becoming the local chess champion, or deny reality by escaping into his daydreams? Does he regress into childish dependency— and do his mother and sisters reinforce his behaviour, compensating for their own loss by regarding him as still their 'baby'? Does he express his frustration and anger in rages and verbal abuse of his parents and the nurse? Does an extrovert personality help him to establish new kinds of social relationships or does an introvert personality increase his risk of social isolation? Are there strong personality traits such as persistence and determination which will help him to cope?

Since John Davis is a fictional character, one can only speculate, but the answers to similar questions are an important part of the nurse's assessment of each individual patient in her care.

References

1. Muller H. J. (1943). *Science and Criticism*. New Haven: Yale University Press.
2. Altchul A. (1975). *Psychology for Nurses*, 4th edn. London: Ballière Tindall.
3. James D. (1970). *Introduction to Psychology*. Harmondsworth: Penguin.
4. Koos E. (1954). *The Health of Regionville*. New York: Columbia University Press.
5. Mechanic D. (1968). *Medical Sociology: a selective view*. New York: Free Press.
6. Balint M. (1964). *The Doctor, his Patient, and the Illness*. London: Pitman.
7. Parsons T. (1951). *The Social System*. London: Routledge & Kegan Paul.
8. Erikson E. (1965). *Childhood and Society*. Harmondsworth: Penguin.

Further Reading

Altchul A. (1975). *Psychology for Nurses*. London: Ballière Tindall.

Antonovsky A. (1979). *Health, Stress and Coping*. San Francisco: Jossey-Bass.

Argyle M. (1967). *The Psychology of Interpersonal Behaviour*. Harmondsworth: Penguin.

Baron R. A., Byrne D. (1984). *Social Psychology: understanding human behaviour*. Boston: Allyn and Bacon.

Bee H. L., Mitchell S. K. (1986). *The Developing Person—A Life Span Approach*. London: Harper and Row.

Berne E. (1968). *Games People Play*. Harmondsworth: Penguin.

Black N., ed. (1984). *Health and Disease*. Milton Keynes: Open University Press.

Goffman E. (1969). *The Presentation of Self in Everyday Life*. Harmondsworth: Penguin.

Hall J. (1982). *Psychology for Nurses and Health Visitors*. London: Macmillan.

Chapter 4

People in Groups

John Donne wrote:

> 'No man is an island entire of itself. Every man is a piece of the Continent, a part of the main'.

Human beings are social beings; they interact with one another in a social world. An individual's behaviour is determined both by his own mental processes and also by the behaviour of other people in the world around him. He responds to their behaviour as they respond to his in the activity called *social interaction*. Just as psychology provides a way of understanding behaviour in terms of individual mental processes, sociology provides a way of understanding behaviour in terms of its social context. Both perspectives are important to the nurse.

Mr Evans, for example, is unique, but he is also a member of several groups—his family, his work group, his trade union, the group of friends whom he meets at the local pub on Friday nights, the local football club—which influence what he thinks and the way he behaves, and must, therefore, also be taken into account in planning his care. These *primary groups* overlap and interact with one another in larger units such as his neighbourhood and his community, which in turn overlap and interact within the overall group which we term *society*. Each group, for example the Evans family, is a social system which can be viewed in the same way as a physiological system such as the digestive or respiratory system, that is as a collection of interrelated parts and the relationships between them. We can also talk about the educational system or the political system as social systems within a particular society, or we can use the term 'the social system' to describe society as a whole.

Groups in this sense are more than mere collections of people; the key characteristic of a social group is the fact that its members interact with and behave towards one another in ways which other members of the group encourage, respond to and expect.

The way Mr Evans behaves towards his wife and children within the family group would not be the appropriate way to behave towards his boss and his colleagues at work. Each group has its own *values* and *attitudes* which guide its members' behaviour. The expected patterns or *norms* of behaviour are learned: for example, from the day a child is born he or she begins to learn the kind of behaviour which is expected within the family, and parents will, consciously and unconsciously, teach their children by encouraging some behaviours and discouraging others. This process of social learning is called *socialisation*. By this means, the pattern of expected behaviour is passed on from generation to generation, gradually changing and developing all the time. The totality of the expected behaviour patterns which a society develops, incorporating attitudes, beliefs, morals, laws and customs, is called its *culture*. Although individuals are unique and endowed with what we call 'free will', their patterns of behaviour depend very greatly on their social and cultural background; they cannot escape entirely from its influence, and some would argue that they are the product of it.

Cultural differences

Because our culture is so much a part of us we tend to take it for granted, assuming that our expectations and patterns of behaviour are normal, inevitable, and 'right' while other patterns are abnormal or 'wrong'. We also tend to assume that our particular patterns of behaviour are common to all mankind, whereas any individual's behaviour patterns come primarily from the group and culture into which he is born, and these are not the same for everyone. It is important for nurses not only to recognise that there are social and cultural differences between people which affect the way in which they behave when they are ill or when someone near to them is ill, but also to respect the differences and to take account of them in planning and giving care.

This is particularly important in a multiracial society such as exists in Britain today, where nurses and patients will quite commonly be of different cultural backgrounds. About 6% of the population of the United Kingdom were born overseas;

in addition there is an increasing number of second-generation immigrants whose parents were born abroad but who were themselves born and brought up in Britain—this is true of the Johnson family. People migrate from one country to another for a number of reasons. Some have come to Britain as refugees from wars or political pressures in their own countries; examples in this century include German Jews, Hungarians, and Ugandan Asians. Others are drawn by economic factors such as better job prospects and opportunities for their children. At different times different groups of immigrants have been the focus of interest and concern; for example, in the censuses of 1901 and 1911, special efforts were made to assess accurately the large number of foreign-born Jews who had emigrated to the UK as a result of the political pressures in their own countries at the end of the nineteenth century.

The new immigrants to a country bring with them the culture—including religion, which in some countries is a major determinant of life style—and the behaviour patterns of their country of origin. For many present-day immigrants to Britain the process of *integration*, which is the process by which an immigrant group modifies its old culture and absorbs the culture of its new home, involves a change from life in a simple rural society to life in a complex urban society. There is an enormous difference between life in a small village in northern India and life in a large industrial city in Britain. People's responses to the change differ; some want to preserve as much as possible of their old culture and to pass it on to future generations, while others, although their own patterns of behaviour are established as the result of their former cultural experiences, are anxious to adopt British ways and are particularly anxious for their children to do so. In both groups the second-generation immigrants, for example the teenage daughters of Asian immigrants, may experience conflict between the old culture and the new. An understanding of these factors is particularly important to the district nurse because it is within the home and family setting that cultural differences are most marked; among the most fundamental differences are those relating to family roles (especially the role of women), child-rearing practices, and food habits.

There are also important culturally determined differences in sickness behaviour. The subjectivity of the definition of illness was discussed in Chapter 3, and clearly the response to sickness of a western European who believes that the 'cause' of his misfortune is a particular disease will be different from say, an Arab who may believe it to be the will of Allah. Such differences affect the decision to seek help in the first place, who to seek it from, and whose advice to follow; the antibiotic cream and the sterile dressing so carefully applied by the nurse may be quietly removed as soon as she has left the house and replaced by a home-made herbal concoction prescribed by the community's traditional healer. Cross-cultural research has also demonstrated significant cultural differences in the prevalence of various diseases, responses to mental stress and responses to pain.

Religion is a very important aspect of culture, and religious beliefs and practices also influence sickness behaviour and patient care. Like the more general cultural differences, religious differences affect both patient and nurse; for example, Roman Catholic nurses are not required to participate in abortions, but have to find other solutions when they are caring for a patient who has had an abortion or who is seeking contraceptive advice. In some societies, religious belief is a major determinant of the whole way of life; for example, the Muslim holy book, the Koran, specifically lays down dietary restrictions, codes about the regulation of marriage, family roles, dress, and many kinds of social activity. Religious rites associated with death are very important and the district nurse must make sure that she understands her patient's beliefs and wishes. Religious festivals which may involve fasting, such as the Muslim Ramadan and the Jewish Yom Kippur, have implications for planning patient care. Many religious sects have other beliefs which affect specific aspects of health care, for example the Jehovah's Witnesses' refusal of blood transfusion and the Christian Scientists' rejection of drugs.

Social positions and social roles

The terminology which is used to describe the way in which people behave in groups is the language of the stage: each person is an *actor* who is given a part (a *social position*) and when he acts according to his part he is said to be performing a *role*. An individual occupies many social positions and plays many different roles, even within the same group. Within his family, for example, Mr Evans is a husband, a father, and his mother's son; at the same time he plays other roles in other groups—as an employee and perhaps a shop steward in his work group, as a member of the local football club, and, temporarily at least, as a patient. Just as the groups interact and overlap so do the roles of individual actors within them. Figure 4.1. shows Mr Evans' social network and some of the roles he plays in relation to other people.

The diagram shows that role relationships are reciprocal—husband and wife, father and child, employer and employee; it is difficult to play the role of husband to someone who does not play the role of wife. Tensions also arise when something prevents a person from playing the role he wants to play or plays it differently from the way other people expect. In the Fisher family, for example, Mr Fisher's physical handicap will interfere with the way he plays the role of husband; one aspect of the traditional 'husband-wife' role relationship is reversed in that Mrs Fisher goes out to work leaving her husband at home all day, and is likely to become the main breadwinner. Mrs Fisher, like most people, has multiple roles—as wife, carer and schoolmistress, and these roles may sometimes conflict—for example, if the caring role which she wants to adopt to her husband had prevented her from taking the opportunity for promotion at work.

The concept of social class

In all societies people are differentiated by social as well as by biological criteria into categories which imply that there are not only 'differences' between the groups but also 'inequalities', since the groups can be arranged in some sort of social hierarchy. In ancient Greece and Rome, the basic distinction was between citizen and slave; in India people were differentiated by caste; for Marx the distinction lay in people's relation to the means of production. In an industrialised society occupational status is a convenient and useful indicator of social position, and it began to be used as a criterion by which to 'sort' information about the health of the population from the middle of the last century. In

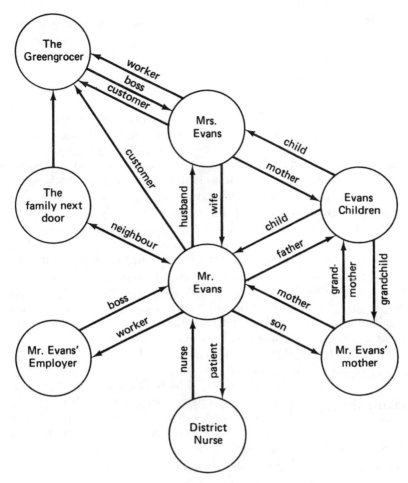

Fig. 4.1. Mr Evans' social network.

1911, the Chief Medical Statistical Officer in the General Register Office, T.H.C. Stevenson, developed a comprehensive classification system based on occupation to analyse infant mortality. With relatively minor modifications his scale has survived to be the major classification of social class used today:

Class I   Professional (e.g. accountant, doctor)

Class II	Intermediate (e.g. manager, school teacher, nurse)
Class III (n)	Skilled non-manual (e.g. clerical worker, shop assistant)
Class III (m)	Skilled manual (e.g. bus driver, coal miner, carpenter)
Class IV	Semi-skilled (e.g. agricultural worker, postmen)
Class V	Unskilled (e.g. labourer, dock worker)

This system is used to classify all census data, and in spite of some inherent problems, such as the classification of married women and retired people, it has proved to be an extremely powerful epidemiological tool. One of the reasons why it has proved useful is that it has been shown to differentiate between people on other social characteristics such as education, income, life styles, linguistic codes and even attitudes, values, and norms of behaviour. For this reason, it is a useful way of differentiating between social classes defined in the more general sense as 'segments of the population sharing broadly similar types and levels of resources, with broadly similar styles of living and some shared perception of their collective condition'.[1]

In interpreting data which has been classified in this way, however, it is important not to impute a *causal* relationship between class and the factor which is being considered: correlation does not necessarily imply causation. While it may be reasonable to infer a causal connection between certain occupations such as coal mining and certain causes of death such as pneumoconiosis on the basis of what is known about the aetiology of the disease, in many other cases the relationship is likely to be much more complex; it may even happen that—as has been argued in the case of the epidemiology of schizophrenia—the variable in question is the cause rather than the effect of the social class classification. In social statistics and epidemiology, unlike in some other branches of sociology and political theory, social class is a statistical concept for classifying data, not a means of explaining why or how social differentials exist.[2]

Social class is also *subjectively* defined, usually in the more general terms 'upper class', 'middle class' and 'working class'; this subjective classification is often applied to factors associated with the 'class culture', such as attitudes, values and life-styles. Within this rather less precise classification most people assign themselves either to the 'middle class' which broadly corresponds to the Registrar General's classes I and II, or the the 'working class' which broadly corresponds to classes III, IV and V; the term 'upper class' is usually applied to the traditional aristocracy.

Some important research studies have analysed the relationship between social class and particular factors, including:

Education
Child rearing practices
Infant feeding practices
Contraceptive practices
Linguistic codes
Family roles
Health

A number of studies of more general class-based differences are included in the suggestions for further reading; a summary of the 'working-class' and 'middle-class' perspectives revealed by one classic study[3] is shown in Table 4.1.

Social class health and health care

Differences in life chances and health patterns between the different social classes begin at birth or even before, and continue throughout life. The baby of an unskilled manual worker (social class V) is twice as likely to be stillborn, twice as likely to die during the first month of life, and five times more likely to die between then and his first birthday than the baby of an accountant or lawyer (social class I). The difference persists throughout childhood although it is slightly less for girls than for boys. During adulthood the overall difference is less marked although there are dramatic differences in death from particular causes. Overall the chances of premature death (that is death before retirement) are 2½ times as great in social class V as in social class I, and the life expectancy for a baby born into social class V is 5 years less than that of a baby born into social class I.

Information about sickness patterns, as was mentioned in Chapter 2, is more difficult to obtain and to assess, but such

Table 4.1 Working-class and middle-class perspectives

	Working-Class Perspective	Middle-Class Perspective
General beliefs	The social order is divided into 'us' and 'them': these who do not have authority and those who do. The division between 'us' and 'them' is virtually fixed, at least from the point of view of one man's life chances. What happens to you depends a lot on luck; otherwise you have to learn to put up with things	The social order is a hierarchy of differentially rewarded positions: a ladder containing many rungs. It is possible for individuals to move from one level of the hierarchy to another. Those who have ability and initiative can overcome obstacles and create their own opportunities. Where a man ends up depends on what he makes of himself
General values	'We' ought to stick together and get what we can as a group. You may as well enjoy yourself while you can instead of trying to make yourself 'a cut above the rest'	Every man ought to make the most of his own capabilities and be responsible for his own welfare. You cannot expect to get anywhere in the world if you squander your time and money. 'Getting on' means making sacrifices
Attitudes on more specific issues	(on the best job for a son) 'A trade in his hands'. 'A good steady job' (towards people needing social assistance) 'They have been unlucky'. 'They never had a chance'. 'It could happen to any of us' (on Trade Unions) 'Trade Unions are the only means workers have of protecting themselves and of improving their standard of living'	'As good a start as you can give him'. 'A job that leads somewhere' 'Many of them had the same opportunities as others who have managed well enough'. 'They are a burden on those who are trying to help themselves' 'Trade Unions have too much power in the country'. 'The Unions put the interests of a section before the interests of the nation as a whole'

Source: Goldthorpe J. H., Lockwood D. (1970). 'The changing national class structure. In *The Sociology of Modern Britain* (Butterworth E., and Weir D.). London: Fontana.

information as is available reflects the general picture of mortality. Rates of 'long-standing illness' reported in the General Household Surveys are approximately 2–2½ times as high among social class V as among social class I, and the average number of days lost through illness or accident among unskilled manual workers is nearly 5 times as great as the number lost by professional men. There are marked differences in the type of illness experienced by people in different classes; for example, respiratory diseases are much more common in social class V while cirrhosis of the liver is more common in social class I. Psychiatric illness has been shown to be 4 times as common among working-class women compared with middle-class women, although it may be less frequently reported or treated.[4]

Differences between the social classes in the availability and use made of health services are also important. Tudor Hart[5] has suggested an 'inverse care law' which states that 'the availability of good medical care tends to vary inversely with the need of the population served'. He argues that in areas with most sickness and death, general practitioners and hospitals have more work, larger lists, the least adequate buildings, and less staff and equipment. The removal of such inequalities was one of the stated intentions of the National Health Service; it has never been achieved, although the use of RAWP formulae for the allocation of funds to health authorities is an attempt to begin to do so.

Even when the need is evident and the services are available, however, differences persist in the extent to which people use them. The Black report *Inequalities in Health*[1] concluded that, although working class adults consulted general practitioners more and were heavier users of hospital beds than middle-class adults, when their increased morbidity was taken into account they made relatively less use of health services, were typically more sick than middle-class patients when help was sought, were less likely to seek medical help for their children, and in particular made much less use of the preventive health services. Similar patterns have also been shown in the use of family planning services, dental services, and cervical screening. These differences offer a particular challenge to all those concerned with health education, including district nurses.

Finally, the evidence suggests that there are differences in the quality of care received and in the patient's response to it. For example, studies of the work of general practitioners have shown that working-class patients have shorter consultations with their general practitioner. A number of sociological studies have suggested that the social distance between patients and health care professionals—doctors are defined as belonging to social class I and nurses to social class II—affects the care given, and that differences in the type of language which they use inhibits doctor–patient communication.

The relationship between health and social class is easy to demonstrate, but extremely difficult to interpret, partly because the concepts 'health' and 'social class' are themselves extremely complex. Sometimes causal factors can be reasonably inferred: for example, some diseases can be directly related to occupation. The ten-fold increase in the risk of death from fire, falls and drowning among boys of social class V compared with their peers in social class I can be related, at least in part, to environmental factors; the prevalance of respiratory diseases can be related to housing conditions; housing conditions can be related to income levels and both are closely related to social class. Income levels and material resources such as access to a car and a telephone may also explain some of the differences in patterns of usage of health services; education has also been shown to be an important factor. Cultural behaviour patterns and perspectives such as those which were shown in Table 4.1, and the subjective definitions which were discussed in Chapter 3, are clearly important but are difficult to interpret. What is important from the district nurse's point of view is that she should be aware of the differences and should take account of them in preparing appropriate and realistic care plans for individual patients.

The family

The group that exerts probably the greatest influence on an individual's behaviour is the family, partly because the attitudes and behaviour that are developed in early childhood within the context of a family group become an integral part of an individual's personality and life style; and partly because for most people the family (although in adulthood it may be a different family) is the group with which they have most frequent and prolonged contact.

Fletcher[6] has suggested that the functions of the modern family are as follows:

To regulate sexual behaviour.
To give a legitimate basis for the procreation and rearing of children.
To provide a home for its members.
To serve as the primary agency for socialisation.

To these functions a district nurse would undoubtedly add:

To provide the primary social context for the care of the sick at home.

It is for this reason that district nurses need to understand the sociology of the family, and though some of the most important points are outlined here it is important that this outline should be 'filled out' by reading some of the wealth of specialist literature on the subject; a few of the most useful books are included in the suggestions for further reading. This section concentrates specifically on family responses to illness and the family's role in care.

The family unit

It is common to discuss family structure in terms of two 'ideal types': the *nuclear* family, consisting of a mother, a father and their children living together, and the *extended* family in which grandparents, parents, siblings, aunts, uncles and cousins (or various combinations of these) live together as a single family unit. Other terms used include the *family of origin*, meaning the family into which a person is born; the *family of marriage* meaning the family which is created by marriage; the *consanguine family*, meaning the family of blood relations; and *kin* or the *kinship network* which is the 'rest of the family' formed by the interlocking network of related nuclear families. The *extended* family is often represented as the 'original' family type, which was economically and socially self-supporting, meeting functions such as obtaining the necessities of life, child-rearing, housekeeping, and caring for sick and other dependent members from within its own resources. The *nuclear* family is represented as the 'modern' family, produced by the consequences of industrialisation in which social and geographical mobility split up extended families and the welfare state took over most of its functions. The extended family type tends to be associated with agricultural communities, immigrant groups, and the working class; the nuclear family type tends to be associated with towns, suburbia and the middle class. Ideal types, however, rarely exist in the real world. There are, and have always been, other kinds of groups in which people live, such as single-parent families, communes of various kinds, unmarried people living alone, and elderly people (often widows and widowers) living alone. The extended family was never as universal as is sometimes suggested, and the modern nuclear family is rarely as isolated.

The social changes described in Chapter 2 have had a significant effect on the structure and life style of the modern family. In general, families are smaller and more socially and geographically mobile; political, legal and economic emancipation of women has profoundly affected traditional male–female, husband–wife, and mother–father–child roles and relationships; social policies in work, housing and welfare services and the development of transport and communications technology have substantially altered social networks between kin.

Many of these factors can be identified in the stories of the seven families. The rural setting has not protected Mr and Mrs Adams from separation from their kin; they, like many other elderly people, do not have children to care for them. The Bakers, as a single-parent family, represent one in ten of all families with dependent children. Mrs Cray, her daughter, son-in-law and grandchildren do not live under the same roof, but the family has close contact with their kin which may provide to a lesser or greater degree the same kind of support network as the 'ideal type' extended family was said to provide. The Johnson family, although not originating in this country, have a similar family network; however, the grandparents are in the West Indies which can present a conflict of loyalties at times and perhaps accentuates the close family ties of those within this country. Family roles within the Davis family probably follow traditional lines; the husband–wife roles of the Fishers were probably different, even before Mr Fisher's illness.

The ideal types of family structures and life styles may offer a useful framework within which the district nurse can assess a family's social dynamics and coping methods, but it is important to recognise that, as with individuals, the complexities of the family system make each family and its needs unique.

The family and illness

The family is not only the context within which illness occurs; the family has a direct influence on the illness and its management, and the illness has a direct consequence on the family.

From the district nurse's point of view the ability and willingness of family members to assist in the care of their sick relative is a major factor in the nurse's care plan (Chapter 8). Thus although John Davis' handicap and need for physical care are at least as great as Mr Fisher's, it may be that the district nurse will spend less time with John because a greater part of the burden of care has been accepted, willingly or reluctantly, by John's parents than by Mrs Fisher. The way in which the carers approach their task will also influence the patient's response; for example, will the devotion of John's mother make him more dependent than he needs to be, or make him emotionally as well as physically dependent?

Disturbed family relationships may actually cause illness, especially mental illness. Laing[7] has argued that family pressures are a direct cause of the schizophrenic's withdrawal from reality, and Brown[8] has shown that they are an important cause of relapse and readmission. Family tensions may cause psychosomatic illnesses as specific as a gastric ulcer or as general as 'tension headaches'. Disturbed parent–child relationships are associated with a wide range of disorders in children including failure to thrive, asthma, vomiting, developmental retardation and accident proneness. There is increasing evidence that psychological stress acts as a trigger factor which precipitates or increases susceptibility to diseases such as coronary thrombosis, rheumatoid arthritis, and even infections such as tuberculosis and streptococcal throat infections. The most dramatic example of the effect of family disruption on physical illness is the increased mortality and morbidity which follows bereavement.[9]

The effect of illness on the family

The effect of illness, particularly long-term illness, on a family is considerable. The practical implications of the 'burden of care' include additional financial expenditure—often at the same time as a reduction in income; having to do too many tasks in the time available—especially if the carer works outside the home and has to manage the home as well as caring for the patient; particular problems such as extra laundry or special food; and the sheer physical fatigue produced by the demands of the day followed by disturbed nights, often for weeks or months without respite. The practical problems are lessened if they are shared among several family members, but it is not uncommon for the burden to be borne almost exclusively by one person—for example, the mother of a handicapped child, a spouse, or the single daughter of elderly parents. Sometimes, the sharing of the common task unites and strengthens a family; often, especially if the demands continue over a long period of time, the stress may become too great, the individuals involved may break down or become ill themselves, and the family as a unit may begin to disintegrate. One might wonder how long Mrs Fisher will be able to cope with the demands of a responsible job, managing the house, and caring for an increasingly disabled husband; quite apart from the demands on her own health, such a situation will impose considerable strain on the marriage.

The practical problems also have social costs. A letter to the woman's journal quoted by Quinn[10] gives some indication of the social cost to the unmarried daughters who even nowadays are often expected to care for their elderly parents:

> 'I've looked after my mother since she had a heart attack soon after my father's death. She is now 77 and is a wonderful person which makes my duties lighter. But I've no friends or other relatives to turn to for a break, and I feel isolated and lonely. I'm 47 and the only man I ever loved was unwilling to have my mother in our future home, so I lost him. Can you help?'

One might consider the social cost to Sarah, Mrs Baker's eldest daughter, in terms of her 'lost adolescence', for Sarah is unlikely to have the time, money or social contacts to enable her to enjoy many of the activities which her former schoolmates enjoy.

Similarly, the social costs of enabling John Davis to live with his family outside an institution will include the loss of any career aspirations that either of his parents might have had and most of the social activities that they might have enjoyed together. Such costs are borne not only by the adults who have at least some choice, however limited; one might also imagine the price paid by Rose Johnson's brother and sister as the result of the amount of time and attention which their mother has had to give to Rose. One of the most important, and the least appreciated, costs is the stigma which is still attached to physical and mental handicap, and especially to mental illness.

Illness also disrupts individual roles within the family. Sickness will deprive the patient of some of his normal family roles—for example Mr Evans is temporarily not the main breadwinner of his family—and these roles will have to be taken on by others. This change may not be easy for either the patient or the family to accept. Mr Fisher may not take kindly to the role-reversal implied by the fact that his wife goes out to work every morning while he stays at home and prepares supper. Mrs Baker will not have found it easy to be father as well as mother to her three children, but the prospect of Sarah trying to be both mother and father to her young brother and sister is even more worrying.

The family's role in care

The miracle is that in spite of these very considerable difficulties, families do care for their sick members and often do so magnificently. The way in which the caring role is played varies according to the family's own resources, and also with the type and stage of the illness. It is important that all health professionals, but especially nurses, recognise that they have no exclusive prerogative to care; care is a partnership between the health professionals, the family, and the individual patient himself.

The community

It is unfortunate that in talking about health services, the word 'community' is sometimes used in antithesis to the word 'hospital'. In one sense the hospital is part of 'the community'; in another sense the hospital is a community in its own right. The word community implies having something in common; the original usage of the word, as the modern usage of the word 'commune', implies the sharing of goods, interests, and values in a face to face situation. We apply the word community to a number of different kinds of social groups and networks based sometimes on occupation, sometimes on shared interests and purposes, but most commonly on shared locality.

For a geographical area to be called a community, however, implies a certain social as well as geographical cohesion. The degree of cohesion varies. For many people living alone or in nuclear family units in an urban area, the 'local community' means no more than the collection of homes and families around them; in other areas families living within a particular locality are bound together by a strong sense of common identity and share the same cultural background. Families with like characteristics tend to live together in the same neighbourhood. The like characteristics may be race, religion, occupation, income or social class, and the coming together may be either a matter of choice or a lack of any alternative, but the result is a 'consciousness of kind' which gives the neighbourhood a certain social cohesion.

Neighbourhoods, especially in city areas, may change, sometimes quite rapidly, as the result of social policy and planning decisions, for example slum clearance and development programmes. Much of the housing in city centres consists of large houses built by the wealthy during the last century. As they moved outward their large houses, too expensive for a single working-class family to afford, were divided into flats and rooms so that one house was occupied by several families; some of the problems which this causes were discussed in Chapter 2. Neighbourhoods may also change because of patterns of immigration. As a new immigrant group settles in a neighbourhood and begins to expand, the former residents move out, and as these immigrants prosper and integrate, they move to better neighbourhoods making room for new and sometimes different groups.

As in the case of families, communities are often analysed in terms of ideal types, and a number of sociological studies have described the ways in which different types of community, and the family and kinship groups within them, function; some are included in the suggestions for further reading. While very few communities in reality conform exactly to the ideal type, the framework which the ideal types provide can help the nurse to appreciate and understand the structure and dynamics of the community within which she works.

Rural communities

A rural community is small in scale with few social groupings so that there is frequent face-to-face contact among its members; everyone knows everyone else, their activities and their attitudes. Residents have often lived in the village for many years, sometimes for several generations; the extended family is more common, and the kinship and neighbourhood networks provide considerable social support in time of need. Social institutions such as the local church and the local school, and 'village activities' like the annual fête, foster 'togetherness'. Cultural traditions are strong and slow to change, and considerable time may be needed for new residents to become integrated and accepted as 'members' of the community.

Urban communities

Population density in cities and towns produces communities on a larger scale. The population is often more mobile, so that families are separated and the kinship network is less strong. Because a large community can support a large number of social organisations, especially occupational and recreational organisations, social networks may be based on these groups rather than on kin, and these networks do not usually carry ties of mutual obligation as strong as those between kin. One problem of urban life is that many individuals are isolated from their original family and neighbourhood groups, but do not become members of new groups, and are, therefore, at risk of loneliness and social isolation; Mrs Cray is one such example. On the other hand, large cities may contain smaller communities where social cohesion, which is often based on the extended family or on occupation, is just as strong as the most tightly knit rural community; an example of this kind of community is the neighbourhood in which Rose Johnson's family lives.

Suburban housing estates

In the past the strongest influence on a residential pattern was a man's occupation. He had to live near his place of work. The development of public transport and the growth of car ownership, however, now allow people to work in the city but to live outside. In most of our great cities the popualtion of the central area is decreasing while the population of the 'surburban ring' around the city is increasing.

One of the characteristics of many suburbs, especially where large new housing estates have been built, is the relative homogeneity of the population in age and income; in some areas the population may consist entirely of young married couples or families with small children. The new estates may be at a considerable distance from people's original homes, and nuclear families are thus separated from their kin at what may be a very vulnerable stage in family development.

In local authority estates these difficulties may be exacerbated by the fact that the council tenant does not have the same degree of choice as the home owner. By slum clearance or through housing shortage the council tenant has to live wherever there is a house or flat available for which he is eligible, and near neighbours whom he does not know and did not choose. The social adjustment which this makes necessary may give rise to many problems, especially when the estate is new.

Retirement areas

At the other extreme, but sharing the characteristics of homogeneity of population, are the 'retirement areas' such as the towns of the south coast to which elderly people like to move on retirement because of the pleasant surroundings and climate. In some areas up to half of the population may be over retirement age. These elderly people are isolated from their kin at an equally vulnerable period, and their problems of social isolation may be exacerbated by bereavement and increasing frailty due to age.

However, recently retired people often enjoy good health and have considerable energy which can be committed to the development of a lively and supportive community.

New towns

New towns differ from other neighbourhoods in that they are deliberately created and planned; housing, jobs, recreational facilities and social services are balanced to provide a planned 'social mix'. Some of the housing is available for private ownership and some is owned by the public authorities through the development corporation which is responsible for controlling the development and expansion of the area.

Conclusion

The term 'community care' implies a caring community, and assumes that 'the community' is a cohesive entity capable of thought, decisions and action. The dangers of this assumption should be recognised, for, as has been shown in this chapter, communities are made up of individuals, and as the previous chapter showed, individuals respond differently to the various aspects of their environment.

Sociology is the study of groups, of social interaction and social behaviour. The concepts of sociology enable us to identify and understand in a patient those social experiences which most affect his behaviour, symptoms, perception of illness, and the strategies for coping with it. But it is important always to remember, as was stressed in Chapter 3, that in each individual the particular combination of these factors is unique.

References

1. Black D., Morris J. N., Smith C., Townsend P. (1980) *Inequalities in Health. Report of a Research Working Group*. London: HMSO.
2. Central Statistical Office (1975). Social Commentary: Social Class. In: *Social Trends 1975*. London: HMSO.
3. Goldthorpe J. H., Lockwood D. L., Bechofer F., Platt J. (1969). *The Affluent Worker in the Class Structure*. Cambridge: Cambridge University Press.

4. Brown G., Bhrolchain M., Harris T. (1975). Social class and psychiatric disorder among women in an urban population. *Sociology*; **9**,2:225–55.
5. Tudor Hart J. (1971). The Inverse Care Law. *Lancet*; **i**:405–12.
6. Fletcher R. (1966). *The Family and Marriage in Britain.* Harmondsworth: Penguin.
7. Laing R. D., Esterton A. (1964). *Sanity, Madness and the Family.* Harmondsworth: Penguin.
8. Brown G. W., Birley J. L. T., Wing J. K. (1972). The influence of family life on the course of schizophrenic illness. *British Journal of Psychiatry*; **121**:241–58.
9. Parkes C. M., Benjamin B., Fitzgerald R. G. (1969). Broken heart: a statistical study of increased mortality among widowers. *British Medical Journal*; **i**:740–43.
10. Quinn S. (1981). Promise to care. In: *Readings in Community Health* (Clark J., ed.). Edinburgh: Churchill Livingstone.

Further Reading

Black N., ed. (1984). *Health and Disease: a reader.* Milton Keynes: Open University Press.

Bond J., Bond S. (1986). *Sociology and Health Care.* London: Churchill Livingstone.

Central Statistical Office (published annually). *Social Trends.* London: HMSO.

Chapman C. (1977). *Sociology for Nurses.* London: Baillière Tindall.

Cuff E. C., Payne G. C., eds. (1979). *Perspectives in Sociology.* London: Allen & Unwin.

Dominian J. (1980). *Marriage in Britain.* London: Study Commission on the Family.

Health Education Council (1987). *The Great Divide.* London: HEC.

Henley A. (1979). *Asian Patients in Hospital and at Home.* London: Pitman.

Luker K., Orr J. (1985). *Health Visiting.* Oxford: Blackwell Scientific.

Rapoport R. N. *et al.* (1982). *Families in Britain.* London: Routledge and Kegan Paul.

Worsley P. (1977). *Introducing Sociology.* Harmondsworth: Penguin.

Chapter 5

The Primary Care Setting

District nursing is not hospital nursing in a different environment. While the basic function of the nurse and many of the skills she uses are the same, the setting has a profound effect on the approach to care.

The role-reversal of community care

The concept of 'role' was discussed in Chapter 4 and the role which the patient plays as a 'sick person' was outlined in Chapter 3. It was suggested that social roles were learnt through the process of socialisation, the most important part of which was childhood experience in the family setting. The roles of patient, nurse and doctor, however, are learnt mainly in the setting of the hospital, and the setting itself largely determines the way in which the roles are defined and played. The role styles of the hospital, in which the professionals are all-powerful and the patient is a passive recipient, are, however, inappropriate for the community setting and have to be modified.

In one sense the roles of patient and nurse are actually reversed, for in the hospital setting the nurse is the 'host' and the patient the 'guest' while in the community setting the opposite is true: the patient is in his own territory which the nurse enters by invitation, not by right. This changes the locus of control; while it may be possible in the ward for a nurse to insist on a particular treatment and difficult for a patient to refuse, in the home a much more subtle approach is required. The patient is king of his own castle, and the nurse who fails to win the confidence and cooperation of the patient on her first visit may next time find the door shut in her face. Apart from the equipment she brings with her, all the equipment she uses—drugs and dressings prescribed by the doctor as well as the table on which she lays out a dressing pack—is the patient's personal property, not the nurse's. The nurse would do well to remember this before ruining the french-polished table by a carelessly placed spirit swab.

The isolation of a private home means that the district nurse carries a greater responsibility because there is no one on the spot to whom she can immediately refer; she has to make her own decisions based on her individual professional judgement. Because she is frequently working single-handed she has to adapt such things as her lifting technique. Specialist services such as physiotherapy may not be available outside hospital and the district nurse may have to extend her role to fill the gaps; she may find herself playing the roles of physiotherapist, dietician, occupational therapist, home help and social worker, all rolled into one.

A third difference in role style arises from the fact that the nurse has continuous responsibility for the nursing care of her patients even though she is not with them all the time. In the community it is often the relatives who provide most of the nursing care between the nurse's visits. The nurse has to learn to share her role and the teaching component becomes relatively much more important.

The settings of district nursing

A considerable proportion of the district nurse's work is carried out in the setting of the patient's own home, but district nurses also work in community hospitals, in clinics of various kinds, in general practitioners' surgeries and treatment rooms, and in residential homes administered by social services departments. In each case the nurse's role changes slightly with the setting.

The most important part of the concept of the *community hospital* is that it is seen as a part of the community services and not an attempt to reproduce in miniature the activities of the specialist services of district general hospitals. Medical advice is provided by general practitioners not hospital consultants, and although most of the nursing staff may be appointed to work only in the community hospital, in some areas district nurses work on a rota basis partly in the hospital and partly outside. Ideally the community hospital provides services for patients needing full-time nursing care—including holiday admissions for those normally nursed at home—but not the specialist services of a district general hospital. Such hospitals may provide day-care services and rehabilitation services, and may be linked to the health centre at which the general practitioners, health visitors and district nurses are based.

Clinic-based services of various kinds are provided by health authorities either in their own premises or those belonging to general practitioners, and also by general practitioners themselves. The district nurse may, depending on her specialist skills and interests and on local facilities, find herself giving immunisations in child health clinics, participating in family planning clinics, and—especially where her work-base includes a treatment room—running her own clinics for special purposes such as the treatment of varicose ulcers.

Most health centres, and an increasing number of general practitioner premises, include a treatment room, and sometimes a specialist treatment room nurse is employed to undertake nursing treatments such as dressings, removal of sutures and ear syringing, and increasingly, a variety of preventive measures and screening programmes. Sometimes the 'treatment room service' is provided by the district nurse, sometimes by the practice nurse employed by the general practitioner.

As the average age of residents in old people's homes increases, and with it their frailty and need for nursing care, an increasing number of the district nurse's patients are nursed in this setting. In one sense the residential home is the patient's own home, but this setting also provides opportunities for work with groups of people—both 'treatment room services' and many forms of rehabilitation and health education.

The district nurse is employed by the health authority and works in close cooperation with the general practitioner in all these settings. The organisational framework, however, varies, and with it some of the nurse's role relationships. Traditionally, district nurses were responsible for providing care for patients living within a defined geographical area. Increasingly since the mid-1960s, however, district nurses have worked as members of a team of doctors, nurses, health visitors and sometimes other specialists, providing services for all the patients who are registered with a particular general practitioner. This system is known as *attachment* to general practice, and the people who work together in this way are collectively described as the *primary health care team*. It is important to recognise, however, that these two concepts do not necessarily go together; this issue is discussed later in this chapter.

Primary medical care

When medical help is sought, the person whom the patient first approaches is normally the general practitioner. Because it is the point of first contact, this part of our system of health care is called *primary medical care*. The general practitioner may request assistance in diagnosis or treatment in the form of special investigations or the opinion of a colleague, or may refer the patient to another doctor who is a specialist in the relevant field of illness. The specialist services, based on the hospital, to which the primary care doctor may refer the patient form the 'secondary' part of medical care. When intensive treatment at the secondary level has been completed, the patient returns to the primary level for continuing health supervision and care.

The system of primary medical care which has developed in this country is quite different from the system in other countries; in the USSR, for example, patients go to the nearest polyclinic, while in the United States they decide for themselves which specialist they need and approach the specialist directly.

General practitioners are not directly employed by health authorities as are other staff in the NHS, but are independent contractors who contract with the local family practitioner committee to provide general medical services to people who register with them. They may also accept private patients in addition to NHS patients. Part of their income is in the form of basic allowances similar to salary, but a considerable proportion is made up of fees for 'items of service'; the money comes out of the central NHS budget but is channelled through the family practitioner committees and not through the health authorities. This gives the general practitioner considerable independence to decide the way in which services will be provided; for example he may build and equip his own premises and employ his own staff, including nurses, over whom he therefore has direct control.

More than 80% of general practitioners work with other

general practitioners in groups of between two and ten, although there are still many single-handed practitioners, especially in urban areas. A group practice enables a more comprehensive service to be provided because doctors can deputise for one another for off-duty periods and facilities such as premises, equipment and staff can be shared.

About one-fifth of general practitioners work in *health centres* owned by health authorities. One of the responsibilities laid on local health authorities by the NHS Act 1946 was to build health centres at which facilities would be available for general medical (general practitioner), general dental, and pharmaceutical services, and hospital outpatient sessions, together with the (then) local authority health and welfare services. For various reasons health centres were at first slow to develop, but by 1980 there were over 1000 health centres in operation in the United Kingdom.

Primary health care

Primary medical care is, however, only part of primary health care. Primary health care has been defined in several ways, e.g.

1 Services provided by the core members of the primary health care team.
2 The family practitioner services (medical, dental, pharmaceutical and ophthalmic) provided through family practitioner committees.
3 Health services provided outside hospitals, services which are the point of first contact with the health care system.

The *Declaration of Alma Ata*[1], which committed all the member states of the World Health Organisation to the goal of 'health for all by the year 2000' through the development of primary health care, defined primary health care as:

'essential health care based on practical, scientifically sound and socially acceptable methods and technology made universally accessible to individuals and families in the community through their full participation and at a cost that the community and country can afford to maintain at every stage of their development in the spirit of self-reliance and self-determination. It forms an integral part both of the country's health system, of which it is the central function and main focus, and of the overall social and economic development of the community. It is the first level of contact of individuals, the family and the community with the national health system, bringing health care as close as possible to where people live and work, and constitutes the first element of a continuing health care process.'

This definition, which is far broader than a list of specific services, describes an approach to health care incorporating values and beliefs that have important consequences for the role of the nurse.

The primary health care team

The aims of primary health care have been described as:

1 The promotion of health in its broadest terms, through education, support and the encouragement of self-care.
2 The prevention of ill-health by prophylaxis, early diagnosis, education and advice on the value of early contact with the primary health care services.
3 The care, treatment and rehabilitation of those who are acutely or chronically ill.
4 The referral of patients to specialist services where necessary, and the provision of continuing care following specialist treatment.[2]

The fact that these aims are far too wide to be achieved by any one person or any one discipline has led to the development of the concept of the multidisciplinary primary health care team. A BMA working party on primary health care teams[3] listed the advantages of team care for both givers and receivers of care as follows:

1 Care given by a group is greater than the sum of individual care.
2 Rare skills are used most appropriately.
3 Peer influence and informal learning within the group raise the standards of care and the corporate status of the team in the community.
4 Team members have increased job satisfaction.
5 Team working encourages coordinated health education.
6 Team working lowers the prevalence of disease in the community.

7 The individual gets more efficient and understanding treatment when ill.

It would be difficult to prove some of these contentions, and some people would disagree with some of them, but it is reasonable to assume that a service provided by a team would be at least more comprehensive than a service provided by a single individual or by a single discipline. The Cumberlege Report[4] noted that 'nurses are at their most effective when they and general practitioners work together in an active primary health care team'. This report was a review of community nursing services in England only published in 1986 as a consultative document.

The members of the primary care team

The most effective composition and size of the nucleus of a team is much debated; in reality, the size depends considerably on the number of general practitioners in a group practice and on what health authority staff are available. Nationally the ratio of district nurses to general practitioners is 1 to 1.7, and the ratio of health visitors is 1 to 2.4. The BMA[3] has distinguished between the 'nucleus' team composed of doctors, nurses, health visitors, social workers and medical secretaries, and the wider team which includes allied professions such as physiotherapists and pharmacists, the administrative auxiliaries such as receptionists and practice managers, and other services provided by hospitals, local authorities and voluntary agencies. Within the multidisciplinary team is the nursing team, the core of which consists of the health visitor, the district nurse and the treatment room or practice nurse.

The *health visitor* is the team's expert in preventive health care. She* is required to be a registered general nurse (RGN), but some health visitors would argue that because of its historical independence and different approach from hospital nursing, health visiting ought to be regarded as a separate profession. She has a statutory responsibility to visit every baby born in her area or registered with the general practice to which she is attached,

---

* Until 1973 only women were allowed to become health visitors; the proportion of men in health visiting is still very small.

and to watch over each child's health and development until school age. But she is also a family visitor who is concerned with the health of the whole family whether there are young children or not, and a considerable proportion of her work may be with elderly people. She visits families in their own homes either on her own initiative or at the request of other members of the team, other health and social agencies, or the family itself, or patients may come to see her at her work base or at the child health clinic. Her job is defined[5] as 'health education and social advice'—that is, to assess the individual or family's health needs, to offer advice or counselling, and to mobilise the resources of other services where necessary. Unlike the district nurse, most of her clientele is independent of the doctor's referral, and in addition to her work within the practice she is also responsible for work in child health clinics, formal health education in schools and other places, and, in many areas, for school nursing.

The *district nurse* is the expert in the care of the sick at home, although increasingly she also works in other settings such as residential homes for the elderly, health centres and general practitioner premises.

The district nurse, who is often referred to as the district nursing sister, is responsible for deciding the nursing care which each patient needs and for ensuring that it is carried out. She is the leader of a nursing team which may include district enrolled nurses and auxiliaries, and sometimes registered general nurses (RGNs) and enrolled nurses working in the community prior to undertaking the relevant education and training courses. The district nurse delegates work as appropriate to the other members of the team, but in addition to her own work she remains accountable for the work delegated to them.

The district enrolled nurse (DEN) therefore may have her own caseload, but she remains accountable to the district nurse for the care given to patients. This issue has been much disputed among district nurses and DENs. Hockey[6] found in 1972 that although enrolled nurses did more basic nursing than RGNs there was nothing that the RGN did that was not at some time done by an enrolled nurse, the level of responsibilities fluctuating in response to expediency. Following this report attempts have been made to produce a clearer delineation of the role of the district enrolled nurse; in particular the Panel of Assessors for District Nurse Training in 1980[7] produced the following definition:

> The enrolled nurse is a member of the district nursing team. He/she is accountable to the district nurse for carrying out part or all of the nursing care programme for individual patients and their families, recording his/her findings and reporting back to the district nurse.

Hockey's report also highlighted areas of work that did not require professional nursing skills and more nursing auxiliaries were employed. However, with the increased complexity of district nursing the skill mix in the district nursing service is now constantly under review.

Since 1947 male nurses have been accepted for district nurse training but they comprise only a small proportion of the total district nursing workforce. Depending on the number available within a health authority they may be attached to group practices or work on a geographical basis. Although many have as their main responsibility genitourinary work with male patients, it is becoming increasingly common for the male nurse to care for female patients; before this is planned, however, it should be agreed with the patient concerned, recognising and respecting different people's prejudices and cultural backgrounds.

Some health authorities provide a 24-hour nursing service in which the evening and night hours are covered by nurses specially recruited for this purpose. The number of staff available is usually small so care in the selection of patients for referral for night care is essential. Where there is no special service the district nursing team will meet patients' needs as far as it is possible to do so by staggering their working hours or by 'on-call' rota systems.

The factors which the district nurse must consider in allocating the work among the various members of her team are discussed in more detail in Chapter 8.

In a few very rural areas the work of the health visitor, the midwife and the district nurse may be undertaken by one person, who is often called a 'triple-duty' nurse. Occasionally the duties of district nurse and midwife are combined. The nurse who undertakes combined duties must be appropriately qualified in each speciality.

The *treatment room nurse* may be employed by the health

authority and attached to a general practice in the same way as the health visitor or district nurse, or she may be directly employed by the general practitioner under the terms of service[8] which allow him to employ 'ancillary staff' and to be reimbursed for 70% of their salaries; the directly employed nurse is usually called the *practice nurse*. Reedy[9] has studied the historical development of the private employment of practice nurses, and has compared their work and their occupational characteristics with those of attached district nurses.

During 1986, the government's consultation on primary health care led to considerable debate on the role of the practice nurse. It became clear that many practice nurses were expanding their role far beyond delegated medical tasks, and some, it was argued, were undertaking work for which they had not been adequately trained. The professional and financial implications of direct employment of nurses by doctors, the 70% salary subsidy, and the open-ended general practice budget compared with the cash-limited district health authority budget, were hotly debated. The Cumberlege report recommended that practice nurses should be integrated into the neighbourhood nursing team and that the salary subsidy paid to general practitioners should cease.

In some areas a *social worker* employed by the social services department is attached to general practice in the same way as nurses. There is still a good deal of mutual distrust between doctors and social workers, and social workers have been less ready than nurses to accept the concept of attachment because they see it as a threat to their professional autonomy. However, a number of notable accounts[10] have demonstrated the contribution that social work can make to patient care within the context of the primary health care team.

Without the support of *administrative staff* the professionals in the primary health care team would be unable to function. This group of staff includes receptionists, secretaries, and in some large practices practice managers. Sometimes tensions arise between lay staff and nurses where a member of the lay staff such as a receptionist—who is sometimes an ex-nurse—takes on what the nurses perceive as nursing duties or offers patients advice on matters which the nurses believe to be more appropriate to professionals.

The wider team

The wider team with whom nurse members of the nucleus team must maintain close contact includes:

Midwives
Other community-based nurses
Specialist nurses
Hospital nurses
Volunteers

The *midwife* is the expert in the care of mothers before, during, and immediately after the birth of their babies, and in the care of the newborn baby. Midwives increasingly work in integrated maternity services which straddle hospital and primary care services, and in this sense could be regarded as part of the 'wider' team rather than the nucleus; but within the primary health care team they play an important role in the provision of antenatal and postnatal care in cooperation with the general practitioner who specialises in obstetrics.

Other community-based nurses include school nurses, clinic nurses, family planning nurses, community psychiatric nurses, community paediatric nurses, community mental handicap nurses and others. They also include nurses working in occupational health services which, although they are outside the administrative framework and finance of the NHS, make an important contribution to community-based health care.

Specialist nurses include, among others, the community psychiatric nurse, the domiciliary family planning nurse, the specialist paediatric nurse and the stoma therapist. The district nurse works with patients of all age groups who have a wide range of medical and surgical conditions and a variety of nursing problems, and she must recognise that she cannot hope to develop and maintain expertise in all specialist fields. She will therefore need to seek advice from others with up-to-date specialist knowledge, using them as 'consultants' both for advice and referral, similar to the ways in which general practitioners use hospital consultants; the other disciplines represented within the primary care team are a resource which should be used in the same manner.

The Society of Primary Health Care Nursing of the Royal

College of Nursing identified two groups of patients needs which can best be met by specialist intervention: those where a different basic training is required, and those where the problem concerned is relatively rare in general district nursing practice.[11] An example of the former kind of specialist is the community psychiatric nurse (CPN) who provides support and specialised care for patients with a psychiatric illness; the CPN may provide care to those who have received treatment as inpatients but have now returned home, those who are receiving treatment as day patients or outpatients, and those who can be treated by the general practitioner in the community without hospital referral. An example of the latter kind is the stoma therapist who offers an advisory service to patients with a colostomy, ileostomy or an ileal conduit. This kind of specialist nurse is usually based in the specialist department of the hospital, but although most of her work is carried out in the wards and outpatient department she may also make follow-up visits to former patients in their own homes.

The use of specialist nurses in primary health care is an issue which provokes considerable debate. The district nurse needs to be aware of the availability of such services in her locality and should be willing to seek advice or to transfer care where appropriate. Concern is however felt, as noted in the RCN report, where specialist nurses are used 'to give a type of care which it should be possible for every district nursing team to give, provided that the size of caseload allows the time to give each patient of this type the appropriate level of care.[11] Equally, specialist nurses should work in partnership with the core members of the primary health care team. The Cumberlege report suggested that specialist community nurses should wherever possible be part of the neighbourhood nursing service, and that where this was not possible, the relationship between the services should be made explicit in a written service agreement.

Another group of nurses who are hospital based but whose role is different from that of the specialist nurse are *liaison nurses*. These nurses are appointed specifically to promote continuity of care between hospital and community when patients are discharged from hospital. They are often associated with a speciality such as paediatrics but do not usually provide direct care as such. Their role is to visit the wards on a regular basis, to collect information concerning the nursing care of patients who are about to leave hospital but who will require continued care or supervision, and to relay this information to the nurse member of the primary care team who will be responsible for providing this care.

Even if such liaison staff are available, however, and particularly where they are not, the nursing members of primary care teams need to maintain close contact with their hospital-based colleagues. The district nurse needs to be able to *give* information to hospital staff about patients for whom she has been caring before their admission to hospital, and also to *receive* information directly from ward staff to enable her to continue care after a patient has been discharged.

This 'wider team' also includes *volunteers*. The contribution of the family and neighbours to care, and the importance of the nurse's willingness to share her role with them has already been stressed. In particular, 'night sitter' and 'good neighbour' services are invaluable in meeting needs which are far beyond the resources of the statutory services.

The concept of a team

A team is more than a collection of individuals; it implies that a number of people are working cooperatively together to achieve a common goal. MacIntosh has defined a team as 'a group of people with diverse but related knowledge and skills who associate for the purpose of directing, coordinating and developing the separate parts as well as the sum total of their expertise in order to create new, and maximise existing opportunities for achieving their common goals'.[12] It has been pointed out that the attachment of nursing staff to general practice does not itself constitute the creation of a primary health care team, and that teamwork can be encouraged but it cannot be created by managerial decision.[2] In their study of the work of the nursing team in general practice sponsored by the Council for the Education and Training of Health Visitors, Gilmore *et al.*[13] commented 'there is a widespread assumption amongst administrators and practitioners that when health visitors and district nurse have been attached to general practitioners, teamwork will automatically evolve. The findings of this study suggest that such a development may not occur without conscious planning based on the promotion of awareness amongst all team members of what is involved in teamwork and of the factors which hinder and accelerate the process'. Some twelve years later the Cumberlege report suggested that this lesson had still not been learnt.

The dynamics of teamwork

The effectiveness of multidisciplinary teams, including the primary health care team, is much debated; it would seem that the characteristics of good teamwork are well known but inadequately applied. The Harding report,[14] which examined the problems of creating primary health care teams, listed four basic requirements:

1   A common objective for the team, accepted and understood by all team members.
2   A clear understanding by each team member of his/her own role, function and responsibilities.
3   A clear understanding by each team member of the role, function and responsibilities of other team members.
4   Mutual respect for the roles and skills of each team member, allied to a flexible approach.

The Chief Nursing Officer's letter on primary health care nursing[1] adds a very important fifth requirement:

5   A mutually agreed system for communication and referral both within the team and between the team and other agencies.

Common purpose and goals

Teamwork involves the definition of common goals and the development of a plan of action in which each member makes a different but complementary contribution towards the achievement of the team's aims. In a primary health care team this includes general goals related to meeting the needs of the practice population and specific goals related to the care of individual patients. Because the perspectives and values of the various professions differ, there will sometimes be disagreement over the goals to be set at both levels; for example the doctor may not welcome the extra workload which the health visitor's case-finding activities create. Conflict is not necessarily destructive, but problems have to be talked through frankly for agreement to be reached, and it is not helpful if team members deal with it, as Gilmore *et al.* found, by simply going their own ways. Each individual professional must set his or her own goals for patients within their care, but in doing so must take account of and share in the achievement of team goals.

The Cumberlege report suggested that to establish and be recognised as a primary health care team each general practice should make a written agreement with the neighbourhood nursing service which would specify the membership of the team (which should not be changed without consultation), the team's objectives and priorities, procedures for referrals and information sharing, and an annual review.

Understanding different roles

Professional roles are learned alongside the appropriate knowledge and skills during the process of professional training, and the process of socialisation which takes place during this time is as influential in respect of professional attitudes and behaviour as are the experiences of childhood in other attitudes and behaviour. Unfortunately, because the different health-care professionals have quite separate educational programmes, their understanding of one another's roles may be very limited.[2] Moreover, at the same time as student professionals are learning their own roles, they are also developing ideas about the roles of other people around them—as they see them performed in the setting in which the learning takes place. Medical students and nursing students learn the roles of doctor and nurse in the setting of an acute general hospital where their goals and values will reflect the purpose of the institution—which is curing patients afflicted by serious acute illness; and their relationship with each other is one of 'director' and 'assistant' in the function of curing. Although these role styles are no longer appropriate in the primary care setting, where the illness conditions and the needs of patients are very different, they may persist. Thus the doctor may regard the health visitor's routine surveillance of healthy children as 'a waste of time', the health visitor may regard the district nurse as 'incapable' of social assessment and health education. Gilmore *et al.* and Milne[15] have found that serious misconceptions about one another's roles abound among team members.

Unless each member of the team understands and appreciates the roles and functions of the others, there will be gaps, duplications and inconsistencies in the care available to patients. It is inevitable that roles will overlap, and it is important that they do, but there must be agreement, based on discussion among team members, about who does what in what circumstances, and there must be sufficient trust to enable a patient to be 'shared' or referred.

Pooling knowledge and skills

Each professional has his or her own particular area of expertise, but there are many tasks, e.g. supportive counselling and referral to other agencies, which can and should be undertaken by whichever member of the team is in direct contact with the patient. Close liaison is essential to avoid conflicting advice, and each member of the team should be able to use the expertise of the others by using them as consultants.

One mechanism for pooling knowledge and skills, and ensuring at the same time the close liaison which is necessary to avoid duplication and gaps, is the *case conference*, in which the members of the team involved with a particular patient discuss their individual assessments of the patient's needs and the possible strategies for meeting them, and agree a common plan of care.

Team management

If a team is to function as a cohesive unit it must have the ability to manage itself as a unit, including the mechanisms for achieving this; this aspect might be called the team's internal management. The need for common aims and policies, which can be arrived at only by discussion and agreement between members, has already been stressed. A critical questions, however, is 'Who leads the team?' The role of leader is closely linked with status, authority and power. A difference in status between doctors and nurses is often felt by both and acted upon in a way which inhibits the achievement of true professional partnership and a complementary approach to patient care; for example Gilmore *et al.*[13] found that in team discussions nurses initiated less, spoke less, and rarely disagreed with doctors. In the primary health care team the doctor often takes the leadership role on the assumption which is made both by doctors and by nurses that it is 'natural' and 'right' for him to do so. Doctors tend to justify this situation—if they think about it at all—on the basis of their comprehensive responsibility for patients, but the real reason often lies in the role perceptions learnt by both doctors and nurses in the hospital setting. Leadership within any team is a matter for the team itself to decide, and it is important that the issues of leadership, authority, and coordination of team action are consciously considered rather than taken for granted.

Although nurses are members of the team and are directly involved in its internal management, they are also, as employees of the health authority, managerially responsible and accountable to a nurse manager who is usually outside the team. Sometimes this causes tensions within the team, especially where the general practitioner (who is not managerially accountable to anyone because he is an independent contractor) does not understand the nursing management structure or the differences between nursing and medical services which make it necessary, or the differences between management, administration and supervision. The tension may be increased, and the role relationships become even more complex, if the team includes attached nurses who arc managerially accountable to a nursing officer, and a practice nurse who is managerially accountable to the doctor because she is directly employed by him. It is usually in the determination of priorities or the allocation of work that these tensions become visible, not in the area of direct patient care.

Such conflicts can only be resolved by frank discussion perhaps followed, as the Cumberlege report suggested, by an explicit agreement between the members. The Cumberlege report included a 'model agreement'; but probably the best guideline is given by Henderson in her well-known discussion of the role of the nurse.[16] 'No one member of the team should make such heavy demands on another member that any one of them is unable to perform his or her unique function . . . All members of the team should consider the person (patient) served as the central figure and should realise that they are all "assisting" him'.

Communication

The necessity for good communication among team members is implicit in the need to agree common purposes, to understand one another's roles, to pool knowledge, to develop coordinated plans of care for individual patients, and to resolve tensions and conflicts. In other words, achievement of all the characteristics of good teamwork which have been discussed depends upon good communication. Good communication requires not only a willingness to communicate and a recognition by all the team members of the importance of communication, but also appropriate and easy-to-use channels for communication, and—perhaps most important of all—time. One of the advantages of a health centre or good practice premises is that members of the team are on the same premises and this facilitates informal face-to-face interaction, but it is often assumed—wrongly—that this obviates the need for more formal communication. It is important that there are recognised systems and mechanisms, including time specially set aside for the purpose, for meetings of the team and of subgroups within it both for joint discussion of individual patients and for discussions relating to the policies and management of the team as a whole.

An important issue in team communication is the use of records, and in particular the problems of confidentiality which this raises. These problems are discussed in more detail in Chapters 9 and 22. Access to one another's records is important for the planning and implementation of a coordinated plan of care for an individual patient, and in some teams all the notes relating to a particular patient are kept together and the whole team records information on the same document.

Conclusion

The extent and methods of inter-disciplinary cooperation in primary health care vary greatly from one part of the country to another. The development of primary health care teams is poor where, for example, the numbers of nursing staff employed are insufficient, where general practitioners do not accept this concept of care, where they work in single-handed practices rather than group practices, where it is impossible to provide adequate accommodation to enable staff of different professions to work from the same premises, where there is considerable overlap of the geographical areas covered by general practitioners, and in inner city areas where there are special health and social problems.

It is important to recognise that teamwork does not necessarily depend on attachment, and equally that attachment does not itself create teamwork. Whatever the local and practical difficulties, the importance of the concepts of a multidisciplinary approach to patient care and of cooperative patterns of working is undiminished.

References

1. WHO (1978). *Declaration of Alma Ata*. Geneva: WHO.
2. Department of Health and Social Security (1977). *Nursing in Primary Health Care* (CNO(77)8). London: HMSO.
3. British Medical Association Board of Education and Science (1974). *Report of the Panel on Primary Health Care Teams*. London: BMA.
4. Department of Health and Social Security (1986). *Neighbourhood Nursing: a focus for care* (Cumberlege report). London: HMSO.
5. Ministry of Health, Department of Health for Scotland, and Ministry of Education (1956). *An Enquiry into Health Visiting* (Jameson report). London: HMSO.
6. Hockey L. (1972). *Use and Abuse?* London: Queen's Nursing Institute.
7. Panel of Assessors for District Nurse Training (1980). *Report of the Education and Training of District Nurses (SEN)*. London: DHSS
8. Department of Health and Social Security (1972). *NHS (General medical and pharmaceutical services) Regulations*. Schedule 1 Part 1, 16 (?). London: HMSO.
9. Reedy B. *et al.* (1980). The social and occupational characteristics of attached and employed nurses in general practice and a comparison of the activities and opinions of attached and employed nurses. *Journal of the RCGP*; **30:** 477–89.

10. For example: Forman J., Fairbairn E. M. (1968). *Social Casework in General Practice*. Oxford: Oxford University Press.
    Goldberg E. M., Neill J. (1972). *Social Work in General Practice*. London: Allen and Unwin.
11. Royal College of Nursing (1980). *Primary Health Care Nursing: A Team Approach* (Report of a working party of the RCN Society of Primary Health Care Nursing). London: Royal College of Nursing.
12. McIntosh J. B. (1974). Communication in teamwork: a lesson from the district. *Nursing Times*; **1970:** 85–88.
13. Gilmore M., Bruce N., Hunt M. (1974). *The Work of the Nursing Team in General Practice*. London: Council for the Education and Training of Health Visitors.
14. Department of Health and Social Security (1981). *Primary Health Care Teams* (Harding report). London: HMSO.
15. Milne A. (1979). Students views of the primary health care team. *Nursing Times* (Occasional Papers); **75,** 28: 113–16.
16. Henderson V. (1960). *Basic Principles of Nursing Care*. Geneva: ICN.

Further Reading

Barber J. H., Kratz C., eds. (1980). *Towards Team Care*. Edinburgh: Churchill Livingstone.

Department of Health and Social Security (1981). *Primary Health Care in Inner London* (Acheson report). London: HMSO.

Department of Health and Social Security (1986). *Neighbourhood Nursing—a focus for care (Cumberlege Report)*. London: HMSO.

Department of Health and Social Security (1986). *Primary Health Care: An agenda for discussion*. London: HMSO.

Gilmore M., Bruce N., Hunt M. (1974). *The Work of the Nursing Team in General Practice*. London: Council for the Education and Training of Health Visitors.

Hockey L., ed. (1983). *Primary Care Nursing*. Edinburgh: Churchill Livingstone.

Section I described the setting in which the district nurse works. This section considers approaches to care at home. Florence Nightingale wrote in 1859:[1] 'I do not pretend to teach her how, I ask her to teach herself, and for this purpose I venture to give some hints'. Following this precedent, guidelines and principles are offered, but not details of techniques nor a prescriptive approach.

Chapter 6 considers the question 'What is district nursing?' and gives an outline of the approach of care adopted in this section. The authors are aware of the sensitivity surrounding the term 'nursing process' but make no apologies for using it. It is used interchangeably, both in this text and by others, with the 'problem-solving approach' which some argue implies that all problems can be solved; or 'individualised patient care' which can be seen to have limitations as care in the community needs to focus on the patient and his family or other carers. Others use the phrase 'a systematic approach to nursing care'. The jargon should not be allowed to obscure meaning; what matters is the underlying principles.

Whichever phrase is used, it simply implies a method of nursing in which decision-making is on a more systematic and scientific basis than it perhaps has been in the past. Such an approach is not unique to nursing and is used by most professional groups. No attempt is made to give a detailed account of the process itself, as most readers will be familiar with this, and the references and further reading at the end of the chapters will direct them to explore ideas in greater depth.

During the past ten years there has been a proliferation of literature on the use of theories, models and conceptual frameworks in nursing (again the different terms are often used interchangeably although there are subtle differences between them). Recently considerable attention has been given to the development and use of specific models for nursing. The use of any one specific model has been deliberately avoided although several are mentioned as examples, and some more detailed work is included in the suggestions for further reading.

It was no accident that the nursing process was chosen as a framework for the *Curriculum in District Nursing for State Registered Nurses and Registered General Nurses*[2]; it was adopted because it was felt that this method would increase the standard of care provided by the nursing team. It must be remembered that this curriculum was developed in 1976 and in many ways was ahead of its time; however, training institutions, in interpreting the curriculum, have taken into account the many recent developments in nursing, medical and technological knowledge.

Chapters 7 to 10 focus on the commonly recognised four stages of the nursing process. The case histories of the seven patients described in Chapter 1 serve as examples, but it is only possible to identify a few of their nursing care needs and it would be a useful exercise for readers to identify other problems that may arise and consider possible nursing care. Section III devotes more attention to some of those with special needs who require care at home.

Some health authorities/boards will have established the nursing process in the district nursing service, others will be in the early stages of its development, while others may not have begun. The introduction of a new system of care requires a commitment from all concerned, but it is worthwhile taking trouble to gain this commitment because it eventually leads to an improvement in the quality of care. Change is often uncomfortable and initially time has to be spent on discussion, and a critical evaluation of the current nursing practice showing that this is not change for the sake of change is essential.

When change is being inaugurated, it is wise to look at what is good and worth preserving in the present system and to see if there is a present foundation on which to build a new system. Many district nurses have always used some of the skills required for the nursing process, but some will need to develop certain new skills and attitudes in the provision of care.

References

1. Nightingale F. (1859, facsimile ed. 1970). *Notes on Nursing*. London: Duckworth.

2. Panel of Assessors for District Nurse Training (1978). *Curriculum in District Nursing for State Registered Nurses and Registered General Nurses*. London: DHSS. *Note* This curriculum has now been adopted by the four National Boards for Nursing, Midwifery and Health Visiting.

Chapter 6

The Nature of District Nursing

The 'patient profiles' at the beginning of this book give examples of patients and their families requiring the services of a district nurse. Most district nurses will 'recognise' these patients and know, for instance, that the apparently straightforward care required by Mr Evans may turn out to be complicated, and that in the case of John Davis she may find she has a minimal role because of the part played by the patient and his parents. Care provided by the district nurse may be relatively simple or involve not only physical needs but a whole range of psychological and social needs, as could well be the case with Mrs Baker and her family.

Before discussing the methods of care for these and other patients it is important to consider first what district nursing is. There have been many attempts to capture the elements of the very complex activity of nursing in a simple definition. Florence Nightingale[1] wrote 'I use the word nursing for want of a better' but provided a definition which still has relevance:

> It ought to signify the proper use of fresh air, light, warmth, cleanliness, quiet and the proper selection and administration of diet—all at the least expense of vital power to the patient.

Probably the most widely accepted definition is that of Henderson[2]:

> The unique function of the nurse is to assist the individual, sick or well, in the performance of those activities contributing to health or its recovery (or to peaceful death) that he would perform unaided if he had the necessary strength, will or knowledge. And to do this in such a way as to help him gain independence as rapidly as possible.

Two other definitions that complement Henderson's are those given by Orem[3] and Rogers[4]. Orem states that:

> The condition which validates the existence of a requirement for nursing in an adult is the absence of the ability to maintain for himself continuously that amount and quality of *self-care* which is therapeutic

in sustaining life and health, in recovering from disease or injury, or in coping with their effects . . . Self-care is an adult's personal continuous contribution to his health and well-being.

Self-care, therefore, is the care that everyone requires each day, which includes the care of the person and where appropriate the following of medical directives.

Rogers' definition states that:

Nursing aims to assist people in achieving their maximum health potential. Maintenance and promotion of health, prevention of disease, nursing diagnosis, intervention and rehabilitation encompasses the scope of nursing's goals. Nursing is concerned with people—all people—well and sick, rich and poor, young and old.

There are several factors common to each of these definitions. First, the implication that nursing is *assisting* the patient with those activities he would normally do for himself, which itself implies complementing the person's abilities and compensating for his disabilities. Such assistance may involve:

Acting for or doing for the patient
Guiding the patient
Supporting the patient physically, psychologically and socially
Providing an environment that promotes personal development
Teaching the patient and the family

All of these activities involve working *with* the patient, who may be deficient in quantity or quality of self-care; and these deficiencies may be physical, social or psychological. Assisting the patient with the activities he would normally do for himself implies that the care for each person must be planned on an individual basis and in order to do this the nurse must tactfully find out how the patient usually lives.

Shetland[5] describes nursing as a process which is:

. . . one of interaction. The nurse enters imaginatively and sensitively into the lives of the people she serves in order to understand their health needs, determine the perception of their needs, reconcile the difference between the two sets of perceptions and institute appropriate nursing measures in interaction with the recipient(s) of her service.

Means of interaction with patients will be discussed subsequently but this definition again shows the importance of working *with* the patient and his family. For example if Mrs Adams believes that it is best for her husband to be left in bed and the district nurse believes it is preferable for him to be turned regularly and sat out of bed for part of the day there will be conflict until the varying points of view are reconciled. It is obviously not always possible to make all the decisions about care with the patient and/or his family but it is important they are involved in the planning whenever possible. Such involvement is always desirable but is particularly important when the patient is cared for in his own home because most of the care is provided by the patient himself or his family.

Figure 6.1 shows how much a patient and his family were involved in his care following amputation of a limb for diabetic gangrene.[6] Apart from the immediate postoperative period the patient and his family 'gave' more care than any other person. This would appear to be a typical picture for the majority of patients cared for at home; the district nurse may visit once, twice or even three times a day and during her visit may give intense nursing care, but this is a small part of the 24 hours.

Common to the three definitions of nursing is the fact that the nurse is not only working with the sick but also with the well, and that she has a role in the prevention of ill-health and the promotion of health. The district nurse is invariably in a good position to carry out this aspect of her work, with the people directly under her care and also with their families or with members of the wider community. The preventive aspect is stressed by the well-known definition of health by the World Health Organisation which states: 'Health is a state of physical, social and mental well-being, not merely the absence of disease'.

People's perceptions of health may vary according to their experiences, expectations, age, activities and interests (Chapter 3); for example John, in spite of his disability and with his considerable degree of dependence, may say he feels 'well' once he has adapted to his limitation, whereas Mr Evans may complain of feeling 'poorly' with far less physical disability because he has not adapted to the breakdown in his usual health pattern which limits

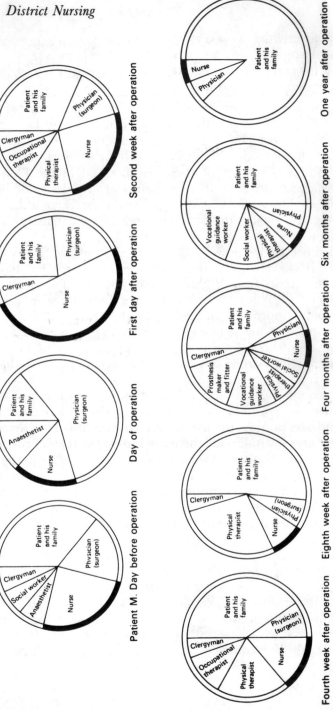

Fig. 6.1. The changing importance of the nurse's role as rehabilitation progresses in the case of a young man having a leg amputated.

his normal activities. This comparison emphasises the need for an individual approach to care for each patient.

McFarlane and Castledine[7] state that the practice of nursing is shaped by the values and ideas which nurses and others hold of their own function. Nursing is such a complex activity that it is virtually impossible to find a simple definition for so wide a range of actions.

All these theories and definitions have in common certain key concepts which constitute what Florence Nightingale called the 'elements' of nursing. The concepts include care, self-care, activities of living, stress adaptation, interaction and several others. Some theorists emphasise one, others another; it is the combination of these concepts in a way which shows how they can explain or guide the activity called nursing that constitutes a 'nursing model'.

McFarlane[8] suggests that nursing models have a value for practice in a number of different ways. She states they may:

1   Serve as a tool which links theory and practice.
2   Clarify our thinking about the elements of a practice situation and their relationship to each other.
3   Help practitioners of nursing to communicate with each other more meaningfully.
4   Serve as a guide to practice, education and research.

Many authors propose the use of a nursing model which helps to order and operationalise the theory of nursing so that all care can be rational and specific for the individual patient and for the wider context. Thus a model forms a framework within which nursing care is assessed, planned, implemented and evaluated. Aggleton and Chalmers[9] state that nursing models are likely to have something to say about the following aspects of patient or client care:

1   The nature of the person receiving (or about to receive) nursing care.
2   The cause of problems which are likely to require nursing intervention.
3   The nature of the assessment process.
4   The nature of the planning and goal-setting process.

5   The focus of nursing intervention during the implementation of the care plan.
6   The nature of the process of evaluating the quality of the care plan.

In the three examples given at the beginning of this chapter the authors describe the nature of the patient in marginally different ways. According to Henderson[2] individuals receiving nursing care are human beings sharing certain fundamental human needs; Orem[3] sees the person as a functional, integrated whole with an overall motivation to achieve self-care; and Rogers[4] argues that the person should be seen holistically, believing individuals to be more than the sum of individual parts. Others, for example Roy[10] and Clark,[11] see the person as a system adapting to or coping with stresses in the environment. Some of the work of these nursing theorists is included in the suggestions for further reading; in particular Clements and Roberts[12] consider several of these models as they apply to family health care and nursing in the community.

Individual care and the nursing process

Many would argue that because the district nurse visits one patient at a time her care is individual, but this is not necessarily so, for the care given may be centred on the disease or the task in hand and be merely ritualistic. However, in order to fulfil the criteria outlined above, more is required; it is necessary to discover the patient's normal life style, habits and preferences, and then identify his problems. The next step is to set the goals of care *in conjunction with the patient*, then plan to meet these goals; subsequently carry out the care and, finally, check that the goals have been achieved. This is the approach known as the nursing process and a brief outline follows.

Jones[13] states that the nursing process is 'an interactive, problem-solving, decision-making procedure for assessing, identifying, selecting and implementing approaches and evaluating results in relation to the care of the ill or potentially ill person'. It can be seen that this definition provides a logical framework for nursing care and is based on four main stages:

1 Assessment
2 Planning
3 Implementation
4 Evaluation

The assessment stage involves the nurse in gathering, analysing and synthesising pertinent information from all sources, and from this information identifying the problems that are amenable to nursing action. Having identified the problems the nurse can then, in conjunction with the patient, determine the desired goals of care and plan to achieve these. The planning stage is followed by the implementation of the specific measures decided upon, and the final step is the evaluation and determination as to whether the goals have been achieved. The evaluation may result in new information being available, leading to a modification in the initial assessment, and this might change the problems identified and require a restatement of goals and a subsequent change of plan. Thus the nursing process needs to be seen as an ongoing cyclical process rather than one that neatly proceeds from one stage to the next.

This problem-solving approach is an orderly and systematic way of providing nursing care. It should not remove any spontaneity from care giving, in fact if a plan for care is carefully made it can save time and allow for the unexpected. The nursing process can be used for patients requiring short-term care, but is of particular value for those patients needing long-term care, who tend to predominate in the caseload of the district nurse. If this systematic approach is used universally the quality of information will be improved and faults in communication when transferring patients to and from hospital will be diminished.

Through the use of the nursing process the district nurse can identify her unique contribution, plan the patient's care and be master of her work. This accords with Henderson's[2] comment: 'This aspect of her work, this part of her function, she initiates and controls; of this she is master'.

The role and function of the district nurse

The role and function of the district nurse can now be clarified. Her *role* is the part she plays in relation to other members of the caring team and her *function* is the job she does, which can be summarised as the provision of skilled nursing care for any person living in the community. The following definition of the district nurse, modified from that given by the Chief Nursing Officer at the DHSS,[14] emphasises the many aspects of her role and function:

> The district nurse is an RGN who has received post-basic training in order to enable her to give skilled nursing care to all persons living in the community including in residential homes. She is the leader of the district nursing team within the primary health care services. Working with her may be RGNs, DENs and nursing auxiliaries. It is the district nurse who is professionally accountable for assessing and reassessing the needs of the patient and family, and for monitoring the quality of care. It is her responsibility to ensure that help, including financial and social, is made available as appropriate. The district nurse delegates tasks as appropriate to other nursing staff, who can thus have their own caseload, but who remain wholly accountable to the district nurse for the care that they give to patients. The district nurse is accountable for the work undertaken by nursing auxiliaries who carry out such tasks as bathing, dressing frail ambulant patients, and helping other members of the team with patient care.

The role and function of the district nurse outlined above accord with the definition of a 'primary nurse' now increasingly being used as a method of staff deployment. Primary nurse should not be confused with the nurse working in primary health care. According to McFarlane and Castledine,[7] the primary nurse is so called because she is primarily responsible for the care of the individual patient. She assesses problems, plans care and evaluates it, retaining accountability for his care throughout his 'stay'. Like the district nurse, the primary nurse will often need assistance with implementing the care plan and will delegate appropriately but retain accountability.

The Scottish Home and Health Department, in a report on the work of the district nurse in 1978,[15] listed the following capabilities that were required in addition to professional knowledge and skills:

Making independent professional judgements
Taking decisions on nursing matters

Accepting responsibility and exercising authority
Taking action in an emergency pending medical intervention
Acting independently
Establishing and maintaining good personal relationships
Reflecting objectively and logically
Thinking in abstract and planning ahead.

These two accounts of the work of the district nurse complement one another; both emphasise her responsibilities and her accountability for the care carried out by herself and others in the nursing team, and both show the need to develop and maintain good personal relationships and managerial skills.

The district nurse has several roles in the giving of care. She has an independent role where she is responsible for the initiation of nursing care; for example, she makes a nursing decision that Mrs Baker's mouth needs care because it is dry due to an inadequate fluid intake. On the other hand for some work she has a dependent role when she gives medication prescribed by the general practitioner. Above all she has an intermediary role when working in collaboration with other workers—for example, many services and personnel will need to be coordinated in the provision of care for John Davis.

The district nurse works with other members of the primary care team and is also often involved with hospital and social service personnel, as well as voluntary workers. Within the team the contribution of any particular member may predominate at any time according to the circumstances; for example, the district nurse is the paramount person in the care of Mrs Cray while her ulcers require intensive treatment, but if these heal the social worker may well play a more significant role. In the case of Rose Johnson the health visitor may be the person to provide continuous support for the family but in an acute episode the role of the district nurse may become crucial. The independent, dependent and intermediary roles may all be integrated in the care of a single patient. The district nurse may make independent decisions about the positioning of Mr Fisher in his wheelchair to prevent pressure sores from occurring; his steroid injections prescribed during relapses of the disease are determined by the general practitioner; and the district nurse liaises with the personnel from the social services department to discuss the provision of aids and adaptations to the home.

It is important that district nurses, as members of a team, work out a personal philosophy for themselves concerning their various roles, for only when they have done this can they develop a commitment to care. Traditionally in hospital as nurses become more senior they perform the more complex technical tasks; however, the district nurse is in the unique position of having only one patient to care for at a time, and carries out the whole range of care. Much of the work of the district nurse is what is commonly called 'basic nursing care', which in hospital all too frequently is left to junior nurses or auxiliaries; but what can give more satisfaction to the nurse, and benefit to the patient, than to be able to give and receive total care from one person. This is quintessential nursing.

References

1. Nightingale F. (1859, Facsimile edn. 1970). *Notes on Nursing*. London: Duckworth.
2. Henderson V. (1960, revised 1969). *Basic Principles of Nursing Care* pp. 12–13. Geneva: International Council of Nurses.
3. Orem D. E. (1983). *Nursing Concepts of Practice*, 3rd edn., pp. 2, 6. London: Collier Macmillan.
4. Rogers M. E. (1970). *An Introduction to the Theoretical Basis of Nursing* p. 86. Philadelphia: F. A. Davis.
5. Shetland M. L. (1965). Teaching and learning in nursing. *American Journal of Nursing*; **9:** 112.
6. Henderson V. (1966). *The Nature of Nursing*. London: Collier Macmillan.
7. McFarlane J. K., Castledine G. (1982). *A Guide to the Practice of Nursing using the Nursing Process*. London: C. V. Mosby.
8. McFarlane J. (1986). The value of models for care. In *Models for Nursing* (Kershaw B., Salvage J., eds.). Chichester: John Wiley.
9. Aggleton P., Chalmers H. (1984, 1985). A series: models and theories. *Nursing Times*; October 1984–March 1985.
10. Roy C. (1986). In *Essentials of the Roy Adaptation Model* (Andrews H., Roy C.). New York: Appleton-Century-Crofts.
11. Clark J. (1986). A model for health visiting. In *Models for Nursing* (Kershaw B., Salvage J., eds). Chichester: John Wiley.
12. Clements I. W., Roberts F. B., eds (1983). *Family Health: A Theoretical Approach to Nursing Care*. New York: Wiley.

13. Jones C. (1977). The nursing process—individualised care. *Nursing Mirror*, 13 October 1977: 13–14.
14. Department of Health and Social Security (1977). *Nursing in Primary Health Care*. CNO (77); **8**: 2.
15. Scottish Home and Health Department (1978). *District Nursing in Scotland*. (Chairman: Hockey L.), p. 18. Edinburgh: HMSO.

Further Reading

Chapman C. (1985). *Theory of Nursing—Practical Application*. London: Harper & Row.
Hunt J. M., Marks-Maran D. J. (1980). *Nursing Care Plans: The Nursing Process at Work*. Aylesbury: H M & M.
Kershaw B., Salvage J., eds (1986). *Models for Nursing*. Chichester: John Wiley.
Kratz C. R. (1979). *The Nursing Process*. London: Baillière Tindall.
Marriner A. (1978). *The Nursing Process: A Scientific Approach to Nursing Care*. 2nd edn. St Louis: C. V. Mosby.
Mayers M. G. (1978). *A Systematic Approach to the Nursing Care Plan*. 2nd edn. New York: Appleton-Century-Crofts.
Pearson A., Vaughan B. (1986). *Nursing Models for Practice*. London: Heinemann Medical.
Roper N., Logan W. W., Tierney A. J. (1981). *Learning to Use the Process of Nursing*. Edinburgh: Churchill Livingstone.
Roper N., Logan W. W., Tierney A. J. (1983). *Using a Model for Nursing*. Edinburgh: Churchill Livingstone.
Roper N., Logan W. W., Tierney A. J. (1985). *The Elements of Nursing*, 2nd edn. Edinburgh: Churchill Livingstone.
Tierney A. J., ed. (1986). *Clinical Nursing Practice*. Edinburgh: Churchill Livingstone.
Tinkham C. W., Voorhies E. F. (1977). *Community Health Nursing: Evolution and Process*, 2nd edn. New York: Appleton-Century-Crofts.

Chapter 7

Assessment of Need

In order to provide realistic care it is important to get to know the patient, his family and the community in which he lives. For example, Mr Adam's care will be different from that required by a 56-year-old with the same degree of physical disability cared for by a young, fit wife living in a bungalow with all modern facilities. Differences between patients, with regard to their families, their environments and their lifestyles, affect and determine the care to be given. The district nurse needs to find out about these details in order to plan and give the best possible care, and assessment is the first stage of the nursing process. It begins with the collection of all the information about a patient having implications for nursing action and ends with a statement of the patient's problems. The aim of the assessment stage is to obtain sufficient information on which to plan a programme of care designed to meet the physical, social and emotional needs of the patient.

Information required

The collection of the information required should reflect the chosen framework, and to make a realistic plan of care it is necessary to remember the aims of district nursing. If it is agreed that those aims include 'assisting the patient in those activities which he would normally do for himself' it is clearly necessary to know what those activities were. Therefore it follows that the most important information is that which concerns the patient's normal daily routine and behaviour, for only when this is known can a programme acceptable to the patient be drawn up. If Mrs Cray always had her main meal at night it is of little avail trying to persuade her to have 'meals on wheels' in the middle of the day. Although Mr Adams has difficulty in communicating, his wife can tell the nurse about the fluids he normally drinks; if the nurse does not find out this information she may well be advising something like 'plenty of milk', which he abhors.

Apart from the physical and environmental needs of the patient, the assessment should include information about possible psychological and social needs. John may well need counselling on his enforced lack of sexual activity, and if the district nurse has not the will, ability or training herself to deal with this problem then she has a duty to ensure that advice is given by another appropriately qualified person. The emotional and financial needs of patients may very well be interrelated with their physical needs, and it is important that in dealing with the complex problems of the Baker family that all aspects are taken into consideration; concentration on the physical needs at the expense of other factors means failure to give total care.

A complete assessment involves information gathered by the district nurse, which forms the nursing history. In addition the assessment should include information from medical records, referral notification from hospital, information from other health workers and information gathered by observation of the patient, family and environment.

The nursing history

District nurses are in a unique and privileged position to gain information about the patient, his family and his environment. Visiting the patient in his own home enhances a free exchange of information, and the district nurse probably gains more knowledge about the patient and his family than most health workers. But for the information to be of use it needs to be written down and available to others involved in the care of the patient.

The nursing history differs from the medical history in that it is required to form a basis for planning *nursing* care and concentrates on the effect of illness rather than on the illness itself. Nevertheless, the medical history and the nursing history should be complementary to one another. The actual taking of a nursing history enables the district nurse to learn about the patient and his normal lifestyle and is a beginning of the nurse–patient relationship. If this is done well time will ultimately be saved, as the information obtained will be available to others caring for the patient.

To be sure that all aspects of need are considered it is advisable to use a recognised layout which will probably be a printed form or Kardex, the design of which will differ in various health authorities. It is important that the design of such a form is developed by the staff using it, since it needs to reflect their philosophy for care and local idiosyncrasies and reflect the chosen framework.

Henderson[1] lists 14 needs of all people which she feels form the components of basic nursing care. The nurse may need to assist the patient with these functions or provide conditions that will enable him or her to:

1 Breathe normally.
2 Eat and drink normally.
3 Eliminate by all avenues of elimination.
4 Move and maintain desirable posture (walking, sitting, lying and changing from one to the other).
5 Sleep and rest.
6 Select suitable clothing, dress and undress.
7 Maintain body temperature within normal range, adjusting clothing and modifying the environment.
8 Keep the body clean and well groomed and protect the integument.
9 Avoid dangers in the environment and avoid injuring others.
10 Communicate with others in expressing emotions, needs, fears etc.
11 Worship according to his or her faith.
12 Work at something that provides a sense of accomplishment.
13 Play, or participate in various forms of recreation.
14 Learn, discover or satisfy the curiosity that leads to 'normal' development and health.

If it is agreed that this list covers the needs of each person then it is possible to use these 14 components as headings on the patient assessment chart, and under each heading there will be a record of how the patient is coping with the activity in question. It is important that all staff understand what each heading includes; for example, although integument is primarily the skin it also includes coverings such as the mucous membrane, hair and nails.

The terminology in the Henderson list is American but it does have the advantage of covering the range of physical, psychological, spiritual and social needs of all people.

A British example which develops Henderson's theory is that of Roper[2], who describes the patients' needs in terms of 12 daily living activities—that is, observable behaviours based on needs. Roper, Logan and Tierney[3] develop the model further; they consider the patient's state on a continuum from totally dependent to totally independent, and in making an assessment chart each activity along this continuum.

In both these examples the nurse in making her assessment needs to question whether the need or activity is currently satisfied and if not, why not.

This links with Maslow's[4] hierarchy of needs where he suggests that an individual operates on ascending levels and that once the lower needs have been satisfied they lose their urgency and then the person requires his needs to be met at a higher level (see Fig. 7.1).

When a person is ill it is generally the physiological needs that take precedence, but it is important that all these needs are recognised; for example, with Mr Adams it would be all too easy to concentrate on his problem of immobility and incontinence, but it is equally important to preserve and respect his dignity as a

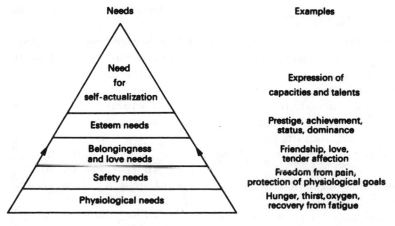

Fig. 7.1. Maslow's hierarchy of needs.

person of worth. In the case of John, means must be found for him to achieve a state of self-fulfilment, but to do this other levels in the hierarchy must first be dealt with such as helping him to cope with his incontinence and problems of immobility.

Besides giving information about the patient's physical, social, psychological and spiritual needs, the nursing history should also include personal data about the patient and his family, and an assessment of the strengths and weaknesses of the various people giving care. It is also helpful to find out and note what the patient and family understand about the illness and their expectations of care. Wolff and Erikson[5] use the 'assessment man' in Fig. 7.2 as a visual reminder of what needs to be considered when making an assessment.

An assessment using the Orem[6] model will consider the balance between the individual's ability to achieve self-care and the reasons, which may be varied, for being unable to achieve this goal.

All of these models share an approach which identifies a deficit in the functions of the individual. Such a deficit may be for physiological, psychological or social reasons. In this way the need for nursing care is identified. Clements and Roberts[7] draw together and illustrate many other approaches such as an interaction model, an adaptation model and a humanistic model.

Gathering information

Adequate information on which to base care is essential, and therefore the skills needed to acquire this are important. The most important single source of information is the patient; taking his nursing history allows the district nurse to begin to establish a positive nurse–patient relationship, to observe the patient's condition and to obtain information from the patient and where applicable from his family.

If the nursing history is to be used as a basis for planned care it needs to be taken as soon as possible. Apart from recording the condition of the patient and estimating how much information is needed to give optimum care, it is important to note how much information the patient or his family are willing to divulge on their initial contact with the nurse, for the reasons for withholding

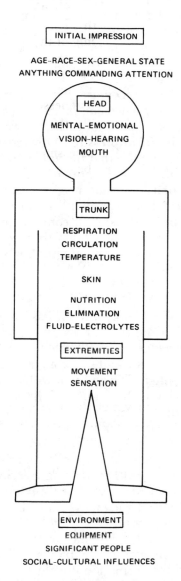

Fig. 7.2. The assessment man (based on a figure from *Nursing Outlook*, **25** : 2 (1980); copyright American Journal of Nursing Company.

information may be an unwitting part of the nursing history. John would be unlikely to discuss his sexual problems on the first visit and Mrs Adams may have been so anxious about her husband that she disclosed nothing more than the bare details. On the other hand anxiety and insecurity may make some patients or their relatives over-talkative.

The district nurse may recognise that it is not necessary to take a full history, for instance when one visit is all that is needed, say to remove sutures from a clean wound. However even in such a case the nurse, from her initial impression of the patient, his family, or the environment, may realise that the full history is required. It is important to remember that the nursing history is not static and completed at the first visit but needs constant addition and modification as new information is revealed or the situation changes. As Shetland[8] states: 'the content and context of the interaction are kaleidoscopic rather than static and change constantly as one factor in the total situation changes'.

Before the first visit

The district nurse should make sure she has sufficient information to enable her to plan the time of her visit and its approximate length, some knowledge of the patient's condition and the treatment he has received, and—of course—the accurate name and address of the patient. The patient will feel more confident if the nurse obviously knows his name and the care he requires, and the district nurse will feel more confident if she knows about the patient. Before visiting a patient for the first time the district nurse may be able to get information from the doctor and the patient's records in the surgery. She may also obtain information from the hospital or from other health and social service personnel. For example, in the case of Mrs Baker the nurse will approach her with greater confidence if she knows that Mrs Baker is aware of her condition and her prognosis. For the patient who has been in hospital following a cerebrovascular accident the district nurse would need to know how much the patient can do for himself. If she does not have this information the patient may regress in the stage of rehabilitation.

When the district nurse finds she has not sufficient *nursing* information about a patient who has been in hospital she should try to visit the ward sister. Such a visit may well be helpful in clarifying the role of the district nurse and helping the ward sister to realise what information is necessary for a district nurse to carry out planned care. Personal contact with nursing colleagues is time well spent.

The first visit

The importance of the initial encounter between the nurse and the patient cannot be overstressed since it may form the basis of a relationship lasting for years. The standard for care to be given is also set at this visit. If the patient does not have all the equipment required by the nurse such as separate towels and flannels the nurse needs to explain tactfully that these will be required on subsequent visits. The nurse should always remember she is the guest in the patient's home, albeit usually a welcome guest; but nevertheless there may be a conflict of roles and the nurse needs to be enough of a guest to enable relatives and patients to feel that they are the master or mistress of their own home. At the same time she must remain a skilled professional and exert sufficient influence to establish her own authority in respect of nursing care of the patient.

It is important that the district nurse who is accountable for the care of a particular patient makes a first visit to the patient. If for some reason this nurse is not available another district nurse needs to make this initial assessment.

Interviewing

To collect a nursing history the nurse must be skilled in the art of interviewing, which is a goal-directed activity aimed at encouraging the patient to express ideas, feelings and facts that help to identify his immediate and long-term needs. The quality of the interview is partly determined by the climate the nurse creates, and if she seems to be hurried the patient will not feel free to explore his feelings. For this reason the timing of the interview is important. Depending on information she has received the nurse may feel it is preferable to leave a first visit until the afternoon when she is less rushed. On the other hand it may be that an initial visit is made in order to cope with an immediate nursing emergency, as when Mr Adams first had his stroke and became incontinent. Then the immediate nursing need for the visit would be life-preserving measures and dealing with his basic hygiene needs. Mr Adams would not be able to give information and his wife would be anxious, so further information would have to be collected on a subsequent visit.

Interviewing is more than a question-and-answer session, it is also an observational technique. The interviewer should listen most of the time and watch for facial expressions and gestures as well as listening to the way the words are said. It is important to listen to what the patient is trying to tell you, not just what he is saying, as in the old jingle:

'A wise old owl lived in an oak
The more he saw, the less he spoke;
The less he spoke, the more he heard.
Why can't we be like that wise old bird?'

Many nurse have a tendency to talk too much and listen too little. When trying to find out what others think and believe, the nurse should keep her questions and comments brief and to the point. She should not have to concentrate on her Kardex to the extent that she is unable to listen to answers. This is why it is important to have a layout the nurse can memorise.

The nurse may use a series of direct or open-ended questions. Such information is factual and merely requires checking (such as name and address) and can be dealt with by the direct question. Other questions need to be open-ended, such as 'how are you managing with your housework?'—and when open-ended questions are used the patient will usually feel freer to reveal any matters of concern.

The interviewer must first clarify the purpose of the interview and explain why she needs the information. She also needs to maintain the momentum by such comments as 'you hadn't finished telling me that'; 'can we go back to that again?' To draw a line between redirecting tangential conversation, and not cutting off important elaboration is difficult. It is a skill which can be only acquired with practice. Above all the nurse needs to create an atmosphere in which the patient and his family feel free to talk. To do this she must feel at ease and this she may not feel if she is worried about filling up the information sheet or she feels is prying into the private life of the patient.

Barriers to communication

The patient's condition may militate against information giving and getting, and in some circumstances the relatives may not be cooperative. The patient may have a preconceived notion of what the nurse needs to know and this may inhibit the giving of extended information. At the same time differences in age or in the experience of the nurse and patient, and differences in cultural, social and ethnic backgrounds, can all impose difficulties. Other difficulties include such things as other people in the room or the noise of the television or radio. It is important in talking to the patient to use language he understands, and this may well be linked with age, culture and social background. For example, 'How often do you pass water?' may be preferable to 'How often do you pass urine, or void?'

It must be remembered that people, particularly when anxious, may not understand what is said to them and there can be considerable distortion between what the nurse has told the patient and the message received by the patient. In a state of anxiety the patient often only hears what he expects to hear, so the nurse should validate the answers: 'Is that how it seems to you?'—'Is that correct?'

The nurse may not be able to start her interview where she wants. She wants to gather information systematically but if visiting a patient suffering from constipation, for example, she may find the first thing the patient wants to talk about is 'my bowels' so the interview starts there. She also needs to be aware of her own prejudices and values, as this may influence what she asks and how she interprets the answers. She needs to show understanding and acceptance, and refrain from making moral judgements.

Measurement

Accurate baseline measurements, from which progress or

deterioration can be determined, are essential, and include the recording of temperature, pulse and respiration rates, blood pressure and urinalysis. These should be recorded when making the assessment of the patient and thereafter recorded with discrimination. If there is a doubt about a patient's fluid intake and output, means of measuring and recording these must be found and this will probably involve the cooperation of relatives.

Accuracy in the assessment of the size of a pressure sore or varicose ulcer is necessary for the subsequent evaluation of progress. This measurement can be done by use of graph paper, drawing on a clear film held over the area, or a comparative description such as 'the size of a 10p piece'; but with the latter method it is necessary to remember that people's perceptions of size may vary considerably.

The Norton pressure sore rating scale[9] (Fig. 7.3) is a tool all too rarely used by nursing staff, and although the study described was carried out in the hospital setting, the findings are equally appropriate for patients at home. By simply scoring using the scale it is possible to assess those patients most likely to develop pressure sores, but other factors such as availability of relatives to help the patient, and the provision of aids such as a ripple bed or

Phys. Cond.		*Mental Cond.*		*Activity*		*Mobility*		*Incontinent*		
Good	4	Alert	4	Ambulant	4	Full	4	Not	4	Total
Fair	3	Apathetic	3	Walk/help	3	Sl. limited	3	Occasional	3	Score
Poor	2	Confused	2	Chairbound	2	V. limited	2	Usually/Ur.	2	
V. Bad	1	Stupor	1	Bed	1	Immobile	1	Doubly	1	

Patients with a total score of 14 or less are liable to develop pressure sores and when the score is lower than 12 the risk is very great indeed.

Fig. 7.3. Patient assessment form (scoring system).

sheepskin, will also need to be taken into account. Such measurements may well be required to make a case for priority of need.

Assessment of the environment

It is important that the district nurse gets to know the community in which she carries out the majority of her work. When she first visits a house she should note the type of neighbourhood it is in. Knowing the resources available, the location of the social services' offices, any relevant voluntary organisations, and the location of the chemist's shop and post office may be essential when advising patients and their relatives. The nurse needs to know the community sufficiently well to be able to assess the community atmosphere, because on this may depend how much she can involve neighbours if she is seeking help.

The type of dwelling in which the patient lives may be significant, but it is important that the nurse does not jump to the wrong conclusions. Because Mrs Cray lives in a high-rise block of flats is she necessarily lonely? Many people are so pleased with the modern facilities provided by a new flat that these may outweigh what seem to be disadvantages. Although in some cases the property may look neglected this is not necessarily due to apathy, but may be due to a variety of reasons such as a lack of finance, illness, or an unwilling landlord. Likewise an overgrown garden may not be a source of distress to the patient (if it is the district nurse may find a voluntary group to deal with this). Therefore, when making an assessment of the environment it is necessary to note not only the state of the environment but also how the patient interacts or reacts to it.

The observation of the immediate environment in which the patient is being cared for may give many clues to the nurse, and among questions the nurse should ask herself are 'Is it a suitable place in which to provide care?'; 'Is it adequately heated?'; 'Is it safe?'; and finally 'Will using it for nursing care disrupt the life of the rest of the family?' It should be remembered that although it is apparently a safe environment for the patient, it could be dangerous to others if drugs or equipment are left around. It may be that the room is not very clean, and with careful discussion and observation it should be possible to establish whether this is of recent origin because of the illness, or is the usual pattern. When washing her hands or collecting water from the kitchen the nurse should notice if there is food, how it is stored, and what are the cooking facilities and the general state of cleanliness.

The nurse should use her sense of smell. She may detect a smell of stale urine although the patient or relatives have not admitted that the patient is incontinent, or she may be aware of the smell of a discharging wound. Although the patient or his relatives may not mention these facts it is up to the nurse to try and find out as tactfully as possible if this is causing distress. If so, this should be noted under the appropriate assessment heading that deals with the patient himself.

Assessment of the patient

From her observations the district nurse will get a first impression of the patient's general state, and should observe whether the patient is thin, showing signs of recent loss of weight, or is overweight; whether he is pale or flushed; and, if the patient is up, his degree of mobility. At the same time she should notice the patient's general mental condition, and look for such signs as a furrowed brow, the avoidance of eye contact, a reddening of the face and neck or clasping and unclasping hands, all of which can be indications of anxiety, embarrassment, or more serious mental disability.

Dependent on the reason for visiting, the amount of physical assessment will vary. However if the nurse uses the structured approach from head to toe she will ensure that she considers all aspects of the patient's condition. The nurse does this more easily if she is actually carrying out care for the patient, for instance when she is with Mr Adams she will notice the condition of his eyes, ears, mouth, skin and movement of limbs, the degree of incontinence and the level of his comprehension.

From what has been said it should be clear that at each visit the nurse should observe any clues about the patient's mental state, his physical condition and the environment in which care is being given. She should do this by using her senses of sight, touch, smell and hearing. Many of the patients being cared for by the district nurse are long-term patients requiring daily visits, and, she should be aware of the danger of 'familiarity breeding contempt' and of the need for the same rigorous observation of patients whose condition is apparently static.

Assessment of the carers

The carers may be relatives, but quite often are neighbours or friends. The contribution of such people to the care of sick people at home is frequently not fully valued. It is therefore important that the district nurse takes an interest in and encourages the care they provide, for if the carers become unable or unwilling to help, then the district nurse will need to increase her visits or the patient may require residential care.

Again, first impressions given by the relatives at a visit may give much information. How Mrs Adams greets the nurse in the morning may indicate her degree of anxiety. If she doesn't look as smart and is more curt than usual the nurse needs to find out discreetly, whether this is because she has had a difficult night with her husband, whether the caring is becoming too much, or whether she just over-slept. It is also important to observe the physical condition of the relatives who are giving care, and to notice whether there are signs of anxiety or signs of not being able to cope. Observation of how the patient and carers interact with each other is also important; for example, the district nurse may notice that Mrs Baker's elder daughter who gives every attention to detail in the care of her mother is looking pale and tired herself and is irritable with the younger members of the family. This should indicate to the nurse that she must offer further help and it also gives her an opportunity for health teaching.

The first part of the assessment stage is complete when a comprehensive picture of the patient and family has been built up by interviewing, observation and measurement. The district nurse then has a nursing assessment on which to base her plan of care.

To summarise, a comprehensive assessment should:

1   Have a layout that allows the nurse to collect information systematically in a short time, based on an agreed framework.

2   Include information that will help the nursing team plan a realistic programme of care for the individual patient and his family.
3   Provide a baseline of information from which subsequent progress can be measured.
4   Be concise, and not duplicate information collected by others in the health team unless the focus is different or that information is not available to the nurse.

The following chart gives an example of what may be included in nursing history; this does not use any one particular model.

Page 1

PERSONAL DATA	Initial history taken by *J. Smith*	Date *6.9.87*
Surname: *Baker*	Marital status: *Divorced*	

Forenames: *Phyllis Ann*	Likes to be called: *Ann*

Address: *7 High Street*	

Date of birth: *8.5.39*	Age: *48 years*

General practitioner: *Dr Black*	Hospital consultant: *Mr Jones*

Referred by: *GP*	Reason for referral: *Patient constipated. Assess for other help required*

Medical diagnosis: *Carcinoma of liver. Spinal metastases*

SOCIAL HISTORY Occupation:	*Shorthand typist on leaving school Recently school meals supervisor Not worked for past 6 months*

Family composition:	*Sarah—17 years—shop assistant (not working at present) Paul—14 years—at St James school Angela—12 years—at St James school*

Next of kin:	*Sarah. Mr John Baker (brother) lives in Australia*

Other Carers:	*Neighbour—Jane, 5 High Street—calls in at approx 8.0 am and in evenings—at work all day*

Environment: *Semi—well equipped—signs of recent neglect*
                         Bathroom/WC upstairs. WC downstairs
                         Immersion heater

Hobbies/interests: *Knitting. TV. Rarely has social outings since divorce*

Religious practices or beliefs: *Non-practising RC*

Other agencies involved: *None at present. Home help offered but refused*

HEALTH HISTORY *(From GP's notes)*   *Nil of note until 1 year ago—then*
                                             sudden loss of weight.
Relevant medical history: *Jaundice—nausea→hospital*
                                             Metastases present
                                           Discharged 1 month ago

---

Medications: *dihydrocodeine 1 tab (30 mg) 4-hourly*
                 nitrazepam 2 tabs (10 mg) bedtime
                 7.9.87 prochlorperazine maleate 1 tab (5 mg) 6-hourly

---

Patient/family understanding about illness: *Patient has been told diagnosis and given prognosis of approx 6 months. Ann does not wish children to be told yet.*

Patient/family reaction to illness: *Ann 'accepts' illness but anxious about children—she thinks it will be longer than 6 months. Sarah realises mother is very ill—tries to cope. Angela—does not seem aware. Paul—probably not coping—goes out a lot.*

Page 2

ASSESSMENT   *Thin, frail lady. Yellow tinge to skin*
General assessment on admission: *and conjunctive. Looks anxious.*
                                        Up and dressed, sitting on settee.

BASIC PHYSIOLOGICAL FACTORS
Activity/movement: *Manages to get up and downstairs once daily.*
                      Inclined to stoop. Moves slowly around living room.
                      Tires quickly.

Rest/sleep: *Board under mattress*
              Sleeps on 3 pillows
              Sleeps approx 6 hours after nitrazepam
              Naps during the day

Nutrition: *Looks thin, obvious weight loss.*
             Eating very little. Nauseated
             (?Sarah understands need for small tempting portions)

Elimination/continent state: *Passes urine × 3/4 daily.*
Urinalysis NAD.
Concentrated—no discomfort. BNO for 6 days—normal pattern daily.
No menstruation for 1 year.

Fluids/electrolytes: *Drinking 'small amounts'—poss. only 100 ml. 2-hourly.*
Usually likes tea, coffee but these now nauseate. Looks a little
dehydrated—skin dry—eyes sunken.

Breathing/circulatory state: *Respirations shallow. No cyanosis.*
Extremities cold to touch but patient not complaining. (T 36.6 °C P88 R22)

Sensory state: *Vision √ (glasses for reading) Smell √ Touch √ Speech √ Hearing √*
Pain—soreness in back sometimes 'like a knife'. Dihydrocodeine
relieves. Finds hot water bottle comforting.

Skin condition: *Dry. Slight reddening over sacrum. Heels √ Elbows √ Norton Score*
16 Mouth dry, lips cracked. Hair greasy, sparse. Nails brittle.

EMOTIONAL STATE   *Very talkative.? frightened that we will talk about illness in*
front of Sarah.

PROBLEM LIST

Date	No:	Date	No:
6.9.87	1 Pain due to metastases	6.9.87	3 Constipation due to poor diet
6.9.87	2 Inadequate fluid intake		and inadequate fluids
	due to nausea	6.9.87	4 Anxiety re children
		7.9.87	5 ? children feel neglected

Where to keep the assessment

It is difficult to give specific advice regarding this as the organisation of district nursing varies from area to area. The nursing history may be kept at the group practice, the health centre or the district nursing centre, and in some authorities the nurses may carry the histories with them on their rounds; but the main criterion is that the history is available to whoever is visiting the patient. It is therefore important that histories are kept where there is ease of access, at the same time ensuring that they will only be seen by properly designated professional colleagues. However, if the patient has told the nurse something in confidence and expressly desired that it should not be repeated then it should not be written down.

Increasingly, computers are being introduced into general practice and it may be that opportunity to use these for district nursing records will develop; their usefulness should be explored bearing in mind the aspect of confidentiality.

Identification of problems

Collecting information about the patient and family is a means to an end. The nursing assessment is not an end in itself but an aid to identifying problems which are amenable to nursing care. The initial assessment should culminate in a mass of information from which the nurse must select that which indicates the patient's problems. In this book the term 'patient problems' is used to mean those problems with which the patient requires help. Other writers sometimes use terms like 'nursing diagnosis', 'nursing needs' or 'nursing problems', but the authors of this book feel that 'patient problems' is more explicit and focuses on the patient himself.

The most common classification of problems is into actual, potential and possible problems.[10] An *actual* problem is one that exists at the time of the assessment; *potential* problems are difficulties or concerns that a patient has an unusually high risk of developing or experiencing, and identification of these problems enables the district nurse to take preventive action; *possible* problems are situations requiring more information before being ruled in or out as actual problems. A clear statement of a problem is essential as this is the guide to the planning of care.

When attempting to identify problems the nurse may find that there is information she needs that is not available, or there are inconsistencies in the information she has received from the patient and the family. For example Mrs Baker may say she has little pain yet her daughter is worried because she felt her mother did not sleep because of pain.

Precision in describing the problems is necessary, and it is important to establish where possible the cause of any problem, as this then indicates the nursing care required; for example, the patient's constipation could be due to a consistently low fluid intake, inadequate roughage in the diet, poor mobility, or haemorrhoids. The nurse must be aware of normal body development and functioning to be able to identify any deviations from the normal, and base her decisions on a sound knowledge of the biological and social sciences. If she is in any doubt she should seek advice.

Examples of the problems of particular patients are set out below:

Mr Adams

Actual problem:	Difficulty in communication due to slurred speech and confusion.
Potential problem:	Pressure sores due to immobility and incontinence.
Possible problem:	Inadequate finance due to extra money being spent on heating.

Mrs Baker

Actual problem:	Pain due to spinal metastases.
Potential problem:	Inadequate fluid intake due to nausea.
Possible problem:	Young children feel neglected because of mother's poor condition.

Mrs Cray

Actual problem:	Obesity due to lifetime habit of over-eating and immobility.
Potential problem:	Lack of healing of ulcers due to excessive heat from fire.
Possible problem:	Social withdrawal and confusion.

John Davis

Actual problem:	Urinary incontinence due to leaking condom.
Potential problem:	Urinary tract infection due to inadequate fluid intake and poor mobility.
Possible problem:	Sexual frustration due to his immobility.

This list of problems is in no way complete, but it is used to show how the nurse can analyse information gained during her assessment, and identify problems for which nursing intervention is required.

It is at this stage that the nurse recognises and rules out problems. For example, the district nurse visits once a week to reassess that Mr and Mrs Fisher are coping, and her initial impression may be of a severely handicapped man who needs help in coping with his general hygiene needs, dressing and undressing. However, he and his wife have learned how best to deal with this, so these can be ruled out as problems at this stage, but as the disease progresses and the patient becomes more disabled these may become problems for which the district nurse will need to provide care. This shows the need for continuous reassessment of the patient and the family and it also emphasises the need to explore with the patient what the nurse and he see as being problems, because there may be different perceptions which could cause conflict.

Problem identification therefore needs to be carried out thoughtfully and where possible this should be done in conjunction with the patient and his family. When the district nursc has gathered the initial information, she will need to share this first with the patient and his family, and then with her colleagues. Together they will determine the problems for which they will need to provide care.

Conclusion

The assessment stage has two main phases: the drawing together of information from various sources, particularly from the patient and family, and the use of this information by the nurse to identify the problems with which the patient needs help. Time spent at this stage is time well spent, as thorough and accurate assessment will mean that the nurse can realistically plan care for the patient and his family.

References

1. Henderson V. (1966). *The Nature of Nursing*, pp 16–17. London: Collier Macmillan.
2. Roper N. (1982). *Principles of Nursing*, 3rd edn. Edinburgh: Churchill Livingstone.

3. Roper N., Logan W., Tierney A. (1985). *The Elements of Nursing*, 2nd edn. Edinburgh: Churchill Livingstone.
4. Maslow A. H. (1943). A theory of human motivation. *Psychological Review*; **50**: 370–96.
5. Wolff H., Erikson R. (1977). The assessment man. *Nursing Outlook*; **25** No 2: 103–7.
6. Orem D. (1983). *Nursing: Concepts of Practice*, 3rd edn. New York: McGraw Hill.
7. Clements I. M., Roberts F. B., eds (1983). *Family Health: A Theoretical Approach to Nursing Care*. New York: Wiley.
8. Shetland M. C. (1965). Teaching and learning in nursing. *American Journal of Nursing*; **9:** 112.
9. Norton D., McLaren R., Exton-Smith A. N. (1962). *An Investigation of Geriatric Nursing Problems in Hospital*, p. 225. Edinburgh: Churchill Livingstone.
10. Mayers M. (1978). *A Systematic Approach to the Nursing Care Plan*, 2nd edn, pp. 33–35. New York: Appleton-Century-Crofts.

Further Reading

Andrews H., Roy C. (1986). *Essentials of the Roy Adaptation Model*. New York: Appleton-Century-Crofts.
Bower F. L. (1982). *The Process of Planning Nursing Care*, 3rd edn. St Louis: C. V. Mosby.
Clements I. M., Roberts F. B., eds (1983). *Family Health: A Theoretical Approach to Nursing Care*. New York: Wiley.
Gebbie K., Lavin M. (1975). *Classification of Nursing Diagnoses*. St Louis: C. V. Mosby.
Kratz C. (1979). *The Nursing Process*. London: Baillière Tindall.
Little D., Carnevali D. (1976). *Nursing Care Planning*, 2nd edn, p. 128. Philadelphia: J. P. Lippincott.
McGilloway O., Myers F., eds (1985). *Nursing and Spiritual Care*. London: Harper & Row.
Marriner A. (1983). *The Nursing Process*, 3rd edn. London: Y.B. Medical Publishers.
Owen G. M. (1983). Skills of interviewing. In *Health Visiting*, 2nd edn. London: Baillière Tindall.

Chapter 8

Planning Care

To ensure the highest possible standards of care, as well as economy of time and energy, it is necessary to plan skilfully and to provide an individual plan for each patient at the same time as organising the total caseload. Not only are there more patients to care for, but also, because of the higher survival rate, longevity and early discharge from hospital many are highly dependent. Not to plan is like exploring without a map. The intention of this chapter, therefore, is to suggest ways of planning care for the individual and his family within the context of the total caseload of the district nurse. Tinkham et al.,[1] who give the principles to be borne in mind when planning care, emphasise that plans should be based on the identified desires, needs and interests of the patient, and those involved in carrying out the plan should be consulted. Above all the plan must be realistic and capable of practical implementation.

The nursing care plan

The assessment stage ends with a statement of the problems experienced by the individual patient and his family. The next stage involves making a nursing care plan which the nurse and patient should use to provide an answer to these problems. The assessment directs the planning and the chosen model, such as self-care or stress adaptation, will influence the plan. Just as in the assessment stage there are distinct phases in planning.

In the assessment of the patient's problems it was emphasised that the cause of the problem should also be stated, and this leads to the next step which is the setting of goals of care. Differing terms are used by the various authors, for example, aims, goals, objectives, expected outcomes. In this text the term 'desired outcome' will be used as this implies a statement of the desired or realistically expected correction of the patient's problem.

The desired outcome of care

The desired outcome should be written in terms of the result expected in the patient, not in terms of the nursing action. The desired outcome needs to be brief, concise and specific; for example, to state that a patient should have 'extra fluids' or 'be mobilised' does not clarify how much fluid is needed or the degree of mobility required, but to state that the patient 'will drink 1800 ml of fluid a day' or 'will walk to the front door using a Zimmer frame' gives specific detail of what it is hoped that the care will achieve. When, later, the nurse comes to evaluate care (Chapter 10), it will be clearer why it is necessary to state the desired outcome concisely. As with the assessment phase it is important to involve the patient and family in the determination of the desired outcome. These goals must be unambiguously stated with the nature, quality and characteristics of the outcome being specified. It is also important to state a date by which time the desired outcome should be achieved. This ensures that the nurse and other carers evaluate and reassess the care given at specified times. With some patients a daily check is needed of such things as fluid intake or the degree of mobility, but with many of the long-term patients a weekly or monthly evaluation is sufficient. Setting specific goals is one of the activities that individualises and personalises care.

Using some of the problems identified in the previous chapter, the plan at this stage would look like this:

Mrs Baker

Problem	A/P	Date	Desired Outcome	Check
1 Pain due to metastases	A	6/9/87	Pain free	at every visit
2 Inadequate fluid intake due to nausea	A	6/9/87	(a) Nausea relieved (b) At least 1000 ml fluid intake tolerated daily	Daily

John Davis

Problem	A/P	Date	Desired Outcome	Check
1 Urinary incontinence due to leaking condom	A	5/8/87	Condom drainage will remain patent	Daily
2 Urinary tract infection due to inadequate fluid intake	P	7/8/87	(a) No infection (b) 2000 ml fluid daily	Weekly (Thurs) Daily
3 Sexual frustration due to immobility	Poss.	7/8/87		

In the above examples the problem is set out indicating whether it is an actual (A) or potential (P) problem and the date the problem was identified. The desired outcome is given and the time for checking whether this has been achieved. It should also be noted that whereas a desired outcome can be written for actual and potential problems this cannot be done for possible problems; these need to be identified and recorded but it is not possible to state goals because sufficient information is not available.

It takes time and practice to develop the skill of writing clear and concise goals for each patient but this is necessary if care is to meet individual needs. Kratz,[2] in a study which looked at the long-term care in the community for a group of patients suffering from stroke, showed that some care was given without goals. The aim of care for the seriously ill patient was usually known and this care was focused to meet the observed needs of the patient. At the other end of the continuum, however, the aim of care was not known for the patient who was not getting better. Care did not correspond to the observed needs and was thus diffuse. Although a large proportion of the patients cared for by the district nurse can be put into the category 'not getting better' it is important nevertheless to focus care on clear goals rather than let it become aimless.

Priority setting

At the same time as setting goals for care it is necessary to determine if there is an order of priority for their achievement, and to decide on the best order for nursing care. Maslow's theory of a hierarchy of needs may guide the nurse in setting priorities (see Fig. 7.1, page 115); for example, until John's incontinence has been alleviated it will not be possible to attempt to restore his self-esteem and social contact with his peers.

Nursing action

Having set the goals the next phase is to plan the action required to achieve these; for example, if the desired outcome was that the patient should drink 1800 ml of fluid per day it might well be stated that in every 2 hours from 6 a.m. to midnight he should drink 200 ml of fluid. It must again be emphasised that the decision-making must be based on a sound knowledge of biological and behavioural sciences, normal development, and the disease process.

Another consideration is who is available to provide the prescribed care. In the instance above it may be possible for the patient to supply the drinks for himself, or if he cannot it may be necessary for the nurse to give drinks when she is present, the home help to provide a thermos flask of fluid, and possibly a neighbour to give drinks in the evening. There are numerous variations on this theme which need to be considered for the individual patient. The action, regarding who shall provide the fluid and how often, needs to link with the cause of the identified problem.

The plans for Mrs Baker and John Davis, will now look like this:

Mrs Baker

Problem	A/P	Date	Desired Outcome	Check	Action
1 Pain due to spinal metastases	A	6/7/87	Pain free	At each visit	Explain to patient and daughter need for 4-hourly analgesic. Patient to keep record of pain. Provide backrest

2 Inadequate fluid intake due to nausea	A	6/7/87	(a) Nausea relieved (b) at least 1000 ml fluid tolerated daily	Daily	(a) See GP re drugs for nausea (b) Explain to patient and daughter. Suggest soda water, small amounts frequently, e.g. 100 ml hourly

John Davis

Problem	A/P	Date	Desired Outcome	Check	Action
1 Urinary incontinence due to leaking condom	A	5/6/87	Condom drainage will remain patent	Daily	Teach parents re: positioning
2 Urinary tract infection due to inadequate fluid intake	P	7/6/87	(a) no infection (b) 2000 ml fluid daily	Weekly Daily	(a) 1 Urine test Fridays 2 MSU to lab monthly 3 Penile toilet (b) Advise John and family to monitor
3 Sexual frustration due to immobility	Poss.	7/6/87			Male nurse to discuss

It should be noted that nursing action has been listed for the possible problem although the outcome cannot be forecast, and the problems have been numbered to save having to rewrite when referring to them subsequently.

The patient's role in planning care

The patient and family should be involved in planning his care. How helpful the patient is will depend on his physical and mental state of health, his understanding of the current situation and his past abilities at problem solving. For example Mr Adams will have a limited role in planning his care, but Mr Fisher should be a full participant in constructing his care plan. The nurse will need to help the patient and family to understand this problem-solving approach to care, and together they will consider the assessment, identify the problems and formulate the plan of care. Involving the patient in planning his care is often seen as one of the most difficult parts of the nursing process as it is not traditionally a part of nursing, and so many patients are passive in their attitude to the nurse and do not expect to play an active role.

People who give care

When planning the nursing action it is important to know who will provide the care required, and to ensure appropriate referral or delegation it is necessary for the district nurse to understand the roles of the various care givers.

The patient and his family

The most important care givers are usually the patient and his family and so it is important for the nurse to assess their ability to cope with the care involved and to ensure that they have been taught how to carry out this care (Chapter 9). Other people closely linked with the family who often carry a considerable burden of caring are the friends and neighbours, and again the district nurse must not merely accept at face value that there are such people to provide care but must be sure of their ability, motivation and availability. Some of the complexity of family relationships has been described in Chapter 4.

Nursing staff in the primary care team

The primary care team was described in detail in Chapter 5. When deciding which member of the district nursing staff shall give care to any particular patient it is necessary to consider the status and roles of the different members of staff, their previous experience, their training and education and the policies of the health authority. It is important for the district nurse to remember that she is responsible not only for the care she gives but also for the care she delegates to the enrolled nurse or to the nursing auxiliary. She must, therefore, plan to make the first visit to the patient herself and then if she delegates care she must subsequently make periodic visits to ensure that the quality of care is all that she would wish, and if it is not, to give advice and guidance.

Referral to other agencies

Within the plan of care the district nurse should note care that needs to be provided by someone other than the immediate family or the nursing staff. The patient may be unable to get enough food of the right kind because he or she is unable to shop and cook. In such cases the nursing action may involve arranging for 'meals on wheels', arranging for a home help on days the meals are not delivered and possibly some arrangements whereby relatives or neighbours provide meals at weekends. The nursing action in this case therefore includes contacting the various agencies or people in order to obtain the equipment required. There are numerous voluntary and statutory agencies the nurse may need to contact and details of these are given in Appendices 2 and 3.

Liaison between hospital and community

Skeet, in her study of the home care needs of recently discharged hospital patients, *Home from Hospital*,[3] says that 'care must be planned, and planned before discharge, if it is to be continuous . . .' and she highlights the inadequacies of care occurring because of poor planning. The most glaring fault was lack of communication; not only did the hospital fail to communicate with the community services but in a high percentage of cases no letter was sent to the general practitioner. The patients' greatest need was advice about activity or drugs, many of the elderly have a multiplicity of drugs with no instructions for taking them. Some patients were struggling to do their own dressings and most knew little about the various services to which they were entitled. Many patients needed more help than they could get and two patients spent their day sitting on commodes waiting for relatives to return in the evening to get them off. In many instances the district nurse or other members of the primary care team were not aware that the patient had been sent home from hospital, but it must also be said that district nurses were sometimes at fault. One of the case studies in the book described 'Mr M., age 69, married, subarachnoid haemorrhage, deaf, almost blind, doubly incontinent, sent home to wife . . . a district nurse called once and delivered incontinence pads'.

To avoid such situations occurring it is important that transfer should be as smooth as possible whether the patient is being transferred from hospital to home or vice versa. The channel through which information should be sent will vary depending on whether there are liaison officers and what their function is. Whether a liaison officer is available or not, when a patient needs to be transferred from one area of care to another the nurse must ensure that sufficient information for the continuity of care is sent to the next person responsible for the nursing care of the patient. Increasingly, copies of nursing care plans are being transferred to and from hospitals with patients. It is important to have this nursing information to ensure continuity of care; this is additional to the medical information.

Where to keep the plan

As with the assessment, practice will vary from authority to authority. If the plan has been determined with the patient, and the patient is aware of his role in the care, it would seem appropriate to leave it at the patient's home. However in some cases there will be problems, particularly when the patient is unaware of his diagnosis, and in such a situation it may be preferable to keep the records at the district nurses' place of work. But no matter where the plan is kept, it must always be available to any nurse who may be called upon to give care to that particular patient. As mentioned previously the records may be computerised. If so, it is essential that up-to-date information is fed into the system.

In summary, therefore, the good care plan is specific to the individual patient, it states the problems and causes of the problems and sets the desired outcome of care for each problem and the nursing action necessary to achieve this goal. The nurse, patient and family will need to decide between choices of action and should make decisions by using the assessment, knowledge of the patient's condition and the findings of research. The plan must be realistic and deadlines should be set for achieving goals and evaluating progress made.

Some patients will have only one problem with which they need nursing help; others will have many. In the examples given only a few patient problems have been identified but all these patients have other problems for which care would need to be planned.

Planning work for a group of patients

Having devised a plan for each patient it is next necessary to consider the care of individual patients within the context of the total workload of the district nursing team. The term 'workload' is used here rather than 'caseload' because there are many factors other than the actual number of patients to be considered.

It should by now be obvious that a clear assessment and plan of care gives a better indication of the degree of dependence of the patient and the approximate length of time required for the visit than a statement such as 'general nursing care' indicated. McIntosh and Richardson,[4] in a study which included looking at the workload of district nurses, showed that designation of tasks is not a good indicator of the time taken. For instance they found that the time taken for bathing a patient ranged from 11 minutes to 84 minutes. To give Mr Fisher his steroid injection may only take a few minutes but to make a reassessment of his physical and psychological status will take considerably longer.

By identifying the problems it is possible to sort out priorities of care. There is no absolute rule as to the order in which patients should be visited. Most district nurses like to visit their diabetic patients as early as possible but it may well be that a patient who has an early hospital appointment or one who is in considerable pain needs to be visited first.

While it is not generally advisable to give patients an exact time for visiting it is often helpful to given an approximate time— particularly, for example, if the nurse requires water heated for bathing a patient. It may be decided that the appropriate nursing action for cleansing Mr Evan's wound is a daily saline bath prior to the district nurse's visit to pack the wound; he therefore needs to be given a reasonably precise time for this visit. It is also important that the patient's day is not disrupted too much because this overemphasises the sick role. If patients are able to get out of the house to do their shopping this contributes toward their feeling of well-being, and they should not be kept waiting all day for the nurse; of course, both the nurse and the patients must be prepared for emergencies to occur and for the well-laid plans to go astray. If this does happen every attempt should be made to contact the patient and to explain and if necessary apologise for the delay.

The number of visits the patient requires during the 24 hour period needs to be taken into consideration; the timing needs to be specific for the patient requiring 6-hourly analgesic injections, and in such a case should be planned in consultation with the night staff. Often the number of visits required will depend on the availability of relatives; for example, Mr Adams will need to be visited twice a day because of his incontinence and dependence and the fact that his wife is elderly and has arthritis. With some patients two nurses will be required to give care because of the weight or ill condition of the patient, and in such situations both nurses need to plan their work and arrange to meet at an agreed time.

In planning the day's work, consideration needs to be given to the number of staff available and to their experience, status and training. Apart from selecting the most suitable nurse for a particular patient, account must be taken of the transport available to each nurse, their hours of work and the policies of the health authority concerning the use of the enrolled nurse and nursing auxiliary. The district nurse, however, must never forget that she is accountable for the proper delegation of the work (Chapter 18).

For reasons of economy it is necessary to keep the amount of time spent on travelling by each member of staff to a minimum. One of the disadvantages of group attachment for district nurses may be an increase in travelling time since not all general practitioners zone their practice areas.

One of the privileges in district nursing is the building up of long-lasting relationships with the patients and their families, some of whom will be visited for many years. On the other hand this can mean long-term contact with the difficult or unpopular patient. One advantage of teamwork and the discussion of plans enables some rotation of staff to such patients. This can be as helpful to the patient as it is to the nurse; communications and relationships operate in two directions and it may happen that a patient dislikes a particular nurse for some reason that is arbitrary or unrelated to her professional role. These situations do not occur frequently but it is important to be sensitive to the possibility, and to try to intervene before a crisis occurs.

The nurse needs to plan her day throughout the span of duty and to be sure of regular coffee and lunch breaks to preserve her own health. If she is tired and hurrying to get the maximum work done in the morning this can adversely affect the patient. Besides visiting the patient at home the nurse may carry out some work in the general practitioner's surgery or at the health centre, and time should be allowed for this. It is important to ensure that time in the surgery is also well planned. An appointment system for patients to see the district nurse can be a help in saving the time of both the nurse and the patients and it is worth while spending time thinking this out in order to save time in the future. The amount of time and the period of the day spent in the surgery work needs to be carefully thought out. For example, if the district nurse continually finds she cannot carry out necessary care for ill and incontinent patients prior to surgery time, perhaps the allocation of work needs to be renegotiated with others in the health care team.

Increasingly the district nursing team is required to visit patients in residential homes, either those provided by the local authority or private nursing homes. Residential homes which initially were intended for the frail elderly invariably now are home to the sick, dependent elderly and may well not have a qualified nurse on the staff. This, therefore, is another area of work for the district nurse.

Meeting other members of the team face-to-face is important. Some members of teams rely mainly on informal meetings and as long as the necessary contact with one another is made this may be satisfactory; in other teams formal meetings are arranged. Whichever system is in operation it is important to plan time for these meetings.

Referral of patients to other agencies can be time-consuming but the time spent in meeting other personnel face to face will usually pay dividends by easing future telephone conversations, and will ultimately save time. An understanding of the roles of others and their problems and restrictions is necessary to ensure proper referral. It may be helpful to visit a patient in hospital before he comes home. This not only facilitates continuity of care but it also helps to reassure the patient that his care will be continued when he goes home. It enables the district nurse to check that the appropriate services and aids have been organised. The district nurse needs to be selective in deciding which patients to visit prior to discharge, but this can be time well spent and needs to be programmed into a day's work.

Increasingly, district nurses are required to have student nurses and other personnel accompanying them on their visits. Time for teaching needs to be allowed and this must be seen as an integral part of the district nurse's workload.

A final demand on time, to be considered when planning work for the district nursing team, is the need for all nurses to keep abreast of current knowledge. This means allocating adequate time for attending study days, for demonstration, refresher courses and reading (Chapter 18).

References

1. Tinkham C. W., Voorhies E. F., McCarthy N. C. (1984). *Community Health Nursing: Evolution and Process*, 3rd edn. New York: Appleton-Century-Crofts.
2. Kratz C. R. (1978). *Care of the Long-term Sick in the Community*. Edinburgh: Churchill Livingstone.
3. Skeet M. (1974). *Home from Hospital*, 4th edn, p. 28. London: Macmillan Journals.
4. McIntosh J., Richardson I. M. (1976). *Work Study of District Nursing Staff* (Scottish Health Service Studies No 37). Edinburgh: Scottish Home and Health Department.

Further Reading

Gilmore M., Bruce N., Hunt M. (1974). *The Work of the Nursing Team in General Practice.* London: Council for the Education and Training of Health Visitors.

Hockey L. (1968). *Care in the Balance: A Study of Collaboration Between Hospital and Community Services.* London: Queen's Nursing Institute.

Hockey L., Buttimore A. (1970). *Cooperation in Patient Care: Study of District Nurses Attached to Hospital and General Medical Practice.* London: Queen's Nursing Institute.

Kron T. (1981). *The Management of Patient Care: Putting Leadership Skills to Work,* 5th edn. London: W. B. Saunders.

Mager R. F. (1962). *Preparing Instructional Objectives.* California: Fearon.

Marram G., Barrett M. W., Bevis E. O. (1979). *Primary Nursing—A Model for Individualised Care,* 2nd edn. St Louis: C. V. Mosby.

Parnell J., Naylor R. (1973). *Home for the Weekend Back on Monday.* London: Queen's Nursing Institute.

Roberts I. (1975). *Discharged from Hospital.* London: RCN Publications.

Skeet M. (1974). *Home from Hospital.* 4th edn. London: Macmillan Journals.

Skeet M. (1981). *Discharge Procedures: Practical Guidelines for Nurses.* London: Macmillan Journals.

Stockwell F. (1972). *The Unpopular Patient.* London: RCN Publications.

Chapter 9

Implementation

The third stage of the nursing process is the implementation of the plan, in other words the actual provision of care. Here the inter-linking and over-lapping of the stages of the nursing process are obvious, for although implementation is the carrying out of what has been previously planned the district nurse must constantly reassess the situation and modify the plan accordingly. For example, when visiting Mr Fisher she may find that his wife is unwell and has been unable to assist him with washing and dressing. The district nurse, therefore, will need to help with this basic care and assess whether the plan needs to be revised in the long term. She must ask herself whether Mrs Fisher is now finding it too much of a strain to cope with her husband and her job, or whether this is just a temporary setback.

If the patient and family have been actively involved in planning care they will be more inclined to help with the actual delivery of care. The professional nursing input may be minimal but if this is so it means that a good deal of care must be provided by the relatives, other carers and the patient himself. Thus it is important to consider the teaching role of the district nurse. The family may be very willing to learn and able to cope but the inevitable burden must not be underestimated, and the district nurse needs to give support and counselling to the patient and his family.

The planned nursing action may have involved the district nurse in contact with other personnel to arrange for services or equipment; this will require communication skills and a knowledge of services available (see Section IV). The actual delivery of nursing care by the district nurse frequently requires adaptation of the practical skills learned in hospital, such as aseptic and lifting techniques and the administration of drugs. The principles of these remain the same but the execution may require considerable adaptation for the home situation.

We return again to the philosophy for care and the belief that the district nurse should be assisting the patient towards self-care. This will involve not only teaching the patient, coordinating the services for his care and carrying out nursings tasks for him, but also using skills required to promote his rehabilitation. Therefore it is important to consider the skills of teaching, counselling, communication, adaptation of nursing techniques and rehabilitation. Development of these skills will help the district nurse to implement care that is best fitted to the patient and family.

Practical procedures must be adapted to the particular situation, but a textbook such as this can consider only the principles. A principle is a general law that acts as a guide to action. Principles serve as guides for future investigation and give practical direction for present action. It is not enough to know and state a principle; it is necessary to be able to apply it in varied situations. In her discussion of the principles of asepsis Hunt[1] gives some guidelines that could be applied to any nursing procedure. She suggests that: 'one should be able to assert confidently that the nurse's actions will never endanger the health and safety of the patients and . . . that nursing procedures are always carried out in accordance with the principles on which they are based'.

Learning and teaching

The district nurse is only available for short periods in the patient's day. Many patients are able to cope entirely with their needs for the rest of the day, but others need some care provided by other people; Mrs Adams will need to be taught the best way to care for her husband between the district nurse's visits; John and his parents together need to be taught aspects of his care such as how to use the hoist; although Mr Evans does not require assistance with care once the district nurse has redressed his wound she may take the opportunity while she is there to teach him and talk about the amount of lifting he will be able to do, and give advice about his diet and the care of his bowels.

Teaching opportunities in nursing are boundless and it is important that the nurse recognises and uses such opportunities. However, the person to be taught must also be ready and willing to learn. Learning is a process by which changes are brought about in an individual's response to the environment. The changes may be in knowledge, skills or attitudes. For example, the district nurse may need to increase, and thus change, the diabetic patient's knowledge of his dietary needs, his skill in giving his injections and his attitude to the disease. If these planned changes do occur the patient can be said to have learned. Learning and teaching go side by side, and a useful maxim to remember is that 'telling isn't teaching and listening isn't learning'.

Redman[2] links the learning and teaching process to the nursing process. She identifies five stages:

1   Assessment of the need to learn.
2   Assessment of the readiness to learn.
3   Setting objectives.
4   Teaching and learning.
5   Evaluation and reteaching if necessary.

This process can be used for any teaching situation the district nurse encounters, including teaching patients, relatives, other carers and other nursing staff. These stages will be considered in relation to the patient and his carers. The teaching of students will be looked at separately.

Assessment of the need to learn

When making the initial assessment of the patient and his family the district nurse should have assessed their degree of knowledge and skill, and the attitudes they hold. It may be obvious in discussion that the patient and his family have detailed knowledge of the illness and its implications, but on the other hand they may have totally misconceived ideas. They may have had previous experience of caring for a sick person at home, or it may be an entirely new experience and the patient and his family may be resentful of a situation that changes the family's life style. In her assessment the nurse needs to help the patient and family identify their learning needs because the learner must perceive a need to learn.

Assessment of the readiness to learn

The nurse may realise that the patient and his family lack

knowledge, but unless they are willing, learning will not take place. Various factors affect the readiness to learn, and sometimes the person may not be unwilling but simply too anxious to pay attention and retain the knowledge. A low level of intelligence does not necessarily mean that a person is unwilling to learn, and in fact the reverse may be true.

Setting objectives

The objectives or goals of teaching must be realistic and achievable since success is more motivating than failure. Once determined, the objectives need to be discussed with the learner, and the nurse needs to determine what the patient and his family must, should and could know. For example the diabetic *must* know the amount of insulin to inject, he *should* know the relationship between diet, insulin and activity and he *could* know the pathology of the disease. Teaching needs to proceed from the simple to the complex, from known to unknown, to be broken down into manageable parts and objectives should reflect this.

Teaching and learning

The learning environment affects the rate, amount and quality of learning. Sometimes in the home it is difficult to achieve the ideal learning situation; for instance, it may be difficult to find a quiet place away from the distractions of family activities to obtain the learner's concentration. Interest and motivation increase when the learning experience is seen to have relevance, but it may be difficult to demonstrate that relevance. For example, it is easy for the nurse who has seen pressure sores and contracted limbs to realise the need for pressure area care and passive exercises. However, patients and relatives who have not seen such complications may have dificulty in understanding the need to be taught these activities and indeed they may feel they are actually cruel to the patient.

The learner has certain expectations of the teacher. The nurse is generally regarded by the public as a person knowledgeable about health matters and her opinion is respected. While she must live up to this reputation she can also capitalise on it, as it often means she has a willing learner. An important teaching principle is that learning is more meaningful when the learner is actively involved—as summed up by the maxim, 'What I hear I forget, what I see I remember, what I do I know'. Much of the teaching given by the district nurse concerns the learning of practical skills and such teaching, particularly, demands the involvement of the learner. For example, to change the drawsheet of an incontinent patient with the patient in the bed may have become a simple task for the experienced nurse but will be difficult for the relatives to carry out. To tell them how to do it would be meaningless, to show them would be a good introduction to their learning but the only way they will learn is by doing it for themselves.

Feedback is an essential component of learning. The learner needs to know whether he is performing a skill well or poorly and this is particularly crucial early on so that bad habits are not formed. The district nurse herself should always act as a role model in the care she gives, the organisation of her work and the attitudes she displays to the patient and the family. Teaching the patient self-care may be initially time-consuming, but in the long term it will save time and increase the patient's independence.

Evaluation of teaching

Evaluation should be continuous during the learning–teaching process. The district nurse may need to pick up clues as to whether a person understands, and also she may use questions and answers, and get the learner to repeat the information. Some people are able to tell the teacher what they do not understand, but others have difficulty in perceiving that they do not know. If learning has not taken place there is a need to reconsider the teaching and it is necessary to question whether the goals were realistic and whether the method of teaching was the best.

Health education

The principles of learning and teaching have so far been linked with the care of the sick person, but the district nurse has a unique opportunity to contribute to the promotion of health and prevention of ill-health on an individual basis. The OPCS study

Nurses Working in the Community, undertaken in 1980,[3] showed that district nurses devoted 17% of their time to 'advice, counselling, reassurance and education'. Most of this was identified as 'general reassurance and social conversation'. This seemingly informal conversation must never be under-valued as it is often during this interchange that cues are given to under-lying concerns. Many have criticised what is seen to be a small amount of health education within the district nurses' work, but the method of data collection did not pick up all those opportunistic interactions taking place during the carrying out of a nursing procedure. During the course of such conversation the nurse may, for example, explain about diet, medications and what is happening to the patient's body.

Much of the responsibility for ensuring his own good health lies with the individual but we can all influence by our own actions. Patients and their families are particularly conscious of their health when the nurse is around.

Health education is one of the most important aspects of preventive medicine[4] and Caplan[5] describes three different levels of prevention: primary, secondary and tertiary. The district nurse has a contribution to make at each of these levels.

Primary prevention is taking specific and identifiable measures to forestall disease and injury, and during her visit to a home the district nurse has the chance to observe for health hazards. Many of the patients the nurse visits are elderly and a home that was once considered safe may now be potentially hazardous, so the nurse should observe the physical environment and look for such dangers as poor lighting, frayed flexes, inadequate storage of drugs and unguarded fires.

In teaching relatives, the nurse can prevent illness or injury by stressing the importance of their having an adequate diet and sufficient rest to prevent them from becoming ill or too tired to cope. In this connection the nurse should also teach the relatives about the correct methods of lifting. The district nurse constantly needs to observe relatives and other carers for any signs of breakdown in their health, because excessive tiredness and anxiety may lead to the occurrence of accidents. Again, the nurse should set an example in such matters as handwashing, careful disposal of soiled dressings and storage of drugs.

While visiting an elderly person at home the nurse may observe friction between younger members of the household or she may notice unexplained bruising on a child leading her to suspect non-accidental injury. In this situation she should immediately report her suspicions to the health visitor.

It is sadly becoming increasingly necessary for members of the public, including the district nurse, to be alert to the signs of drug and solvent abuse and alcoholism. The district nurse having access to the home is in a unique position to notice cues and will need to share concerns with the general practitioner, social worker or health visitor as appropriate.

In *secondary prevention* measures are taken to limit or stop the progress of an already established disease or injury, to prevent complications and sequelae and to limit disability. For example, while visiting Mrs Cray the district nurse should teach her about the need for a sensible diet and the need for exercise and rest, in order to maintain her general health and to promote the healing of her ulcer.

An increasing need for health education by the district nurse is in the prevention of hypothermia. This is a particular problem with the elderly, although other groups such as young babies, patients with lowered thyroid function, the poor housebound and those taking certain drugs are also susceptible. Again the important function of the nurse is to look for signs of susceptibility to hypothermia and to look at possible means of preventing its occurrence. Inadequate heating, clothing, nutrition and exercise may all be contributory factors and these may be due to ignorance, apathy or sheer lack of finance. The nurse through her teaching may be able to make improvements or she may well need to seek the provision of other services and extra finance.

Bereavement visiting is another example of secondary prevention and is mentioned in more detail in Chapter 16. Skeet[6] showed the need for much greater intervention at this level for patients discharged from hospital even following relatively minor treatment.

Tertiary prevention involves taking measures to maintain an incurably ill person at the optimum level of activity and to forestall unnecessary suffering. The district nurse is now increasingly involved in caring for the chronically sick, the disabled and the terminally ill at home, and she needs to know how to assist these patients and their families achieve the best quality of life in the time left.

Strehlow[7] identifies a group frequently neglected in health education—the frail elderly. With the increasing numbers of elderly it is important to identify the means and the persons who will be involved in their health education before they become sick. There is a need in part to alleviate isolation and loneliness but at the same time enabling them to retain their individuality.

Most of the health education given by the district nurse will be with individuals and their families, but she may also be involved in group health teaching in a field of particular interest, for example slimming groups or, because of a particular expertise in something such as first-aid measures or promoting keep-fit groups. Group teaching uses the same principles of identifying a need to learn, setting objectives, planning teaching and evaluating the results. Particular points that need to be considered are the size and composition of the group to be taught, the previous knowledge of the group, the time allowed for teaching and the setting in which the session is to take place.

The professional health education officer, usually appointed on a district health authority basis, forms a distinct element of the health services provision and will act as a resource person for the district nurse providing as back-up service and a stimulus.

Teaching other personnel

Increasingly, students and staff from other health and social services, as well as student nurses, are required to gain some experience in the community. Under EEC regulations (see Chapter 19) the student nurse is required to spend at least 2 weeks in the community as part of her basic training and this is likely to increase. Some of this time may be spent with members of the team other than the district nurse. The district nurse has a unique role in sharing her knowledge and skills with these learners and she must ensure that the time spent with her is a true learning experience. To do this she must know at what stage on her course the student is and what previous teaching about district nursing and the community services she has received. The district nurse must define the objectives of the student's experience and remember that the student is gaining an *insight* into district nursing, not learning all about it. To achieve this insight the district nurse must identify the aspects the student needs to experience in order that she may relate her experience when she returns to the hospital. It is often difficult while in a house to highlight the points the student should note, and adequate briefing before entering the house and discussion afterwards are therefore essential.

Although a one-to-one teaching situation can be ideal, it can also be tiring for both the teacher and the learner. Nevertheless there may be advantages of having a visitor accompanying the district nurse on her rounds as she may be able to help with the lifting and care of patients. However the privacy and dignity of patients must be respected and their permission sought to bring a visitor into the house, for although another person is usually welcome, occasionally a third person may break a developing relationship or inhibit a patient from sharing confidences with the nurse. In such a situation it may be preferable to ask the student to wait in the car, and this can then be used as a positive teaching point on the importance of confidentiality and development of relationships.

As well as nurse-learners, the district nurse may be asked to take with her on her rounds health visitor students, social work students, general practitioner trainees or other community workers. The district nurse should use this as an opportunity to teach other workers something of her role and such teaching and understanding should eventually help to improve working relationships and communication between members of the community health team.

Counselling

The district nurse increasingly has a role as a counsellor, a means of giving support to the patients and their carers which may be in the form of a discussion or an interview to help people with their difficulties. Problems for the patient associated with his illness may include a change in life style, limitations in his activities or the need to accept a poor prognosis. The relatives too may have similar anxieties and may need help in sorting out their priorities; for example, there may be the conflicting demands of a young family and a sick elderly relative.

Nurse[8] gives some clear guidance for nurses about their role as counsellor and the use of professional counsellors. She says that counselling differs from teaching in as much as it helps the person to become aware of alternative courses of behaviour, and it is the function of the counsellor to assist the individual to make his own decision among the choices available. Counselling requires a non-judgmental attitude on the part of the nurse, an empathetic approach and a relationship in which the person being counselled can express his thoughts and feelings in such a way as will clarify his problems and his attitude to them.

Counselling takes time and nurses must make time available for this, and be alert to cues from patients and relatives that they need to talk. In order for counselling to be effective there must be a relaxed atmosphere; this is probably best achieved by sitting down with the person or persons concerned and having a cup of tea. Sometimes it may be difficult to find the right environment, particularly if it is the relatives who need the help and they do not want to talk within the hearing of the patient. In such cases counselling may have to take place in the kitchen or garden. The district nurse therefore needs to create an atmosphere where the family feel free to talk about their worries, and to help them find the means of coping with their problems. Counselling does not necessarily mean that the problems themselves can be resolved but that problems can be faced with less anxiety and tension. Sometimes the value of counselling simply involves getting the patient to ask the right question; for example, 'How am I going to adapt my living style?' rather than 'When am I going to get better?'

The need for understanding listening is as important as the giving of actual information and advice. At the same time it may involve elements of comforting, consoling, teaching and correcting or giving information. The nurse should beware of giving false reassurance to a patient and his family for this implies there is little cause for anxiety, and they will mistrust a nurse who says 'don't worry' when they are obviously concerned. To give false hope shows a lack of understanding and sensitivity. The reassurance the nurse can give with conviction is that the patient and family will receive all possible support and that the patient will be kept as free from pain as possible.

Collaboration, coordination, communication

Frequently the nursing action planned for the patient will include contacting other personnel for services or equipment. This involves the use of skills of collaboration, coordination and communication. Collaboration means working with other persons to plan, provide and evaluate aspects of care; for example, to ensure that Mrs Baker remains as free from pain as possible the district nurse, the general practitioner and Mrs Baker together should be planning and evaluating the drug regime. John and his family, together with the nurse and the physiotherapist, should agree his programme of exercises.

The district nurse's role in coordination is rather like that of the conductor of an orchestra, bringing together the many parts to function harmoniously as a whole. The district nurse may assess the need for the patient to have 'meals on wheels' and a home help, but if the patient also attends a day hospital one or two mornings a week she needs to coordinate the provision of the services on the other days to avoid gaps and overlaps. Coordination also requires the collaboration of the various personnel.

Communication, which may be written, verbal or non-verbal, is an integral part of collaboration and coordination. There are three components to any process of communication: the communicator, that is the person sending the message, the message and the recipient of the message. For communication to be effective it is essential that the message is received and understood, and this can be difficult if the message has been sent as a written communication or a telephone message to a third person. Whenever possible direct communication with the person concerned is preferable because personal contact means that alternative approaches can be discussed. For example, if the district nurse is unhappy about the present treatment for Mrs Cray's ulcer it would be helpful if she and the general practitioner met at the patient's home to discuss together with the patient possible changes in treatment. In providing the best care for Mrs

Baker and her family it will probably be helpful to have a team conference involving the district nurse, general practitioner, health visitor and social worker.

Collaboration, which implies freely sharing information and working with other people, is essential in providing a coordinated approach to achieve mutually acceptable goals. To work well with other people requires an understanding of their role and function, as well as being able to convey one's own role and function to other people. The quality of communication between the nurse and the patient, and between the nurse and other workers, has direct bearing on how well the patient's needs are met.

Adaptation of nursing techniques

The district nurse needs to use her previous knowledge of principles of techniques and any new knowledge gained in the community and has a responsibility to remain a safe practitioner. Nurses in the home have fewer technical resources than they would have in hospital, more ambiguity to deal with, and they are also in the anomalous position of not having a clearly defined authority. The district nurse will be called upon to carry out a whole range of techniques ranging from the simple to the complex but it is merely the intention here to describe the adaptation of known principles to a few techniques that are considered by many to be the more difficult to adapt.

Aseptic technique

In a discussion of aseptic techniques in the community, Davison[9] says that 'as long as nurses understand those underlying principles, adjusting to individual circumstances should present no difficulties'. He believes that nurses should develop an 'aseptic conscience' arising from this understanding. Maurer,[10] whilst stating that infection is not a common problem at home, does stress in the case of wounds that no risks should be taken and no microbes should be allowed into an open wound. In addition she says that equipment which is used to pierce or cut the skin or cover a wound should always be sterile. Therefore, although the person may have acquired immunity to the micro-organisms commonly present in his own environment it is important the district nurse takes steps to avoid introduction of new organisms.

It is now easier for district nurses to adhere to these principles because they usually have available to them dressings and equipment from a central sterile supplies department (CSSD). If this is not so, dressing packs can be obtained on prescription and alternate means of sterilising instruments will need to be used. Boiling of instruments before and after use is an acceptable means of sterilisation, and even if disposable forceps are provided it may be necessary to boil ancillary instruments such as scissors and probes. Some authorities provide an antiseptic solution for sterilisation but to soak instruments before and after treatment is time-consuming. Hampshire dressing packs which incorporate sterile gloves rather than instruments are convenient for use at home and are increasingly being provided.

The district nurse has to adapt her technique from that learned in hospital, where frequently there were two nurses to carry out the procedure; now she needs to act as her own 'dirty nurse', pour out the lotions herself, remove the dressings and complete the whole procedure unassisted. To do this she must work out the best method for use in each situation which enables her to adhere to the principles of asepsis.

Handwashing may be difficult in some households. Broome[11] showed that use of a Hibitane-impregnated tissue was at least as effective as handwashing, or solutions such as Hibiscol or Hibiscrub may be used instead. The guiding principle is that hands should, at the least, be cleaned before commencing a procedure and afterwards, and it is up to the district nurse to determine the best way of achieving this. Before commencing a technique it is important that the nurse prepares a clean working surface. She may be offered a clean Formica-topped trolley or a rubbish-strewn table, and it may need considerable tact to get the latter cleared. In choosing the room in which an aseptic procedure is to be carried out a number of things need to be considered. Whilst the kitchen may seem ideal in terms of availability of running water and working surfaces it is not appropriate when there is a discharging wound to be exposed. The nurse must at all times respect the patient's property and protect the furniture used, and pets should be removed from the room.

Nursing bags vary in size, style and contents; but it must always be remembered that the contents must be kept clean and that the nurse's hands need to be cleansed prior to removing articles from the bag. The bag should never be put on the floor but a suitable protected surface found for it. In the majority of households the nurse will find that the patient and/or family are most anxious to make arrangements to suit the nurse.

Disposal of dirty dressings and used instruments is the final consideration when carrying out aseptic techniques. Dressings should be well wrapped and burned if possible, although this is less easy now that few open fires exist. If there are large amounts of offensive dressings to be destroyed, arrangements can be made for their collection by the environmental health service. Disposable forceps should be broken to avoid their re-use and when possible wrapped and put in the dustbin. If the nurse is in doubt about the safety of disposal it may be better for her to wrap the articles concerned and take them back to her work base for destruction. Some instruments need to be returned for resterilisation, and again it is important to ensure these are wrapped to avoid cross infection.

Carrying out an aseptic technique in the home may call for considerable ingenuity on the part of the nurse, but if she bears in mind the principles of asepsis taught in her training it should be possible to do this even in an unsavoury environment.

Use of equipment

Equipment may be obtained from various sources and to arrange for its provision in the home frequently takes time in communicating with the various services. As part of her planning for care the nurse must determine which equipment is required; she should be realistic in this and not order unnecessary items. One very necessary item is frequently a commode or chemical toilet for the patient with particular elimination needs. For some of the aids to daily living it may be useful for the nurse, physiotherapist and occupational therapist together to work out with the patient what is the most appropriate device, but it must be remembered that equipment costs money and once it is no longer required it should be returned. The district nurse has a responsibility to make sure equipment is used correctly, maintained and returned.

The district nurse needs to use much imagination in finding the best means of caring for the patient at home, and frequently it is the patient or his family that devise the best adaptations. Equipment is now always readily available and there may be a waiting list for delivery, but in the meantime patients need care, so household objects may have to be used temporarily as a substitute. For example, an upturned dining chair or a suitcase well padded with pillows or cushions can be used as a backrest, a coffee table or cardboard box can act as a bed cradle and newspaper under a sheet will help to protect the mattress of an incontinent patient until incontinence sheets and laundry can be provided. Economy and thoughtfulness in the use of equipment is necessary, for while it may be ideal to change the patient's clothes and bedding each day the district nurse must consider who is doing the washing. Sometimes aids such as incontinence pads will need to be used to protect the bedding although this is not the treatment of choice. The use of aids also needs to be determined in the light of help available, for example, if it is not possible for a patient's position to be changed frequently it may be necessary to provide a ripple bed or sheepskin to help prevent pressure sores occurring. Mr Adams may need such a bed or a ripple cushion in the chair as his wife cannot move him between the nurse's visit, whereas another patient with a similar degree of disability may not need such equipment because there are enough carers to move him regularly.

The organisation of the nursing environment is important and it is necessary to plan with the patient and family in which room care is preferable. This means taking into account such factors as toilet facilities, stairs and the family activities. The arrangement of the room is crucial; for example, if a patient needs lifting in bed it is obviously easier if the bed is not against the wall, but it is all too easy to concentrate on the sick person and forget the normal family activities. In some households this may be acceptable but in others it can cause resentment. The organisation of the home for John obviously took considerable time and consultation between members of the family, health and social services before he was transferred home from hospital. Time spent planning before discharge from hospital can be of great value in such instances.

Sometimes the nurse needs to find a compromise between the ideal equipment and that preferred by the patient. A notorious problem with district nurses is that of caring for patients in a double bed. Whilst this is obviously not ideal for nursing the psychological comfort to the patient may be preferable to some physical discomfort caused to the nurse and other carers. However, if the patient is heavy, and needs lifting and nursing while in bed, it may be necessary to move him into a single bed. One of the chief considerations is the height of the bed, and a hospital-type bed is preferable to a divan although it may be possible to raise the latter on blocks. On the other hand the hospital-type bed will tend to emphasise the sick role; but this may be inevitable. Many would argue that Mr Adams should not be in his double bed—but if a single bed was recommended where would the double bed be put? Where would Mrs Adams sleep? And how much would it upset both Mr and Mrs Adams to sleep separately after all these years?

Lifting

Lifting is an important area in which the district nurse has to adapt her known skills. She is at particular risk of back injury because she may not have help with lifting; beds and chairs are often low and a large proportion of the patients requiring lifting are elderly and can do little to help themselves. The district nurse will have been taught lifting methods in her nurse training and will need to adapt these methods in the home. The principles of good, safe lifting however remain the same and are:

1 The weight to be moved should be as near the workers hip level as possible, and therefore the height of bed and chair need to be considered.

2 The lifter(s) should stand near the weight to be moved in order to maintain balance and use the large muscles.

3 Legs should be apart to get a broad base and to enable the lifter to shift the weight of their body as the particular object is moved.

4 The weight should be moved toward rather than away from the lifter.

5 The lifter should keep the back as straight as possible, flexing the hips or knees rather than bending the back. This ensures that the large muscles of the thigh and trunk are used rather than those in the arm.

These principles should be applied when lifting any patient and when teaching others to do so.

If possible the nurse should get help with lifting and to do this will need to assess the ability and physical strength of other carers. Not infrequently the carer may also be elderly or disabled; for example, Mrs Adams could not be expected to help with lifting her husband. If the nurse has any doubt about her own ability to lift a patient unaided because he is heavy, very ill or awkward; she should arrange for another member of the nursing team to meet her at the house. This in the long term saves time and energy and prevents injury to nurse and patient. If a relative or other person is to help with the lifting it is important that the nurse teaches that person the best way to lift. Besides being lifted in and out of bed, patients may need to be put into and out of chairs and baths. The latter can cause considerable difficulty as most bathrooms are small with the bath fixed to one wall and with no handles.

Aids for lifting should be used when possible; hoists can be invaluable as long as there is room to manoeuvre them and the nurse can instil the necessary confidence in the patient and the relatives in their use. Lifting poles may be provided to fit some beds and sometimes heavy furniture or a bar fitted to a wall can be used to help the patient lever himself; a rope tied to the foot of a bed can be used for the patient to pull himself into a sitting position. The nurse, patient and family together must work out the best methods of lifting to preserve the health and strength of not only the patient but of all the carers concerned.

Administration of drugs

After the stringent rules in hospital the district nurse may feel the storage and administration of drugs in the community is very relaxed. Drugs are the property of the patient for whom they were prescribed but they may be taken irregularly and haphazardly stored. The district nurse has a responsibility to try to ensure that drugs are taken correctly, that they are effective and that they are stored safely; at the same time she must observe for side effects.

When interviewing the patient the district nurse should check the drugs the patient is taking against the medical notes, and ensure that the patient knows when and how to take the drugs. Drugs should be stored in their proper containers, kept in a safe place and clearly labelled. Patients, particularly the elderly and the confused, should be advised not to keep drugs at the bedside as they may forget they have taken them and then on waking in the night take further drugs, leading to accidental overdosage. The nurse needs to check that the patient understands the need to take a full course of drugs and obtain a further supply when necessary. The district nurse should advise the patient or his family that any unused drugs be destroyed by burning or flushing down the lavatory.

Except where the patient is giving his own injections or having regular injections administered by the nurse, as in the case of a diabetic patient, syringes should not be left in the house. The district nurse should make sure that a used syringe is destroyed in order to avoid any chance of re-use or of its falling into the hands of a drug addict. Teaching regarding the taking of drugs, their storage and disposal is another important aspect of health education.

The district nurse has further responsibilities pertaining to the administration of drugs and the effectiveness of drugs taken. For example if a patient is having diuretic drugs she should observe whether the oedema is reduced and urine output increased, as well as checking if the patient is taking necessary potassium supplements. Side effects should also be looked for, for example by the regular testing of urine for glycosuria when patients are taking corticosteroids.

Many patients have a multiplicity of drugs to take and this is a particular problem with the elderly. They may have difficulty in opening the containers, reading the labels and remembering when to take the various tablets, not to mention the reason for each medicine, so it may be helpful for the nurse to label the drugs in a manner understood by the particular patient. For example, a diuretic may be labelled 'Water tablets, take on getting up'. With some patients the district nurse may need to visit to organise the day's supply or arrange for a neighbour to do this.

If the nurse has actually to administer drugs she should take the usual precautions of checking that she has the correct drug dose and observe for any incipient side effects. When possible the nurse should have written instructions from the doctor but if these have been given verbally she should make sure they are clearly written on the patients' records as soon as possible. Verbal or telephone messages should be repeated back to the doctor to be sure they are interpreted correctly.

Administration of controlled drugs

The patient and family may be responsible for administering oral drugs which fall into the category of controlled drugs as defined in the Misuse of Drugs Act 1971 (modified in 1985).[12,13] In these cases the district nurse should be particularly vigilant in ensuring they are aware of the correct dosage and frequency, and the importance of safe storage.

Specific rules apply for the administration of controlled drugs by district nurses. The person administering must be a trained nurse (a 'trained nurse' according to the Act can be an RGN or an enrolled nurse, but some health authorities may have a policy for it to be RGNs only). As this is different from hospital policy, where a second nurse always checks the drug with the trained nurse, special care must be taken.

In the giving of controlled drugs there must always be a written prescription available in the house, and careful records must be kept. Exceptionally, one dose may be given following verbal instructions but this must be one dose only and must be written up by the doctor as soon as possible. The records must include the stock provided, the amount given, amount left and the signature of the nurse, and most authorities have special forms for this. Disposal of any controlled drugs remaining when the course is discontinued or the patient dies is of particular importance. Again the patient or family need to be consulted, but the nurse must make it her responsibility to try to ensure the drugs are destroyed. Usually the relatives are only too willing for the nurse to organise this, and she should then record the amount of drugs for which destruction has been arranged. The 1985 modifications to the Misuse of Drugs Act 1971 state that *for the purpose of destruction only,* a patient or his representative is authorised to surrender prescribed or supplied controlled drugs to a doctor, dentist or pharmacist who will then be able to destroy them without formality.

Patient's drugs are ordered on a prescription which should be collected from the chemist by a responsible person, and this is particularly important in the case of controlled drugs. Occasionally the district nurse may need to collect prescriptions on behalf of the patient if there is no one else to do so. It is difficult for any nurse to keep up-to-date with the constant changes in drugs available. If the nurse does not know of the drug, its action or side effects she needs to find out by looking it up in MIMS (*Monthly Index of Medical Specialities*) available at the surgery or by asking the general practitioner or chemist.

Concept of rehabilitation

Rehabilitation is often viewed as a speciality with a focus on long-term chronic conditions, when in fact it should be an integral part of all patient-centred care. Mitchell[14] defines rehabilitation as 'the process of restoring persons to their previous capabilities or helping them make the most of their existing capabilities', which ties in with Henderson's definition of nursing,[15] '. . . helping the patient gain independence as rapidly as possible . . .', and the philosophy of assisting towards self-care. Returning also to the World Health Organisation's definition of health as 'a state of physical, social and psychological well being, not merely the absence of disease', it can be seen that rehabilitation needs to include the social and psychological aspects of disease as well as the physical. A major objective is limiting the extent to which a disability becomes a handicap.

Any person who becomes ill or injured needs to be rehabilitated to some extent. There may be only a temporary disability, as for example with Mr Evans, where it should be possible to return the patient to his previous job and capabilities. On the other hand disability may be permanent as in the case of John where he must be helped to make the most of his remaining capabilities. A third category of disability is progressive disability as in the case of Mr Fisher, whose condition can be expected to deteriorate progressively although there may well be periods of remission. His existing capabilities will vary at different stages of the illness and will need to be reassessed constantly. Because a diagnosis of a terminal illness has been made this should not detract from rehabilitation. For example, Mrs Baker needs to be helped to make the most of her capabilities, helped to remain the mother figure and to get the maximum fulfilment in the life that is left to her. Throughout any care there should be an emphasis on prevention of the occurrence of secondary disabilities such as pressure sores and contractures.

With the trend for patients to be discharged from hospital early, few have reached the optimum point of recovery when they return home, so it is important for the district nurse to start a programme of rehabilitation as soon as possible. To do this she needs to bear in mind the principles of rehabilitation as described by Boroch[16] which can be summarised as follows. Rehabilitation:

1 Requires the cooperation of patient and family.
2 Is patient–family centred.
3 Is a continuous process with varying degrees of emphasis on physical, social and psychological needs.
4 Is goal directed.
5 Requires collaboration of all health team professionals.

The district nurse is fortunate in knowing the home where she makes her assessment. She actually sees and experiences the social setting, the family network and the immediate environment in which the patient is being cared for; and she can discover how the family interacts without having to rely on hearsay. It is necessary to have a clear picture of the patient's previous health status and way of living if the aim of rehabilitation is to be to return the patient to his previous state as nearly as possible. Physical, social and psychological rehabilitation need to be carried out concurrently, for it would be fruitless to spend time and effort on producing maximum physical function with John if he is not helped at the same time to accept the limitations of his disability and to feel socially acceptable and economically independent.

The changes patients and their families are able to make in their life styles in order that they may adjust to altered levels of health will depend on their individual ability to cope and adjust as well as their general resources. It is important that the nurse helps families to maximise their strengths in this respect and minimise their weaknesses.

Rehabilitation therefore is a complex operation and to say simply that the goal is to 'rehabilitate a patient' is being too vague. Specific goals need to be set and rehabilitation must be an integral part of total care.

Progress notes

During the implementation stage of the nursing, progress records should be kept, but they do not necessarily need to be made at each visit. If the plan of care has clearly identified what the nursing action should be, the nurse does not need to record that she has carried out what was planned. For example, there should be a clear plan detailing treatment for Mrs Cray's ulcer, and if the treatment had been carried out as planned and there is no obvious change in the state of the ulcer or the patient herself, records need not be made. Repetitious, meaningless recording such as 'dressing renewed', 'general care given' have no place in the progress notes, the purpose of which is to communicate a current situation to someone who is not present and to create a record of that situation.

The frequency with which these notes are written depends on the stability or otherwise of the problem and the relevance of the observations. Progress notes for some patients should be written weekly or monthly, as for example for Mr Adams and John, whereas Mrs Baker's progress regarding pain, nausea and fluid intake should be recorded at each visit. Record keeping is an important component of each stage and a summary of the major points is included in the next chapter.

References

1. Hunt J. M. (1974). *The Teaching and Practice of Surgical Dressings in Three Hospitals*. London: RCN Publications.
2. Redman B. K. (1976). *The Process of Patient Teaching in Nursing*, 3rd edn, p. 24. St Louis: C. V. Mosby.

3. Dunnell K., Dobbs J. (1982). *Nurses Working in the Community.* London: HMSO.
4. Department of Health and Social Security (1977). *Prevention and Health.* London: HMSO.
5. Caplan G. (1961). *An Approach to Community Mental Health.* London: Tavistock.
6. Skeet M. (1974). *Home from Hospital,* 4th edn. London: Macmillan Journals.
7. Strehlow M. S. (1983). *Education for Health.* London: Harper & Row.
8. Nurse G. (1975). *Counselling and the Nurse—An Introduction.* London: H. M. & M.
9. Davison V. (1971). Current dressing techniques. *Occupational Health.* **23:** 287–92.
10. Maurer I. M. (1973). Disinfection and sterilisation in domicilary nursing. *Nursing Mirror,* **136,** 17: 46–7.
11. Broome W. E. (1971). *Dressing Techniques.* London: Butterworth.
12. Home Office: *The Misuse of Drugs Act 1971 (Modification) Order* (SI 1985 No 1995). London: HMSO.
13. Home Office: *The Misuse of Drugs Regulations 1985* (SI 1985 No 2066). London: HMSO.
14. Mitchell P. H. (1977). *Concepts Basic to Nursing,* 2nd edn. New York: McGraw-Hill.
15. Henderson V. (1966). *The Nature of Nursing,* p. 15. New York: Macmillan.
16. Boroch R. M. (1976). *Elements of Rehabilitation in Nursing—An Introduction,* p. 7. St Louis: C. V. Mosby.

Further Reading

Learning and teaching
Anderson D. C., ed. (1980). *Health Education Practice.* London: Croom Helm.
Hinchcliff S., ed. (1986). *Teaching Clinical Nursing,* 2nd edn. Edinburgh: Churchill Livingstone.
Knopke H. J., Diekelmann N. (1981). *Approaches to Teaching Primary Health Care.* St Louis: C. V. Mosby.
Mager R. F. (1962). *Preparing Instructional Objectives.* California: Fearon.
Phillipson C., Strang P. (1984). *Health Education and Older People: The Role of Paid Carers.* Keele: Health Education Council/Dept of Adult Education, University of Keele.
Pohl M. L. (1978). *The Teaching Function of the Nurse Practitioner,* 3rd edn. Iowa: Wm. C. Broom.
Redman B. K. (1980). *The Process of Patient Teaching in Nursing,* 4th edn. St Louis: C. V. Mosby.
Scottish Home and Health Department (1983). *Health Education for Health Visitors, District Nurses and Midwives.* Edinburgh: SHHD.
Thompson W. W., Bridge W. (1983). *Teaching Patient Care and Guidance for the Practising Nurse.* London: Heinemann Medical.
Wilson-Barnet J. (1983). *Patient Teaching.* Edinburgh: Churchill Livingstone.

Counselling

Royal College of Nursing Institute of Advanced Nursing Education (1978). *Counselling in Nursing* (Report of a working party). London: RCN Publications.
Tschudin V. (1982). *Counselling Skills for Nurses*. London: Ballière Tindall.

Nursing techniques

Chartered Society of Physiotherapists (1975). *Handling the Handicapped at Home*. Cambridge: Woodhead-Faulkner.
Hollis M. (1985). *Safer Lifting for Patient Care*, 2nd edn. Oxford: Blackwell Scientific.
Jacka S. M., Griffiths D. G. (1976). *Treatment Room Nursing: A handbook for nursing sisters in general practice, schools and industry*. Oxford: Blackwell Scientific.
Queen's Institute of District Nursing (1965). *Safer Sterilisation of Equipment*. London: Queen's Nursing Institute.
Mandalstram D. (1980). *Incontinence and its Management*. Beckenham: Croom Helm.
Chartered Society of Physiotherapists (1983). *Handling the Handicapped: A Guide to the Lifting and Movement of Disabled People*, 2nd edn. Cambridge: Woodhead-Faulkner.

Communication

Ashworth P. (1980). *Care to Communicate:* London: RCN Publications.
O'Brien M. J. (1978). *Communications and Relationships in Nursing*, 2nd edn. St Louis: C. V. Mosby.
Ellis R., Whittingham D. (1981). *A Guide to Social Skills Training*. Beckenham: Croom Helm.
Ellis R., Whittingham D. (1983). *New Directions in Social Skills Training*. Beckenham: Croom Helm.

Collaboration

Gilmore M., Bruce N., Hunt M. (1974). *The Work of the Nursing Team in General Practice*. London: Council for the Education and Training of Health Visitors.
Roberts I. (1975). *Discharged from Hospital*. London: RCN Publications.
Skeet M. (1974). *Home from Hospital*, 4th edn. London: Macmillan Journals.

Rehabilitation

Field M. (1967). *Patients are People: A Medical-social Approach to Prolonged Illness*, 3rd edn. New York: Columbia University Press.
Johnstone M. (1976). *The Stroke Patient. Principles of Rehabilitation*. Edinburgh: Churchill Livingstone.
Johnstone M. (1980). *Home Care for the Stroke Patient*. Edinburgh: Churchill Livingstone.
Mattingley S., ed. (1981). *Rehabilitation Today*, 2nd edn. London: Update Books.
Wilson-Barnet J., Fordham J. (1982). *Recovery from Illness*. Chichester: John Wiley.
Myco F. (1983). *Nursing Care of the Hemiplegic Stroke Patient*. London: Harper & Row.

Chapter 10

Evaluating Care

The nursing process is incomplete without the stage of evaluation. This is the means by which the care given to the patient and the family is checked. Evaluation can lead to reassessment, and may thus be seen as restarting the cycle which emphasises the dynamic and cyclical nature of the nursing process. Reilly[1] defines evaluation as 'a process concerned with the quality of a substance, action or event'.

The provision of high-quality care must be the goal of all nurses and it is essential that they have a reliable means of measuring the standard of care given. Evaluation is unfortunately often neglected but it is necessary if the nurse is to know whether care should be continued as planned, whether goals and subsequent action need to be changed, or if more information is required. Of course, a thinking nurse is continually evaluating the results of her care while she is actually nursing the patient and helping the family, but a more formal evaluation that is written down is needed. The very process of putting the evaluation on paper encourages critical thought and, once written, the evaluation can be shared.

The nursing profession is becoming increasingly conscious of the need for evaluation and producing evidence not only of effectiveness in caring for individuals but also in the process and system of care. Terms such as quality assurance, performance indicators, and audit are now in common usage. Kron[2] states that quality assurance directs nurses towards a greater accountability to the public in the way they use their professional knowledge when they make decisions about nursing care.

The United Kingdom Central Council Code of Professional Conduct[3] (see Appendix 1) reminds nurses, midwives and health visitors of their responsibility in the safeguard of the public. Clauses 10 and 11 of the code particularly emphasise this. It can be seen that evaluation of the working situation is necessary to meet these areas of accountability.

The skills required for evaluation are the same as those used in assessment: observation, interviewing, communication, analysing, judging and inferring from the clues given by the patient and his relatives. The main difference between assessment and evaluation is that evaluation is undertaken in retrospect after the plan of care has been implemented, or concurrently with the action being carried out.

Evaluation has three elements: the evaluation of the outcome of the planned action for the patient and his family; the evaluation of the actual nursing performance and whether nursing tasks have been performed satisfactorily; and finally the evaluation of the system of care. Evaluation therefore is an attempt to identify the quality of care received by individuals and the quality of care provided by the care givers. These three elements will now be considered in greater detail.

Evaluation of the goals of care for individual patients

The primary function of nursing care is the resolution of patient problems. In the planning stage the desired outcome of care was precisely set out; now, the goals that were enumerated must be checked. For example, in the case of John Davis, one goal set was that he should drink 2000 ml of fluid a day, and whether this goal has been achieved can be seen simply by checking the record which the family have kept of his intake. If the goal had merely been 'extra fluids' it would be impossible to evaluate whether it had been achieved because definitions of 'extra fluids' vary. Similarly, unless the actual size of Mrs Cray's ulcer has been stated it will be impossible to determine by how much it has decreased or increased. Evaluation, therefore, emphasises the need as far as possible to set goals in measurable terms.

Although the desired outcome is set out for actual and potential problems (see page 135) it is also necessary to evaluate the 'possible' problems that were noted in the planning stage and decide whether further information is necessary and whether these problems should now be ruled out, or included as either actual or potential.

Evaluation will not always show positive results, but it is just as important to determine if and when care is *not* producing the desired results, and to ask the reason why. It may be that the assessment was inadequate in the first place and the problems were not clearly defined, or that the information on which the plan was based was either inaccurate or insufficient. On the other hand, the goals set for a patient in that condition or in those circumstances may have been unrealistic, and insufficient regard may have been paid to the available resources for care. Sometimes the failure to set clear and realistic aims is found to be due to the fact that the patient and his family were not sufficiently involved in the plan of care; or for some reasons they did not understand; or they misinterpreted what was expected of them. Finally, and often sadly, the patient's condition or the availability or ability of other carers may change radically, in which case, of course, plans that were once realistic cease to be so.

Changing the plan

There are therefore several reasons for changing the plan of care. First, the goals may have been achieved and the patient's problem solved. If this is so a line should be drawn through this part of the plan and the date by which the problem was resolved should be recorded. It should be remembered that a 'patient problem' is a problem with which the patient requires help; therefore when nursing help is no longer needed and the patient can cope for himself this requirement can be removed from the plan. For example, it is hoped that many of John's initial problems will ultimately not be problems once he learns aspects of self-care and independence. Following nursing advice and teaching he and his parents should be able to cope with the urinary drainage and observation for signs of infection and to inform the district nurse if they have any worries. Similarly, the plan for a diabetic patient, who with the help of the nurse is learning how to manage his own care, will need to be changed as he achieves independence.

Another reason for changing the plan is that information is now available that was not revealed at the assessment. This may include new information about the patient's condition, his lifestyle or his relationships with his family and due to the fact that this information was not originally available the wrong goals may have been set. In some cases the nurse and the patient are too optimistic and this can lead to frustration, while in other cases the nurse, or the patient, or both may have made a wrong assessment of the resources that would be available; they may, for example, have been over-optimistic about the provision of 'meals on wheels' or the supply of home helps.

However, although evaluation may indicate the need to change the plan, one hopes that in most cases it will show that the plan was adequate. For many patients visited by the district nurse the plan will remain the same for a long time. However these cases too must be evaluated periodically; for example, Mr Adams will have a continuing potential problem of pressure sores due to his poor mobility and incontinence. If at the time of evaluation he remains free from sores the plan would be considered appropriate and care would be continued as before.

Evaluation of the carers

If in the initial assessment it was decided that relatives and others could carry out certain aspects of care it is necessary to monitor their ability to do so. For example, the district nurse needs to watch each day how Sarah is coping with Mrs Baker. At each visit to Mr Fisher the nurse needs to evaluate the plans they made, in which he and his wife were to cope with the majority of his care; if they can no longer manage she must reconsider the plan. It may be that the goals remain the same but the plan will need to be changed.

Munley[4] discusses the stress of care givers and includes in this group professional staff. She identifies the care givers' recognition of the tenuousness of their own lives which may also overwhelm them with grief. Stress also arises from the seeming inadequacy of personal and physical resources and feelings of failure.

Most carers make an effort to keep up the image of coping, and judge themselves in terms of how they imagine they are being judged by others (known as the 'looking-glass self'). This effort can lead to the phenomenon colloquially known as 'burn-out'. As a district nurse working in relative isolation the patient and family expect her to be all things to them, coping with their physical, social, emotional and spiritual needs. Everyone learns coping mechanisms such as distancing, but this is generally easier for the professional than the relative. It is vital, therefore, that nurses recognise in patients, relatives, colleagues and themselves when the limits to their ability to cope are being reached.

Responsibility for evaluation of nursing care

The definition of the district nurse[5] states that she is 'professionally accountable for assessing and reassessing the needs of patient and family, and for monitoring quality of care'. Evaluation of care, therefore, is the particular responsibility of the district nurse, although she may have delegated the giving of care to the district enrolled nurse or nursing auxiliary; they have a responsibility to make observations while carrying out care and to report their findings to the district nurse. The district nurse must herself visit patients whose care has been delegated to others and ensure that the quality of care is good and that the plan is still appropriate. If, for example, the bathing of frail elderly patients is delegated to a nursing auxiliary the district nurse herself must visit these patients at least monthly to evaluate the care and to reassess the patient. An ideal way of carrying out this evaluation is for the nurse to perform the bath herself and make a systematic reassessment of the patient, his family and environment.

Care conferences

It is sometimes difficult for the nurse to evaluate care alone, particularly in the case of the patients she is seeing almost every day, because subtle changes in the patient, his family or his environment may easily escape her notice. It is therefore important to involve the other people who have been concerned with the patient to whom the patient may have expressed quite different fears and anxieties. If plans have been formulated clearly at the daily meeting of the district nursing team it should be possible to discuss these plans and to change them if necessary. Although the district nursing team should meet daily, the timing of the meeting will depend on the working conditions and the travelling distance for different members, and on the staff available. Many teams seem to prefer the early afternoon. The purpose of such meetings should be to discuss the progress of patients, highlight problems and plan subsequent care, and also to set aside a definite time for those patients whose care needs to be evaluated on a weekly or monthly basis.

Sometimes it will be beneficial to use the meeting of the team as an opportunity for a wider care conference involving general practitioners, health visitors and social workers. It may be useful to discuss with the whole primary care team whether plans for particular patients are realistic and to gain further information and advice. For instance it will be important to involve the social worker in discussions regarding the Baker family, for when Mrs Baker dies the care of the children will be her concern. Although such meetings do take time, it is time well spent if it produces better care.

Criteria for discharge and termination of visits

Mayers[6] suggests that the criterion for discharge is the achicvement of the long-term goals that were set on admission. It is not always easy, however, to know when patients no longer need nursing help.

One reason for discharging a patient from the care of the district nurse may be that the patient has reached a state of health in which he no longer needs professional help; this may well be the case with Mr Evans. With some patients the needs and problems may be partially resolved and the resources within the family mobilised in such a way that the nurse can withdraw; this situation may eventually be reached with John, with the district nurse remaining available if the family run into any difficulties. Other patients may have been referred to another health or social worker, and unless there are nursing tasks to carry out the district nurse can withdraw her services; for example the district nurse's involvement with Rose Johnson will be intermittent while that of the health visitor may be continuous. It is a waste of manpower to duplicate care unnecessarily.

Other reasons for discharging a patient are that he has moved to another area or has been transferred to hospital. When this happens good liaison is important to ensure continuity of care. Finally the patient may die, but this does not necessarily mean that the district nurse's involvement in that household has ended, for she may need to visit the bereaved family to offer continuing support.

Terminating care in some cases will mean breaking a long-standing relationship between district nurse, patient and family, and the patient may be reluctant to 'let go' of the nurse, and vice versa. The patient needs to be prepared for discharge by encouraging his independence and if other workers are to be involved it may be a good idea to introduce them before the district nurse leaves. The patient needs to be assured that if he encounters any difficulties the nurse can be contacted again.

The district nurse has the responsibility for admitting and discharging patients, and before discharge she must decide whether the desired care has been achieved and if necessary the right referrals have been made. It is, of course, not enough to say that the treatment has been completed or the wound healed, but the nurse must be assured that the patient can cope with his continuing care.

Actual discharge

When it has been agreed that the patient should be discharged, the district nurse should remove the records and take away or arrange for collection of any equipment; however some patients will need to retain certain equipment and they should be told whom to notify when it is not needed. Drugs should be destroyed as described in the previous chapter. The patient and relatives will feel more secure if the nurse leaves a telephone number for them to contact her or other appropriate person if necessary.

When a patient dies the district nurse needs to be sensitive to the needs and wishes of the bereaved, and if she has formed a long trusting relationship with relatives such as she would with Mrs Adams she may well visit several times before saying goodbye or introducing the health visitor. Once Mrs Baker dies, Sarah and her brother and sister will need a great deal of support but this may be best given by the social worker. If Mr Fisher's condition deteriorated and he died his wife might gain her support from work colleagues and friends but because she is articulate this does not mean that she does not need, and would not value, professional support. There is not, therefore, any definite rule about bereavement visiting but the district nurse needs to assess the needs of the bereaved and should plan to visit or to refer to others as appropriate (see Chapter 9).

Observational visits

Periodic visits may need to be made to patients who do not require any nursing intervention but need evaluation of progress. Such visits may be made to a patient who has had care in the past and is coping satisfactorily with the help of his family, but who may be expected to suffer a recurrence of his original condition or perhaps some general deterioration of his circumstances. Visiting such patients may be useful as a preventive measure and will help to support and reassure the relatives in a time of doubt. Another reason for making an observational visit is to establish a trusting relationship with a family with whom nursing needs are anticipated, the obvious example being where a patient has been diagnosed as having a terminal illness but who is at present coping adequately and does not yet require practical nursing help. On such occasions the nurse can act as a general guide in helping the patient to get the best out of life while he can.

Although 'observational' visits may appear 'social', and they should of course appear that way, it is important that they have a clear purpose so the nurse should identify goals and make a systematic reassessment.

Recording the evaluation of nursing care

Progress notes explain the progress of the patient in achieving the stated goals; the frequency of recording these details depends on the condition of the patient, for example Mrs Baker's condition will change on a daily basis and progress notes will be written at each visit, whereas for Mr Adams a full evaluation will be recorded only monthly unless significant changes occur.

Numbering of problems saves repetition and unnecessary writing when recording progress. For example two of Mrs Baker's problems for which goals were set and care planned were (see page 134):

Problem 1 Pain due to spinal metastases.
Problem 2 Inadequate fluid intake due to nausea.

The progress notes will read:

7.7.87 1 Dihydrocodeine taken every 4 hours. Pain less but patient drowsy.
2 Prochlorperazine 5 mg prescribed by GP. Occasional nausea.
Tolerating approx 50 ml fluid hourly. Sarah not yet got soda water.

Similarly two of the problems identified for John (page 135) were:

Problem 2   Potential urinary tract infection due to inadequate
fluid intake.
Problem 3   Possible sexual frustration due to immobility.

Progress notes for John will read:

7.7.87 2 Urine tested NAD. MSU sent.
Father coping with penile toilet. At least 2000 ml fluid per day.
Family aware of signs of infection—will report if any.
Review 7.8.87
3 Male nurse visited. John not concerned at present but will ask to see
male nurse again if he wishes further discussion.

The check date for Problem 2 has now been made for one
month's time so unless the family report any changes further
progress notes will not need to be written for one month. Problem
3 can now be crossed off the problem list and plan. It will be noted
that the evaluation as reported in the progress notes links with the
desired outcome which is derived from the identified problem.

Evaluation of nursing performance

Linked with the monitoring of care for individual patients is the
evaluation of the quality of care given by the nurses. Such
evaluation is necessary for nurses wherever they work but it is
especially important in district nursing where so much care is
carried out in isolation and where it is easy to develop a ritual
approach guided by habit rather than the best interests of the
patient.

Assessment of nursing performance is frequently thought to be
limited to the appraisal of a learner by a trained nurse. While this
is important, it is also necessary to monitor the quality of care
provided by the trained nurse. The most important person to
assess the care given by the district nurse is the nurse herself.

During much of her time the district nurse will be her only examiner and thus she needs to be a severe and reliable judge. Reilly[1] makes some suggestions about the way the nurse should behave if using the nursing process as the method of care, and provides a useful checklist for self-evaluation, but as it uses American terminology and relates to the American care system it has been adapted here.

The district nurse should assess her own abilities in the following areas:

Assessment—
1　Forms good relationships with patient and family.
2　Makes relevant observations.
3　Conducts purposeful interviews.
4　Elicits appropriate information from patient and family.
5　Uses other sources of information gathering, e.g. records, other personnel.
6　Shows understanding of patient's response to health/illness/environment.
7　Accepts the right of families to their own beliefs, moral code and life style.
8　Seeks to avoid interference of own biases when interpreting information.
9　Identifies family resources that can be used in meeting health needs.
10　Identifies patient problems from information gathered.

Planning—
1　Involves patient and family in planning care.
2　Identifies short and long-term goals for care.
3　Selects appropriate nursing care measures.
4　Refers to other members of the health and social services.
5　Determines priorities in care.
6　Organises a caseload.
7　Communicates plan of care to other nursing personnel.

Implementation—
1　Performs nursing care procedures adapted to the home environment.
2　Uses technical skills competently.

3   Cares for and uses equipment appropriately.
4   Encourages patient to use his/her capabilities to the maximum.
5   Preserves the patient's privacy.
6   Helps patient and family to accept realistic limitations imposed by illness.
7   Instructs the patient and his/her family in relation to identified learning needs.
8   Utilises opportunities for health education.
9   Initiates appropriate referrals to other personnel.
10   Records significant information accurately.

Evaluation—
1   Measures the results of nursing action in terms of the outcome of care.
2   Modifies care plan as appropriate.
3   Communicates with others in the primary health care team.
4   Examines individual care planning within the context of the total workload.
5   Evaluates the district nurse's role within the local setting.

This checklist can also be used to assess the abilities of others, but peer evaluation happens whether it is intentional or not; another nurse visiting a patient will inevitably notice the standard of care by observing the availability of equipment, the plans of care, the involvement and attitudes of patient and other carers. Patients and families will often make comparisons between different nurses and this must be accepted; patients too have their favourites. Because a nurse carries out care differently it does not necessarily mean it is worse than that of another nurse but different methods can cause confusion and conflict for the patient—hence the importance of the clear plan which enables continuity.

Kron[2] gives a set of questions for testing whether the nursing performance was adequate. These are:

(a)   Were the objectives worded clearly?
(b)   Were the objectives realistic for the patient?
(c)   Was the original assessment complete?

(d) Was the identified problem a problem to the nurse or the patient?
(e) Did new problems arise that were not recognised?
(f) Was the patient included in the care plan?
(g) Was the nursing action appropriate?
(h) Was there sufficient documentation?
(i) Were changes required in nursing intervention?

She suggests these questions could be used not only for self-assessment but also for peer review and possible client feedback.

Superior and subordinate evaluation

The district nurse who is accountable for the nursing care of a group of patients will need to make assessments of other members of the nursing team and be aware of their strengths and weaknesses.

The nurse manager has responsibility for the standards of care provided by the nursing teams responsible to her and she, too, will visit with the various members of the district nursing team and discuss problems and look at records.

Evaluation is not however confined to the experienced nurse looking at her subordinates; the student visitor will also evaluate care as she sees it. The student may well challenge the district nurse about aspects of her care which may sometimes appear less professional than that given in hospital. While it is right that the student should make such an evaluation it is important that she understands the principles of the caring in the home and remembers that the nurse is a guest and can work only with the patient's consent.

It is important to remember that the purpose of evaluation is not to find fault but to assess the quality of care; if the quality is good then praise should be given as this gives encouragement and helps to maintain motivation and high standards.

Pearson[7] argues that an effective quality assurance programme may need to use a variety of methods and discusses various approaches. He describes the use of Qualpacs (as described by Wandelt and Ager[8]) which concentrates on the process of nursing by considering by direct observation the nursing care given. Goldstone *et al.*[9] have developed the Monitor system to measure the quality of care in acute medical and surgical wards in the UK and this has possibilities for adaptation in other contexts.

Phaneuf[10] describes the nursing audit as being a process-oriented approach to appraise the nursing process as it is reflected in the patients' records and as a retrospective method of quality assurance. Quality assurance moves nurses towards greater accountability to the public by their use of professional knowledge in making decisions about the nursing care of their patients.

Evaluation of the system of care

A nursing audit may be carried out by members of the district nursing team in association with nurse managers and possibly other members of the primary care team in order to evaluate the effectiveness of the whole system through which care is given in a particular locality.

A paramount problem is, inevitably, the way the district nursing team fits in with the primary care team as a whole and a number of problems, some of which have legal consequences, may arise because different members of the team are accountable to different authorities and the doctors are virtually independent. The nurse will look to the doctor for authority in clinical matters, such as the prescribing of medication, but the nurse is employed by the health authority and responsible to them through her nurse manager. The authority may lay down rules about what the nurses should do (or, more often, should not do) or the circumstances in which they may perform certain tasks, with which the doctor may disagree.

The doctor, used to having structural authority over practice nurses, may be genuinely confused about his role and the extent of his authority, while the nurse, anxious to please and seeing no harm in extending her duties, may all too easily carry out the doctor's wishes without realising the confusion and conflict this can create for the team as a whole. Examples of such areas of conflict are the performance by the district nurse of procedures such as immunisation, ear syringing, venepuncture, electrocardiography and assessment visits. The nurse needs to be sure she is conversant with the policies of the health authority/board in relation to carrying out such procedures. Conflict is not necessarily caused by any doubt as to the district nurse's ability to carry out the tasks, but more likely by doubt about the appropriateness of these tasks to the work of the district nurse. This problem must be tackled, not by surreptitiously doing one thing and saying another, but by a frank discussion with the team as a whole, and it may well be that at the audit the two viewpoints can be reconciled. If nurses are needed to undertake extended duties, the nursing management can arrange for those selected and willing to do them to have proper training, and the necessary changes in their employment contracts.

The nursing audit can be used to identify the various problems that may arise within the primary care team due to lack of harmony and consultation between members, lack of resources or poor management and planning. The research of Goldstone and Worrall[11] and Dunnell and Dobbs[12] has confirmed the earlier findings of Hockey[13] and suggests that in the intervening years the planning and work of the district nursing team has not been rationalised. The work load for district nurses varies widely both in the actual caseload and the number of high-dependency patients allotted to each nurse, and there still appears to be no agreement in practice as to which duties are best done by enrolled nurses and which by RGNs, and which nursing duties can be delegated to auxiliaries. Furthermore, many district nurses still spend too much time on travelling and on non-nursing duties.

The whole subject requires more research, but in the meantime the nursing audit can pinpoint local difficulties and by consensus management can try to rectify them. It is, however, up to each nurse to question and analyse how she spends her time and reflect why the help given to one patient is defined as 'nursing' and the same help given to another is defined as 'non-nursing'. For example, when is getting the patient a cup of tea part of nursing and when is it not? The balance between the 'it's not my job' attitude and simply doing tasks to save bother, or because the doctor said so, or there was no one else on hand, is delicate and in the end each nurse must make her own decision. However, the decision is likely to be sound if the nurse remembers to ask, 'Why am I doing this?', 'Could it be done just as well by someone else?'

and 'Am I doing it at the expense of my true nursing function?' She might even ask 'Does it need to be done at all?'

Finally the nursing audit will look at comments and complaints from patients or from team members about difficulties with other agencies. Some of these may be resolved on discussion, but if they cannot be overcome then at least an explanation for the difficulty or complaint should be given to all members of the team involved.

Record keeping

Throughout this section record keeping has been mentioned in relation to the planning of patient care but as each health authority has its own system and design of records no hard and fast rules can be given. Some general principles are, however, considered below.

Patient care records

For each of the stages of the nursing process the type and content of the record to be kept has been discussed and suggestions made as to where these records should be kept. To be sure the records are meaningful it is important that the nurse bears in mind their purpose which can be summarised as follows:

1   To ensure continuity of patient care.
2   As a means of communication between team members—not only nursing staff but with general practitioners and health visitors as well as with the patient and family.
3   To provide a means of monitoring efficiency of the services by checking the outcome of care.
4   To provide useful information for research into patient care, use of equipment, or use of the services.
5   For legal purposes—which is why it is important that they are accurate and say something meaningful.

Other records to be kept

The district nurse will have to keep a variety of records other than those relating to individual patients. Facts will be required for statistical purposes and possibly for local and national research.

The statistical information required will generally include the number of people visited by each nurse, the age group of the patients, the treatment given by the nurse, the medical diagnosis, the source of patient referral, and the outcome of care. The actual information required will depend on the current survey but nurses must recognise that the completion of these details is an important part of their function to ensure that accurate statistics are available about patients' needs and the provision of care so that any overlaps or gaps can be highlighted. Health authorities are beginning to develop data collection in line with the recommendations of the Körner[14] committee and much of this will be computerised.

Apart from records about patients and their care it is also important to keep accurate records of any equipment loaned and services requested from other health and social services. Finally the district nurse will be expected to keep certain records of her personal activities; for example, depending on her duty hours she may need to record evening or weekend duties, and she must also keep accurate records of mileage covered during her working day if she has a car; in some authorities telephones are provided for the nurse at home and calls made for the purposes of her work need to be recorded. Accuracy in record keeping is crucial and all records must be signed; the signature means 'I take responsibility for what precedes my name'.

References

1. Reilly D. E. (1975). *Behavioural Objectives in Nursing: Evaluation of Learner Attainment*, p. 2. New York: Appleton-Century-Crofts.
2. Kron T. (1981). *The Management of Patient Care: Putting Leadership Skills to Work*, 5th edn. London: W. B. Saunders
3. United Kingdom Central Council (1984). *Code of Professional Conduct for the Nurse, Midwife and Health Visitor*, 2nd edn. London: UKCC.
4. Munley A. (1983). *The Hospice Alternative—A New Context for Death and Dying.* New York: Basic Books.
5. Department of Health and Social Security (1977). *Nursing in Primary Health Care*; CNO (77) **8:** 2.
6. Mayers M. G. (1978). *A Systematic Approach to the Nursing Care Plan*, 2nd edn. New York. Appleton-Century-Crofts.
7. Pearson A. (1983). *The Clinical Nursing Unit.* London: Heinemann Medical.

8. Wandelt M. A., Ager J. W. (1974). *Quality Patient Care Scale.* New York: Appleton-Century-Crofts.
9. Goldstone L. A., Ball J. A., Collier M. M. (1983). *Monitor—An Index of the Quality of Nursing Care for Acute Medical and Surgical Wards.* Newcastle upon Tyne: Polytechnic Products Ltd.
10. Phaneuf M. C. (1976). *The Nursing Audit: Self-Regulation in Nursing Practice,* 2nd edn. New York: Appleton-Century-Crofts.
11. Goldstone L. A., Worrall J. (1980). The problems of variations in work patterns of district nurses. *Nursing Times;* **76,** 11: pp. 45–51.
12. Dunnell K., Dobbs J. (1982). *Nurses Working in the Community.* London: HMSO.
13. Hockey L. (1972). *Use or Abuse? A Study of the State Enrolled Nurse in the Local Authority Nursing Services.* London: Queen's Nursing Institute.
14. Körner E. (1984) NHS and DHSS Steering Group on Health Services Information 5th report. *A report on the collection and use of information about services for and in the community of the NHS.* London: HMSO.

Further Reading

DHSS Nursing Research Liaison Group. (1986). *Report of the nursing process evaluation group.* (Chairman: Friend P., Editor: Hayward J.). Kings College, University of London.

Rowntree D. (1977). *Assessing Students: How shall we know them?* London: Harper & Row.

Schoolcraft V., ed. (1984). *Nursing in the Community.* New York: John Wiley.

Veuey J. E., Kaluzny A. D. (1984). *Evaluation and Decision Making for Health Service Programmes.* New Jersey: Prentice-Hall.

Yura H., Walsh M. B. (1978). *The Nursing Process: Assessing, Planning, Implementing, Evaluating,* 3rd edn. New York: Appleton-Century-Crofts.

Special Needs

Systems of health care management have been altered to accommodate changes in the treatment of patients. The turnover of patients in acute hospitals is continually increasing, bringing many pressures to bear on all the health and social services and in particular on the community health services. The increase in the number of elderly people as a proportion of the total population has brought added pressures, especially in relation to patients over 75 years old. Continued development of day facilities for patients, especially the elderly and the mentally ill, together with day-surgery and 5-day wards is particularly encouraging but these trends also have their effects on members of the primary care team.

Panel of Assessors: *Report on the Education and Training of the District Nurse (1976)*

Although the principles governing the nursing process laid down in Section II are applicable to all patients wherever they are nursed, there are nevertheless groups of patients whose special needs cannot be dealt with within the generality of nursing care principles. Therefore, at the risk of some overlap, it was decided that the special aspects of care for the groups most likely to be seen by the district nurse should be the subject for separate short chapters.

The groups selected are to some extent arbitrary, and some patients will fall into more than one group, but by separating off the special needs for groups like those with handicap and disability it is hoped that students will appreciate that the particular may be contained within the general.

The care of the sick child constitutes a minimal part of the district nurse's caseload as the majority of such care is provided by the parents. However, although she may care for few sick children, the district nurse needs to be aware of the special needs of this group when the occasion arises. The children who will require care can be divided into those with acute, short-term illnesses and those with long-term or handicapping conditions.

In the 1920s much of the district nurse's work was involved in caring for children with infectious diseases, but with the advent of immunisation and antibiotics such diseases are less prevalent. Unfortunately, however, with the recent fall in the 'take-up' of immunisation against whooping-cough this disease is once more becoming more common and it can be fatal, particularly for young babies. Similarly, while measles is less prevalent, the complacency of some parents about vaccination has led to the inevitable increase in this disease, which can lead to complications such as otitis media, bronchitis and encephalitis; again the district nurse may need to help in the early stages of the illness. The general practitioner or health visitor may also refer to the district nurse children with other acute illnesses such as upper respiratory tract infections or gastroenteritis. Planned early discharge from hospital of children following surgical treatment will involve the district nurse in procedures such as dressing wounds, removing sutures or caring for the child in a plaster of Paris splint.

Children born with physical and mental handicaps are living longer and parents may need practical help with the long-term care, or in the short term when the child develops one of the childhood illnesses. Others, like Rose Johnson, have a chronic illness such as sickle-cell anaemia and the parents may normally cope with the child's care but during an acute exacerbation of the illness may need help with the administration of antibiotics and the care of the child who may suffer considerable pain. It is sometimes possible and preferable to care for the child with a terminal illness at home and the district nurse may be involved in this inevitably distressing situation.

The district nurse therefore may be called upon to care for or advise parents on the care of sick children with any one of a whole range of illnesses and she cannot be expected to have knowledge of all the diseases, their implications or the care required; if in doubt she must consult hospital staff or a colleague. In a few authorities specialist paediatric district nursing schemes are available for providing care or giving advice and such schemes will be discussed later.

Reasons for keeping the sick child at home

Research into the effects of hospitalisation on the young child (Bowlby[1], Robertson[2], Hawthorn[3]) shows that this can psychologically harm the child, and have long-term effects such as future delinquency and job instability. Hospitalisation frequently leads to other more immediate problems such as regression in walking, feeding and language development, and bed-wetting; it has also been found that wound healing may be delayed and there is always a risk of cross infection. A further problem for the parents may be that many specialist children's hospitals are regionally based and this can involve considerable travelling which is costly in both time and money.

Because of great publicity in the 1950s of the National Association for the Welfare of Children in Hospital (NAWCH), and subsequent government recommendations, most hospitals now have free visiting arrangements and many have living-in facilities for the mother. Some mothers cannot avail themselves of these facilities because of other children at home and this can cause conflict. Other improvements include an increase in play and educational facilities in hospital (as recommended by the Platt Committee[4]) and a policy that children should not be nursed in adult wards but in children's wards with a registered sick children's nurse in charge; but these improvements are not enough and unless it is absolutely necessary hospital admission for the child should be avoided.

Having said that the child should be cared for at home it is important to recognise that this can cause considerable stress to the parents. Harrison, in her study *Families in Stress*,[5] highlights the anxiety incurred by parents caring for two different groups of children at home, those with Perthes' disease and those with cystic fibrosis, and although the pattern of these illnesses is very different, both cause great stress for the families. This would apply equally to families with any sick child and while it may not be possible to avoid stress it is important to recognise that it exists and to give the parents support.

Assessment

Assessment of the child

Firstly, the district nurse needs to assess how much information the child is able to give and what is his reaction to her as a nurse. The degree of fear or cooperation will depend on the child's previous experience of nurses, on what he has seen on television, or on the nurse's particular task; for example, if she is to give him an injection and he understands what this means, she will be unlikely to get much cooperation before this has been carried out as any friendly approaches will be treated with mistrust. Even a toddler can be involved in giving some information such as his name and age, likes and dislikes, and it is important to encourage him to talk; the information can be checked with the mother afterwards. However, the nurse's best ally in assessment will usually be the child's mother as she is most likely to notice any changes in the child's physical condition or behaviour.

Assessment of the child needs the nurse's acute skills of observation since, for example, the child may not be able to locate or describe pain, although the position in which he holds himself may be an indicator. Accuracy in measurement of temperature will be important with the acutely sick child because many children are prone to febrile convulsions and the district nurse should aim at prevention of such a distressing occurrence. Another crucial assessment particularly with a baby is the fluid intake, and the nurse must observe for any signs of dehydration.

Assessment of the carers

The most significant person providing care will normally be the mother, although the father and possibly other children may be involved. The ability of the mother to cope needs to be assessed and this ability may be hampered by her anxiety, sleepless nights, other children to care for, or other commitments such as employment outside the home.

Assessment of the environment

An important consideration is where to nurse the child. If he is to stay in bed it may be preferable to have a bed made up on the settee downstairs to avoid the mother going up and down stairs. In this way the child does not feel isolated and can be constantly observed. The heating, ventilation and safety of the room in which the child is to be nursed are further areas to be assessed.

Most of the information the nurse will gain from the child and the family, and from her observations and measurements, but she should also get information from others who know the family. In particular, the health visitor may be able to give some idea of the family's strengths and weaknesses and their ability to cope in a crisis. It is important that the district nurse refers back to the health visitor anything she feels of importance.

From her assessment the district nurse needs to identify the problems with which the family needs help. Paramount may be the parents' anxiety, and alleviating this may be the nurse's first priority.

Planning care

Goals of care need to be set and the nursing action determined, and this will include teaching parents how to give care. For example, for the child with a raised temperature the desired outcome will be that 'the temperature will subside within normal limits' and the action to this end may involve tepid sponging of the child. The mother should be advised to wash him in tepid water and change his clothes. Care given by the mother will be less likely to make the child fretful than care from a stranger.

An important part of the care plan is ensuring an adequate fluid intake, especially for a baby; the amount will depend on age, the size of the baby and his normal intake. The plan may include the mother giving clear fluids if the baby is reluctant to feed, is vomiting or has diarrhoea. The mother must be given specific instructions about making up these feeds. For example, a 5% sugar solution can be made with one teaspoonful (just over level) of sugar to each 100 ml of water; if the baby is vomiting or has diarrhoea a pinch of salt should be added.

The district nurse may need to help the mother plan the giving of the child's medications in relation to feeds and suggest means of overcoming an unwillingness to take drugs.

When planning care for the child with a long-term illness it is necessary to consider the child's daily routine; for example it is important to establish a routine for the diabetic child that fits in with his normal school day so he does not constantly feel 'different'. An important fact to bear in mind when planning care for the child at home is that it invariably takes longer to carry out any specific procedure such as an injection than it would with an adult, and time needs to be allowed for this.

Special schemes for care

Some urban authorities have a specialised service for the care of the sick child at home.[6,7,8] The first such scheme started in Rotherham in 1954 and the next in Birmingham in 1955, and others have since evolved. Some schemes are organised for all sick children in an area, others are for special groups such as post-surgery or children with spina bifida. These schemes usually employ registered sick children's nurses, who are also qualified district nurses, working in close liaison with hospital paediatric units and the health visitor. The schemes vary in their organisation but the aim is to give specialist high-quality care at home to the sick child, and support to the family. In some areas a night nursing service has been introduced because this is often the time when parents most need support.

The advantages of a specialist service are that there is a nurse available with a wide knowledge of childhood illnesses and the specialist care required; invariably the caseload will be numerically smaller and this means she can plan to give the time required to each child. The nurse can form close links with the hospital units and keep up to date with current treatments. However, a disadvantage of such schemes is that it involves considerable travelling for the nurse. Such a specialist service is at present only feasible in urban areas. Another disadvantage is that the specialist nurse is not attached to a group practice like her colleagues, but with planning this problem can be overcome.

The Court report[9] recommended the formation of paediatric teams including specialist child health visitors and child health nurses to provide a range of child care at home. The roles and relationships of these personnel would need to be more clearly defined but the principle of providing specialist care for this group is clearly spelt out. These recommendations have only been implemented in a very limited way.

Implementation of care

In implementing care the district nurse's role will be primarily that of a teacher but she will also need to counsel and to coordinate services. She must teach the parents how to give the care she advises and frequently she will learn from the parents hints on how best to carry out certain aspects of their child's care; for example, the easiest means of bathing the severely handicapped child or washing and cutting the hair of the child with cerebral palsy who cannot sit still. While it is preferable in the majority of cases for the parents to carry out care the nurse must constantly be aware of the need to relieve the mother to give her a rest. Sometimes nurses have guilt feelings because they are not doing the care themselves; they have to learn that the counselling and supporting role is of great importance as this helps the mother to keep going.

The district nurse's coordinating role is again important. She needs to be sure that the family are receiving all the help to which they are entitled. Links with the appropriate voluntary association can be supportive to the parents, such as the Sickle Cell Society, the Cystic Fibrosis Society, the Spina Bifida and Hydrocephalus Association or the British Diabetic Association. Through such societies families can get help with baby-sitting and holidays, and get ideas about equipment and services available. The district nurse needs to liaise with the health visitor and possibly the school nurse who may arrange for treatment to be carried out at school.

Evaluation of care

A child's condition may quickly change for better or worse and therefore a basic rule is to overvisit rather than undervisit. Acute skills of observation are required for the degree of dehydration, temperature and activity, but above all the mother's opinion should be sought, as she will notice subtle changes in her child.

The nurse needs to evaluate her own and the team's ability to cope with the child and she also needs to consider how to fit the child's care into the total caseload. She must evaluate the quality of her relationship with the child and family, and she will need to consider carefully when she should terminate her visits. In some cases, as for example with Rose, it will be helpful to visit periodically even in her 'good' phases to maintain the relationship with the child and family.

References

1. Bowlby J. (1965). *Child Care and the Growth of Love*, 2nd edn. Harmondsworth: Pelican.
2. Robertson J. (1970). *Young Children in Hospital*, 2nd edn. London: Tavistock.
3. Hawthorn P. J. (1974). *Nurse, I want my Mummy*. London: RCN Publications.
4. Ministry of Health (1959). *Welfare of Children in Hospital* (Platt report). London: HMSO.
5. Harrisson S. (1977). *Families in Stress*. London: RCN Publications.
6. Atwell J. D. (1975). Paediatric day case surgery in Southampton. *Nursing Times*; **71** 22:841–3.
7. Jenkins S. M. (1975). Home Care in Paddington. *Nursing Mirror*; **140,** 9:68–72.
8. Robottom B. M. (1969). The contribution of the children's nurse to the home care of children. *British Journal of Medical Education*; **3,** 4:311–2.
9. Department of Health and Social Security (1976). *Fit for the Future: Report of the Committee on Child Health Services* (Court report) Cmnd 6684. London: HMSO.

Further Reading

Clarke F. (1984). *Hospital at home: The alternative to hospital admission*. London: Macmillan.
Illingworth R. S. (1983). *Common Symptoms of Diseases in Children*, 8th edn. Oxford: Blackwell Scientific.
Weller B. F., Barlow S. (1983). *Paediatric Nursing*, 6th edn. London: Baillière Tindall.

Chapter 12

Handicap and Disability

Handicapped people are first and foremost *people*, with the same basic needs, aspirations and rights as other people, and they are not usually sick. These two premises constitute the two major challenges for district nurses caring for handicapped people.

The words 'handicap', 'impairment' and 'disability' are often used synonymously, but they are not necessarily the same. The World Health Organisation distinguishes between the three concepts as follows[1]:

Impairment is any loss or abnormality of psychological, physiological or anatomical structure or function.

Disability is any restriction or lack (resulting from an impairment) of ability to perform an activity in the manner or within the range considered normal for a human being.

Handicap is the disadvantage for a given individual which results from an impairment or a disability, that limits or prevents the person from fulfilling his or her normal (i.e. appropriate to the individual's age and sex, and social and cultural factors) role.

For example, in the case of John Davis, who became tetraplegic following a motorbike accident, the *impairment* is the loss of sensation and functioning of the muscles below the level of the injury to his spine, the *disability* is his inability to walk (and to do other things), and the *handicap* is the fact that he can no longer do his previous job.

Impairment affects different people differently. The task of the nurse caring for a person suffering from a physical or mental impairment is to minimise the person's disability and the resulting handicap, and to maximise the person's potential for health and a normal life. Perhaps the best approach is to forget the words impairment, disability and handicap, and to focus, as this book tries to do, on the individual's special needs.

The problem of stigma

In addition to their individual special needs, disabled people (whether their impairment is intellectual, psychiatric, or physical) suffer one problem in common—that of being perceived by other people as 'different'. This problem has been called 'stigmatisation'[2] after the Greek word 'stigma', which means 'a mark'.

Because disabled people are seen as 'different', people tend to treat them differently, often in ways which are quite irrational. For example, the title of the BBC radio programme *Does he take sugar?* derives from the way in which a person in a wheelchair is often assumed to be mentally handicapped or deaf and dumb. Similarly, it is often assumed that handicapped people do not or should not have the same sexual needs and desires as other people.

The Harris report,[3] commissioned by the Department of Health and Social Security in 1970, showed that there were in the UK well over a million people who were sufficiently physically disabled to require support, and about 150 000 sufficiently disabled to need specialist care; although the majority were elderly, a substantial minority (about 40%) were not.

A further million people in the UK are mentally handicapped. Following the passing of the Chronically Sick and Disabled Persons Act in 1970 (which placed an obligation on local authorities to inform themselves of the number of disabled people in their areas and to take steps to meet their needs), the International Year of Disabled People (1981), the Education Act of 1981 which has led to the presence of many more handicapped children in ordinary schools, and the shift from institutional to community-based care for mentally handicapped people,[4] there has been an increased awareness and understanding of the needs and rights of disabled people, but the services provided are still by no means adequate.

Types of disability and handicap

This chapter focuses in particular on the needs of the young physically disabled person, using the example of John Davis, but the district nurse will also meet people suffering from sensory impairment (blindness and deafness), from chronic psychiatric disorders (see Chapter 13), and from mental handicap. In the last two cases, district nurses will often be working alongside community psychiatric nurses and community mental handicap nurses.

Mental handicap

The term 'mental handicap' is a great improvement, on previously used terms such as 'mental deficiency' or 'mental retardation', but is still poorly understood, not least because it covers such a wide range of impairments. The basic feature of mental handicap is that it is a life-long condition in which there is limited intellectual functioning; the disability is a learning disability, and the handicap is the restriction which this places on living a normal life, particularly when life is lived in a closed institution such as a large hospital. About one-third of mentally handicapped people have an accompanying physical handicap, often a neurological disorder which may also be the cause of the mental handicap. The move from institutional towards community care for mentally handicapped people is based on the principle of 'normalisation'[5] which should involve what John O'Brien[6] has called the five 'key accomplishments'.

1 Community presence: the right to live in the community, sharing the same facilities as other people instead of special segregated residence and facilities.
2 Choice: including small things (what to eat, what to wear) as well as large things (who to live with).
3 Competence: the experience of developing self-care with whatever assistance is required.
4 Respect: having a valued place among a network of people and valued roles in community life.
5 Community participation: being part of a network of personal relationships which includes friends.

The great shift in emphasis which has taken place over the past decade from a hospital-oriented medically led service to one which is multi-disciplinary and community based, together with the principle that mentally handicapped people in the community should have access to the same range of services as other people, means that district nurses will increasingly care for mentally handicapped people in the community.

Physical disability

For the 15-year-old to 19-year-old age group, the rate of road traffic accidents is nearly twice the rate for the total population, and society is now experiencing an upsurge in the sale of motorbikes and mopeds to young people. Teenagers are more prone to athletic injuries because of their high degree of participation in sports by comparison with other age groups. The growing problem of residual disability in sportsmen is reflected in the advent of the Association of Sports Medicine which advises on and researches into the specialised prevention and management of sport injuries; and its work is increasing.

Cystic fibrosis and spina bifida are no longer conditions confined to children, and the thalidomide victims are now young adults. Improved treatment techniques have increased longevity, so 'new' handicapping conditions present themselves to those caring for young adults. It must also be remembered that the process of ageing itself affects the course of disease and disability, for example in diabetes and asthma. The diabetic regime and the occurrence of asthmatic attacks may be affected by menstruation, especially at the menarche, and later, by the menopause; the effects of long-term drug treatment in these two conditions, which may itself bring about disabling changes, are well documented.

There is a great deal of evidence to suggest that the young adult is disadvantaged in terms of medical provision—and this occurs at the time of the difficult transition from childhood to adulthood, from dependence to independence and self-sufficiency. There are paediatricians for children, and surgeons and physicians for adults, but there are children's wards in which a well-developed 15-year-old would be out of place, and adult wards in which an immature 16-year-old would be equally misplaced; the existing district handicap teams cater only for the needs of children of school years.

Thus, while children and adults can rely upon specialised care, the young adult often cannot. At around 16 years of age the transfer of responsibility for care passes from a child-orientated service to an adult-orientated service and the fact that this transfer is itself inadequate is highlighted by the Warnock[7] and Court[8] reports. The Court committee noted that:

> . . . physical and mental handicap predispose children to psychiatric disorder and in this and other ways may aggravate and prolong the developmental problems facing all adolescents. The constraints to living imposed by handicap affect the adolescent's life at home, at school, in employment and in society. Additionally they are subject to all the stresses of accelerated physical, sexual and emotional development and to the prospect of change in environment and occupation. For the handicapped, adolescence is a period of crisis, yet at the moment of leaving school, there is the danger that they are less supported than at any time hitherto.

The Court report goes on to discuss the need for continuity in care, and stresses time and again the importance of close liaison between all those workers involved in the care of disabled young people. The committee accepted that the team would include specialist and primary care medical and nursing services, remedial services, social services and volunteers, and also welfare and employment agencies and careers services.

The Chronically Sick and Disabled Persons Act (1970) requires that special and separate units for chronically handicapped young people should be provided locally, but the growth of such units is slow and in some areas the chronically disabled adults remain the responsibility of the geriatrician irrespective of age.

Assessment for care

The initial assessment of the disabled person will centre upon the activities of daily living—the ability to eat, wash, dress and use the toilet. With the young disabled, the majority of the needs in these areas will have been met, either because the disability has existed through childhood or, as in the case of John Davis, they have been dealt with by the hospital service, and involved doctors, remedial therapists and social workers. Nothing should be taken for granted, however, and the best-laid plans may be incapable of implementation once the patient is discharged. Preparations were made for John, and the primary care team were involved with the family prior to discharge, but, as the work of Skeet[9] and Hockey[10] demonstrates, there is often a sad lack of preparation for hospital discharge and an even more common exclusion of the primary care team from that preparation.

No assessment can be contemplated without the total involvement of the family of the young disabled person for, as the case histories of John Davis and Mr Fisher illustrate, the contribution of parents or wife to the daily care is immense. The relatives will bear the burden of looking after the young person on a constant day-to-day basis and will thus hold a responsibility for noting behaviour and for monitoring progress or otherwise. In order to do this, the level of ability and the strengths and the weaknesses of the patient must be understood and accepted by the carers. In addition, an awareness of any association between the handicapping condition and existing behavioural problems, or anticipated ones, is essential if change is to be noted or potential problems prevented or detected early. Bearing the burden of care, the parents or the young spouse must be participants in the process of assessment and decision-making, not only in formulating the nursing care plan but in discussions with the doctors, the remedial therapists and the disablement resettlement officers. The relatives must not be seen merely as welcome 'caretakers'.

The teaching and counselling role of the district nurse is of paramount importance here, as is her ability to sit and listen and to accept the advice and the knowledge of the relatives. The teaching role may not only include instructing relatives in therapeutic procedures to be continued at home, such as nursing care, but also advising on physiotherapy and speech therapy. The nurse will need to determine such needs before entering the home, so contact and liaison with all who have been involved in care is essential. Domiciliary physiotherapy services are still few, even though the need is tremendous for such disabled people as John Davis. While the nurse will assess the need for continuing physiotherapy and do what she can, she needs help; the written exercise sheet for the use of both nurse and relatives is invaluable, and, is absolutely essential when physiotherapy is concerned with active treatment as well as prevention: care must be therapeutic.

Assessment of relatives must include an assessment of their ability to cope and to cope continuously. Parents are more often than not anxious to care for handicapped children at home and special schools are available, as are paediatric services and financial support. As adolescence and young adulthood supervene, the 'child' becomes bigger and heavier, the demands, including the financial demands, become greater, the relatives become older, and service provision alters. The burden of caring becomes difficult and even impossible, yet relatives are often reluctant to admit to the burden, and feelings of guilt may be experienced. Where the disability has existed from childhood, such occurrences can to some extent be anticipated and prepared for; for example where a father has previously carried the child up and down stairs to bathroom and bed, alterations to the home can be made in readiness for adulthood, lifts installed or a downstairs toilet added to the home. The knowledge that the patient can be admitted to a holiday home or hospital once or twice every year can do much to relieve the stress experienced by relatives who will know that they can have a break whilst their loved one is being cared for.

Further assessment will identify particular problems. John, for example, is bed and chair bound, he can go outdoors but will only venture into the garden in sunny weather because he worries about his condom drainage. Although he seemed to have accepted his changed bodily image while in hospital among people in a similar condition to himself, or worse, now he is at home he is not really ready to accept the stares of other people. He likes to read and gets through a thriller a day most days; his parents visit the library for him but keep bringing back books he has already read. He used to like the cinema and always attended the home matches of his favourite football team, but he cannot go to these places now because of his concern over his incontinence—and anyway the cinema does not accommodate wheelchairs. Dad would push him to the football ground, but it is unfair to ask him every Saturday when usually he goes down to the allotment, and anyway, there are all those people at football matches.

Apart from the counselling role that will centre upon John's involvement in the assessment and the decision making, the nurse will need to be familiar with the following:

Other safe urinary drainage units.

The availability of a travelling or voluntary services library.
Local facilities to accommodate the disabled at libraries and in
other public buildings.
The availability of volunteers to transport or push the patient to
libraries, shops and football matches and/or football supporter
clubs.
The existence of self-help groups where patients and/or
relatives can meet in similar circumstances to themselves.

Mobility remains a problem for the disabled, in spite of the
responsibility of local authorities to ensure that public buildings
are accessible, and the availability of the mobility allowance. A
number of voluntary organisations try to help by making
available drivers and volunteers.

Any assessment of the needs of the disabled will include
financial considerations. Finances are not always considered by
the hospital team because sickness benefit is forthcoming from the
state and the employer for some time if the patient has been
employed. The financial burden of caring for someone in the home
is great: for example the immobility of the patient means that
heating must be adequate, and John's parents' heating bill will
become much higher as John and his mother spend all day in the
home. Thought needs to be given to applications for financial
assistance, and the relevant DHSS leaflets, available also from
health centres and larger post offices, provide details of the
benefits and allowances that are available.

Planning care

The future for the disabled can be forbidding, and honesty about
any prognosis is usually advocated, but nurses will need to know
how much the patient and the family know before they enter the
home. Honesty about the future can assist in laying the
foundations of the nursing care plan in which patient and family
can be involved.

John, for example, is going to remain largely immobile and very
little can be done about that, but he still has some movement
which can be exploited, and new skills can be learned using what
is available. A start should be made by ensuring that the good
muscles are kept in prime condition and even strengthened with a

view to doing more with them. The useless parts of the body cannot be ignored, however, because pressure sores would cause weakness, vulnerability to infection, and cosmetic disfigurement; exercise and movement of the whole body is therefore important. This involves planning, and planning together, and the emphasis should be on encouraging the patient to concentrate on what he can do and achieve rather than on what he cannot do—on the positive rather than the negative.

The nursing care plan will therefore focus mainly upon preventive measures such as avoiding pressure sores, prevention of further disability, the early detection of indicators to ill-health and early treatment, the maintenance of continence, prevention of accidents and provision of a diet that will prevent obesity where there is immobility.

A district nurse who is suddenly asked to visit a John Davis who is a tetraplegic, recently discharged from hospital and is in need of a daily bath and dressing, might well find herself completely at sea and unable to plan care because she does not know who is doing what with the family. Where then does the nurse begin? John has obviously had a hospital-based social worker working with him and the family since the home has been adapted to meet his needs. Responsibility for continuous assessment for financial benefits, home adaptations and aids for daily living may be referred to a community-based social worker. The team of health care workers surrounding John now includes the hospital specialists, the general practitioner, the social worker and the district nurse; between them they will possess a great deal of information about John, but this will be utterly useless if it is left uncoordinated. Teamwork is essential to avoid the risk of individual team members working to conflicting ends, each having different priorities.

A case conference is one way of ensuring that activity is coordinated and that realistic targets are set. With patients such as John, there is special value in a case conference prior to hospital discharge, but any team member should be able to initiate the case conference if there is a need, be it patient need or the need for information and coordination by health care workers themselves.

Some psychological problems can be anticipated when caring for the disabled and their families. An enforced change of job can lead to loss of earnings and an inability to support the family in the manner to which it has become accustomed. To have no prospect of a job at all is worse still and goes against the work ethic on which our society is based. The inability of a husband and father to carry on working can lead to a reversal of roles where the man stays at home and the wife goes to work. Employment Resettlement Centres enable persons who have lost work skills to undergo assessment and retraining. The disablement resettlement officer (DRO) is trained to undertake assessments and to advise disabled people about the possibility of returning to work or the need for retraining. The DRO often recommends registration as a disabled person because, by law, firms who employ more than 20 people must employ a 'quota' of registered disabled people. Many DHSS financial benefits are also dependent upon registration. For those who are unable to work, diversional and occupational therapy is important, but, as in the case of the elderly, activities should not be designed merely to fill in time. The participant must also experience a sense of achievement. John can read, go to football matches and has his own television and cassette recorder, but where is the sense of achievement and contribution? For him a workshop might be an answer, or encouragement to achieve proficiency in a sports group for the physically disabled.

A particular feeling experienced commonly by relatives is that of isolation—they feel that they are alone in caring, that they are the only couple (or spouse) within their neighbourhood and social group who have a disabled son (or wife). Participation in existing self-help groups and involvement with voluntary bodies can be of value in enabling such feelings to be shared, as well as actually providing support and assistance. Nurses should know what organisations are available locally and the local library, the Community Health Council and Citizens Advice Bureau can usually provide relevant information. Some relevant voluntary organisations are listed in Appendix 3, but those of special interest to the young disabled include:

Central Council for the Disabled, the Disabled Alliance, the British Council for Rehabilitation of the Disabled, British Sports Association for the Disabled and Sexual Problems of the Disabled (SPOD).

Sexual problems can be anticipated; John will never experience a normal sex life but his desires and needs will remain. The arthritic patient, the person with only one useful arm, the cosmetically disfigured, will all experience problems. These problems are now acknowledged and widely discussed, and further reading is recommended. The counselling role of the nurse is important here, as is her ability to discuss sexual needs and to recognise that the available ways of meeting them are normal and therefore acceptable activities, and do not represent perversions or inadmissable behaviour patterns.

Guilt is a feeling that can be experienced by both patient and family. The patient feels guilt because he cannot contribute to the family life as before, physically or financially. The relatives feel guilt when the realisation dawns that they no longer want, or are physically unable, to continue caring.

John's mother has given up work to care for her son, but she may eventually resent his intrusion on her life style only to feel guilty about this very feeling later on. John may feel guilt over his mother actually making changes just for him. The nurse must be sensitive to changes in family dynamics, and where possible prevent disharmony by promoting the continued discussion of problems within the family.

Life styles should not be drastically changed if it can be avoided. Mrs Davis could continue in her part-time job if John's independence was encouraged and care was planned. For example, if the district nurse visits John in the morning, washes him, gets him up and dressed, changes the urine bag and generally meets his needs, surely Mrs Davis would not be missed? If John were to attend a workshop, sports or OT group, or if the home help called in towards lunchtime too, Mrs Davis's continued work might become a realistic possibility. Equipment to assist John in his independence when alone would be important and might include remote control for the TV, a mechanical hand for retrieving items from the floor, a nearby telephone, an intercom system to the front door and even a flask of coffee and a novel on the bedside table.

Relatives who can no longer cope need careful and sympathetic understanding. A holiday break should not be offered unless the answer is that a break is all that is necessary, and if it becomes necessary for the patient to leave home the family should have the reassurance that suitable residential care is available.

Implementation and evaluation

The attitudes of the whole family must be considered and evaluated as any nursing plan is put into practice. Siblings for example may seem fully involved in planning care and express commitment, even excitement, yet in practice jealousy over the disproportionate amount of time spent on and with the disabled family member is almost inevitable.

Dislike of the disabled sibling can arise when his frustration at being disabled and different is converted to anger, which is of course vented on those nearby and those who are really most loved.

Disabled people are in need of care but not to the exclusion of all else and of all other people. Over-protection and over-indulgence are common but families should be urged to avoid this, and to share themselves and material things as equally as possible. The benefits of the nursing plan, as implemented, should be conveyed to the family so that they are encouraged to recognise their own dispensibility and the potential of the patient for a degree of independence.

Evaluation will determine when the needs of the patient have been met and district nursing intervention is no longer required. Complete discharge from care may never occur when the immobility of the patient and the lack of family involvement mean that nursing care must be continuous, and in this case the nurse may decide to undertake continuous preventive health care and so remain involved with the family. This type of case could be passed to the health visitor, but whatever the course of action, patient and family should always have access to professional advice and support when needed. Every effort must therefore be made to ensure that self-referral will occur in case of future need.

References

1. World Health Organisation (1980). *International Classification of Impairments, Disabilities and Handicaps*. Geneva: WHO.

2. Goffman E. (1963). *Stigma: notes on the management of a spoiled identity.* New York: Prentice Hall.
3. Harris A. I. (1971). *Handicapped and Impaired in Great Britain.* London: HMSO.
4. Department of Health and Social Security (1971). *Better Services for the Mentally Handicapped.* London: HMSO.
5. O'Brien J., Tyne A. (1981). *The Principle of Normalisation: a foundation for effective services.* London: Campaign for People with Mental Handicap.
6. O'Brien J. (1987). *A guide to personal futures planning.* In *The Activities Catalog: A Community Programming Guide for Youth and Adults with Severe Disabilities.* (Bellamy G. T., Wilcox B., eds). (In press.)
7. *Report of the Committee on the Education of Handicapped Children and Young People* (Warnock report; 1978). London: HMSO.
8. *Fit for the Future: Report of the Committee on Child Health Services* (Court report; 1976). London: HMSO.
9. Skeet M. (1974). *Home from Hospital,* London: Macmillan Journals.
10. Hockey L., Buttimore J. (1970]. *Cooperation in Patient Care.* London: Queen's Nursing Institute.

Further Reading

Department of Health and Social Security (1971). *Better Services for the Mentally Handicapped.* London: HMSO.

Blaxter M. (1976). *The Meaning of Disability—A Sociological Study of Impairment.* London: Heinemann Medical.

Coping with Disablement. London: Consumer's Association.

Dressing for Disabled People. London: Disabled Living Foundation.

Sex and the Physically Handicapped. London: National Fund for Research into Crippling Diseases.

Royal College of Physicians (1986). Physical disability in 1986 and beyond. *Journal of the Royal College of Physicians*; **20**: 3 (Supplement).

Simes D., Bicknell J. (1985). *Caring for Mentally Handicapped People in the Community.* London: Harper & Row.

Tierney A. J. ed. (1983). *Nurses and the Mentally Handicapped.* Chichester: John Wiley.

Hodges B. (1983). Handicap or special need? In *Community Health* (Clark J., Henderson J.). Edinburgh: Churchill Livingstone.

Chapter 13

Mental Illness

Throughout history, attitudes to people whose behaviour has deviated from normal has varied widely. At times fools and madmen have been regarded as 'inspired' and endowed with special sight, but on other occasions they have been connected with evil spirits and witches. To the confusion of the historian there have been times when both attitudes coexisted.

Because mental health is relative it is often difficult to tell where health ends and disease begins, for what is regarded as mental illness varies, not only from period to period, but also between different groups in the same period. Eighteenth-century rural England tolerated eccentrics like Squire Western or bizarre poets like John Clare more readily than would people in the new industrial towns of that time. On the other hand, the wayward genius of men like Van Gogh and Blake—whether in town or country—today would probably be treated by tranquillisers, group therapy and social rehabilitation. Mass production and the computer age require conformity.

By these tokens it is impossible to say whether mental illness is increasing; some illness, especially that due to infection, has declined. For example, at the beginning of the century one in five admissions to mental asylums was due to syphilis, now it is less than one in 200. Also, due to better living conditions, it is likely that the incidence of schizophrenia has decreased.[1] However, mental illness associated with ageing is increasing, for the simple reason that there are now more old people, and the proportion of elderly with mental infirmity rises rapidly over 75 years.[2] Although it cannot be proved, it seems likely that there is an increase in stress-related diseases and psychoneurotic illness due to the pressures of modern urban life. This begs the question, however, of whether these illnesses have become more common, or whether we have become better at recognising them. And has stress really increased? Living through Tudor inflation and the Reformation, with the Age of Faith crumbling, must also have been quite stressful.

From time to time the district nurse will come across patients, their relatives, or other carers whose behaviour 'interferes with their ability to lead a life acceptable as normal within the context of their social surroundings'[3] and this will impede the nurse's efforts to give total care. She is unlikely to encounter cases of overt psychosis, which comprise a small part of the sum of mental illness, but there is a wide range of deviation from what we call 'normal', ranging through mild paranoia, delusion, amnesia, cyclical depression, aggression and other manifestations of disturbance that do not call for the whole gamut of the psychiatric services, but nevertheless, if the nurse does not make a sound assessment, can cause suffering and untold trouble to the nurse herself later.

Since few district nurses are trained as psychiatric nurses, what can they do to ensure that they are safe practitioners when they encounter mental illness? Above all they should have some basic knowledge of the characteristics, predisposing factors and aetiology of the various groups of psychotic and neurotic illnesses. For example, Mr Adam's disorientation at the age of 85 years is hardly likely to indicate incipient schizophrenia, but a sudden manifestation of delusion or paranoia by John Davis would be cause for alarm. Depression in Mrs Cray would not be surprising; she lives in a high-rise flat and we know that such dwellers consult their doctors with psychoneurotic symptoms more frequently than people who live in houses, and she is in fact already obviously socially withdrawn.

All the cases mentioned in Chapter 1 could be candidates for different forms of stress and each could show different signs and symptoms. However, to be a safe practitioner the district nurse must not only be able to differentiate the signs and signals that may indicate an impending breakdown, she must also recognise at what point she needs help and at the same time know where to get that help.

Assessing the need for care

Mental illness is associated with a temporary or permanent disturbance of the mind characterised by disorders of behaviour and reasoning, and generally occurring in adult life. These disturbances are usually associated with endogenous factors but sometimes the origin is exogenous as with alcohol, drugs or the effect of toxins. It is important that the exogenous factors are excluded before considering psychological factors.

First, it is important to exclude the effect of drugs as a cause of a patient's apparent disorientation. It is well known that patients have been described as suffering from 'senile confusion' when in fact the confusion was due to the injudicious prescribing of sedatives, or that the multiplicity of drugs being taken were interacting in such a way as to cause mental disturbance. It is important to check that the patient is taking the right drugs, in the right doses, at the prescribed times, and, since elderly patients tend to treasure all drugs like a valued rosary, that they are not taking 'pain killers' or 'stomach pills' prescribed by some previous doctor—or not prescribed at all—now hoarded in the bathroom or on the mantlepiece.

Secondly, because severe infection is comparatively rare and the 'delirium of fever' largely confined to Victorian melodrama, it is often forgotten that infection can cause mental disorder. After all, the 'wandering mind' was a symptom of the typhoid state. Infection that is being held at bay by antibiotics may still manifest itself in 'light-headedness', as can a variety of other conditions—including constipation.

Apart from drugs, other poisons may affect the mental facilities, the most important being alcohol. According to E. M. Jellinik, 'alpha alcoholism' is due to an underlying personality defect, but this only accounts for a minority of cases, whereas it is estimated that probably 2% of the population suffer from health effects due to alcohol.[4] To become alcoholic all that is necessary is the availability of alcohol and the incentive. Some occupations are particularly prone; for example, journalists, public relations personnel and publicans. Alcoholism tends to be a problem of the extremes of social class, being comparatively low in the middle classes. Alcohol depresses the function of the brain and makes the subject more accident-prone, and it must be remembered that it can lie at the root of otherwise unexplained aggressive behaviour such as battering and violent family quarrels.

Finally, though rare, a sudden change of behaviour may indicate a brain tumour or presage a cerebral accident, and this possibility should not be ruled out without investigation. Moreover, because a patient already has a personality problem or is thought to be mildly alcoholic, this is not to say that he is not also developing a brain tumour. A wise surgeon once asked: 'If a man says he has a pain in his stomach who am I say to say he has not?'

Most of the mental disturbance encountered by the district nurse will, however, be endogenous, and if she is to pick up the danger signals she must learn to assess vulnerable personalities and situations. Some patients and carers are as stable as the Rock of Gibraltar, but others have personalities that are potentially 'at risk'. These include the introverted and withdrawn, the immature and insecure, the overaggressive and those with poorly developed powers of ratiocination and communication skills. The latter are vulnerable because they are denied the catharsis of 'talking things out', and the former cannot be helped by appeals to reason. Unfortunately it is often the vulnerable personalities that create, or somehow find themselves in, risk situations, which may include trouble with the boss, minor law-breaking, marital quarrels and broken homes. When a number of these factors combine the storm cones might well be hoisted.

Apart from the 'at risk' personalities, there are situations of vulnerability that are the common lot of most people. For example, there are the crisis points in life mentioned in Chapter 3 which include a sudden change in the life style such as marriage, parenthood, redundancy or retirement, bereavement or exposure to some external disaster. With regard to the latter it must be remembered that the effect may be delayed for some time, as was seen with men who had been prisoners of war—a point worth remembering when taking a nursing history.

Since endogenous depression is widespread the district nurse should be alert to its signs and dangers. Most people show some cyclical movement between elation and depression, and when the peaks and troughs are violent this may indicate manic depression. Some people, however, have long depressive phases not warranted by circumstances. This proviso is important. If Mr Fisher's wife leaves him, he loses his job and his sclerosis gets worse, his subsequent depression is not pathological—it is justified. Indeed when people do *not* get depressed or anxious when circumstances warrant it they may equally be displaying a personality disorder. However, if Mr Evans, with no obvious worries, starts sitting with his head in his hands, refusing to speak to his family and complaining of insomnia, the nurse would be right in regarding these as sinister omens for which she needs further advice.

Besides the distress that depressive patients cause to themselves and those around them, the possibility of suicide must be kept in mind. Throughout the world something like a thousand people commit suicide every day, and although in terms of actual numbers the age group over 55 years is most heavily represented, in terms of deaths per 1000 for a specific group the figure is highest for those between the ages of 24 and 35 years.[5] In England there are over 4000 suicides recorded each year and, of course, not all suicides are recorded as such. The upper classes seem more likely to kill themselves than the lower, with doctors having a particularly high rate. Predisposing factors seem to be the availability of the means (such as access to dangerous drugs), highly competitive job situations, and domestic stresses such as marital break-up and divorce proceedings. In women the premenstrual syndrome is important: Strindberg's Miss Julie characteristically cut her throat with a razor when 'her monthly was coming on'. Similarly, hormonal swings are linked with puerperal depression, once the cause of many suicides in comparatively young women.

An important factor in the histories of suicides, and attempted or parasuicides, is a disorganised life pattern—possibly a disorganised marriage, a broken home or unsettled housing, and, all too often, heavy drinking and drug taking. While young adolescents are the most vulnerable group and the district nurse should be vigilant for danger signs among the young carers, numbers of lonely old people take their own lives either because they are confused or because life has become meaningless, or, tragically, because they feel that they have become a burden to those around them. Finally, in this elderly depressive group, is the train of events that so often occurs with bereaved people, where, particularly after the death of a spouse in what has been a long and happy marriage, a surprising number of surviving partners die (sometimes called 'heartbreak death') within a year of their partner's death.

Planning care

Each patient is an individual, and unique. Where the nurse feels that the mental state of the patient, or the carer, is such that those around him are at risk, the doctor should be consulted and probably a case conference called. In an emergency the machinery for compulsory admission can be invoked but it must be remembered that an 'urgency order' is only valid for 72 hours.

Hospital admission will be the exception, and with emphasis on care in the community the patient is likely to be returned home comparatively quickly. In these circumstances the district nurse can get support from other members of the team, one of whom will probably have had some psychiatric experience. However, the nurse's most valuable ally in such cases would be a community psychiatric nurse if such a nurse were available in the area. This group of nurses had their origin in the work of far-sighted psychiatric hospitals in the 1950s. Following the abolition of the Joint Board of Clinical Nursing Studies, courses were organised under the aegis of the National Boards and the number of psychiatric nurses taking these courses increased. A survey conducted by the Community Psychiatric Nurses Association[6] calculated that in 1985 there were 2758 community psychiatric nurses, but their distribution was uneven; over 5 years there had been a rapid rise in the numbers, and the overall population ratio was 23 800 per CPN. The most typical management structure for the CPN services appeared to be a senior nurse (grade 7 or 8) reporting to the appropriate nursing officer which, in the new arrangements, may vary from health authority to health authority. While 37% of the CPNs are still based on psychiatric hospitals there has been a sharp rise in the number based on health centres and general practitioner practices. Experiments show that where such nurses are used there are fewer referrals to hospital, and the whole primary care team has benefited from the opportunity to learn.

The type of help planned for patients with psychological problems will depend on the patient's age, condition, potential and the suspected primary reason for his breakdown. For example, the school nurse might well be consulted about so-called 'problem' children who may be worrying the patient or his carers;

illness in the house sometimes has a disturbing effect on children and it may be necessary to seek help from the child guidance clinic. Social workers with particular experience with youth work may be able to help with difficult adolescents and Mrs Baker's children may well need considerable help in this respect both before and after their mother dies, for being fatherless as well as watching their mother die, they are at risk and may be prey to all sorts of fantasies.

However, while problems concerning children are generally only likely to come to the district nurse in her capacity as 'guide, philosopher and friend', her main concern will be about the psychological overlay that is likely to exist in patients like Mr Fisher, Mrs Baker and John Davis, and their carers. A watchful eye must be kept lest the strain imposed on such families tips over into real depression. Planning care therefore involves prevention; ideally the stress placed on carers should not be more than they can bear, but if it is, then there must be intervention and this will inevitably involve other members of the team, particularly the health visitor, and then probably other agencies.

Implementing the plan

Unless the mental disturbance is such that it overshadows all other aspects of the patient's illness, the plan to meet the psychological needs of the patient or his carers will be integrated into the main plan; probably much of this will be actually implemented by other people, such as social workers or the community psychiatric nurse. Although the causes of mental illness are usually multiple and defy tidy diagnosis there are ways in which mild and temporary disturbances can be mitigated.

It may be that such problems as insomnia and depression or other stress symptoms can be dealt with by drugs; sometimes a short, sharp course will break a bad spell. However it is essential that such courses are properly monitored, for patients react in a variety of ways and for some 'the dreams that come' are worse than the insomnia. For the most part, however, the causes of mental disturbance lie outside the realm of mechanistic medicine, and help must come from elsewhere. How effective that help is depends on how accurately the assessment has been made, how severe the disturbance is, and what resources are available and how easily they are mobilised.

If the primary cause 'seems' to be marital breakdown—'seems' because there is always a cause beyond the cause—then it is possible that help can be obtained from a marriage guidance counsellor. If, on the other hand, disturbance or depression seems to have its roots in a sense of uselessness and social withdrawal— sometimes the accompaniment of retirement—then it is possible that help can be provided from the social services department or through the vocational training services of the Department of Employment; but it must always be remembered that social withdrawal is a symptom as well as a cause. The patients and their carers who serve as models in this book all have different needs and each must be helped as an individual. Mr Fisher may prove himself very useful, and therefore much wanted, as a treasurer to various voluntary societies. John Davis might be helped by some educational course tailored to his capacity which gives him a series of hurdles to overcome—and therefore a purpose to life. Mrs Adams needs a break if she is to continue caring, but her idea of a holiday will not be the same as that of Mrs Davis. Planning this type of care needs imagination, cooperation with other agencies and knowledge of what is available.

Evaluating the plan

In caring for people with mental or emotional problems the best-laid plans are more likely to go astray than in almost any other branch of care. Alas, patients and clients do not always respond to occupational therapy, diversional activity, visits to day centres or courses in music and drama, and some, obstinately, do not respond to drugs in accordance with the claims made by the manufacturers. Because so often the problem resides in the patients themselves rather than in external circumstances, the plan may have to be re-evaluated many times. Success may only be partial, and since from time to time anxiety and depression must be the common lot of man, the nurse must be thankful if she is instrumental in preventing real, and damaging, breakdown when people are exposed to stressful conditions over a long period.

The Greeks saw the needs of the mind and the body as

inseparable, and in planning total care for her patient the nurse needs to return to this concept, bearing in mind that the generalist nurse cannot know all the answers but should at least know where to find them.

References

1. McKeown T., Lowe C. R. (1974). *Introduction to Social Medicine*, 2nd edn, p. 329. Oxford: Blackwell Scientific.
2. Department of Health and Social Security (1978). *A Happier Old Age*, p. 7. London: HMSO.
3. McKeown T., Lowe C. R. (1974). *Introduction to Social Medicine*, 2nd edn, p. 326. Oxford: Blackwell Scientific.
4. Lewin D. C. (1978). Care of the dependent patient: alcohol addiction. *Nursing Times*, 6 April; p. 570.
5. Lock S., Smith T. (1976). *The Medical Risks of Life*, p. 30. Harmondsworth: Penguin.
6. Community Psychiatric Nurses Association (1985). *National Survey*. London: CPNA.

Further Reading

Carr P. J., Butterworth C. A., Hodges B. E. (1980). *Community Psychiatric Nursing*. Edinburgh: Churchill Livingstone.
Community Care: with special reference to adult mentally ill and mentally handicapped people. (Short report; 1985). London: HMSO.
House of Commons Social Services Select Committee Report. H of C papers. London: HMSO.
Simmons S., Brooker C. (1986). *Community Psychiatric Nursing: a Social Perspective*. London: Heinemann.

Chapter 14

Acute and Chronic Illness

All too frequently district nursing is seen to be predominately about caring for the elderly and chronic sick, yet Dunnell and Dobbs[1] showed that 28% of the work of the district nursing team was with the under-65s and 7% was devoted to hospital discharges, a large proportion of which were patients having had relatively straightforward surgery. The Royal College of General Practitioners in 1973[2] found that 65% of conditions seen by general practitioners were minor, that is, self-limiting with no risk to life or permanent disability, as against 15% major life-threatening situations and 20% chronic conditions with permanent disabilities.

It must be remembered that less than half of people with a limiting acute illness go to the doctor so utilisation studies do not give a true picture of the situation. Some people with seemingly minor illnesses will consult the nurse instead of the doctor, probably while the nurse is visiting the home to care for another family member, sometimes by appointment with the district nurse or practice nurse in the surgery. Indeed, there is a small but growing number of people who envisage the development of a nurse practitioner, as pioneered in this country by Stilwell and described by Hall[3] and more recently advocated by Cumberlege[4]. Thresholds for seeking medical care depend on cultural and demographic factors, and upon the availability or otherwise of appropriate services. Of our seven patients, only one (Mr Evans) has what could be described as an acute illness; one in seven would be about the right proportion in the average district nursing caseload.

Patients with acute illness

Acute illness may be defined as an illness having generally a known time span and a known prognosis. The care of patients with an acute illness forms a small but significant part of the district nurse's work. Regrettably nurses and doctors are inclined to dismiss acute/minor illness as being of little importance, yet a patient like Mr Evans may be very concerned about his job, and loss of money and such anxieties can inhibit wound healing. It may be the effects of the illness that are more traumatic than the physical problem itself.

It has been shown that the district nursing service is frequently not used to the full. Hockey and Buttimore[5] found that many patients were asked to return to hospital for suture removal, frequently without thought about provision of transport and whether the patient would feel fit enough for the journey. Skeet,[6] whilst highlighting horrific breakdowns in—or complete lack of—communication between hospital and community for patients with long-term and severe illnesses, also showed that nearly a quarter of patients discharged from hospital who received no formal follow-up would have welcomed a visit to clarify instructions, to receive explanations quietly and slowly, or to provide a chance to ask questions. There was an expressed need for advice on drugs, diet, how much to do; as one patient said, what does 'don't do too much' *mean*? Mr Evans had an infected wound so it was automatic that a district nurse was asked to visit to carry out dressings, but if he had not had this it may have been that her first visit would have been to remove the sutures, which could have been too late to sort out his anxieties.

Gilmore *et al.*[7] made suggestions about the need for general practitioners to identify patients discharged from hospital. However, this is often difficult, as frequently the practice team are unaware that the patient has even been admitted, and by the time the discharge letter arrives he may have been home several days. This is an area that warrants further consideration as the research has shown that early intervention can prevent anxiety and unnecessary suffering. Ways need to be found to achieve an objective of the 1974 NHS reorganisation which is to ensure smooth transfer of care between hospital and community.

Another area of acute, short-term care that is increasing is the development in day surgery. Ideally the district nurse should visit the home prior to a decision being made that a patient is suitable for day surgery. There needs to be careful planning of such treatment; in particular, patients invariably need a visit in the evening following surgery when anxieties become manifest.

Not all patients with acute illness being cared for by the district nurse are those having had surgical procedures or those being discharged from hospital; some will have acute medical conditions and be referred directly from the general practitioner. Whatever the situation, however minor it may appear to the nurse, to the patient and his family it may well present as a crisis that can, albeit temporarily, cause severe disruption and hardship to the whole family.

Assessment for care

The district nurse needs to use her judgment as to how much information is required to enable planning of care. A very detailed assessment, such as that required for Mrs Baker, is probably not needed and in any case that detail is acquired over a period of time. However, it is important to be alert to cues because it may be through having access to the home that other problems (not necessarily with the patient himself) may be identified. If the patient has been discharged from hospital the district nurse should have adequate information provided by the hospital: it is increasingly the practice for a copy of the current care plan to be sent home with the patient.

Planning care

The frequency of visiting will depend first on the medical/surgical condition and whether there is any prescribed treatment such as a dressing, injections or eye drops. Secondly, it will depend on the assessment of how the patient and family are coping and, as described above in the research by Skeet,[6] a visit to see that all is well and give opportunities for questioning can save considerable stress.

Implementation and evaluation

The actual nursing tasks required may be simple or minimal but one of the particular skills required at this stage is making the judgement of when to discharge the patient from the books. This decision should not merely be based on the observation 'the wound has healed', but also on whether the patient and family are coping. It may also be that no further nursing care is required but referral to another agency is necessary, for instance the district nurse may have noticed a child with excessive bruising which would lead her to make the health visitor aware of the situation. A key difference in being involved with patients with acute illness from those with chronic illness is that the nurse is involved with the patient and family for a much shorter time, so she needs to be particularly sensitive to any cues that the patient or his family need further help.

Patients with chronic illness

Chronic illness is characterised by its permanence. The increase in average life expectancy brings with it an increase in chronic illness and disability. Kratz[8] found that chronic illness and long-term care are not synonymous; many people learn to cope with their illness without the help of others. Werner-Beland[9] vividly describes the problems of continually living with chronic health problems and the associated problem of grief not only in the sick person but also in those closely involved.

McCarthy[10] states that chronic illness is not a homogeneous entity and is predominantly found in the following groups: the mentally ill, the mentally handicapped, disabled children and young adults, the elderly, and those with problems of addiction to alcohol or drugs. One of the differences he identifies between these groups is that in the elderly there is invariably multiple pathology, whilst in the young the disease is more frequently a single problem.

Regrettably, there is all too frequently a fragmentation of care for those with chronic illness. This is partly due to the number of organisations involved, a multiplicity of autonomous agencies and, increasingly, a proliferation of specialist nurses. Too often there is no one person to control all the resources needed; this may preclude optimal care for the individual patient, and it precludes any coherent policy of allocating priorities between patients, leading to inefficient deployment of resources. McCarthy[10] describes situations with as many as nine or ten people visiting a household because of demarcation of tasks. Clarke[11] says that much is written about the nursing care of patients with chronic illness, but she regrets that nursing practice seldom approaches the standards promulgated.

The goals and expectations of achievement for the chronically sick differ from those for patients with acute illness. The key consideration is to achieve each patient's potential; some will achieve maximum possible independence and self-determination because of the kind of people they are, for example, resourceful, motivated, emotionally secure and psychologically dynamic. Chronicity depends on many complex factors such as pre-morbid personality, the nature and extent of the disorder, the phase in the life span and psychosocial situation. Some conditions are present from childhood (as with Rose Johnson), others may have an insidious onset such as rheumatoid arthritis. Mr Fisher has a condition which not only has an insidious onset but also is subject to periodicity—with remissions and relapses. The chronic conditions of Mr Adams and John, though very different, were both sudden in onset. The means of onset of a condition may also affect how the patient and family cope with the situation. Bowlby[12] in 1969 indicated that in sickness or calamity adults often become demanding of others, and in 1973[13] he stated that there is not necessarily a direct relationship between the nature of a person's physical condition and the intensity of his behavioural response. A frequent target for the patient's anger is the doctor, the nurse, or those most intimately involved in the care.

As a large proportion of district nursing work is involved in long-term care it is a sad reflection on nursing *per se* that this is so frequently undervalued and unfavourably compared with more dramatic episodes. Stockwell[14] in her study of the unpopular patient found that 'nurses liked patients who cooperated in getting well'—those staying in hospital 3 months or more were less popular. It could be argued that the situation in district nursing will be different when it is known that the larger proportion of patients will require long-term care, yet Kratz[8] found that in a well-defined situation district nurses were competent and gave focused care, yet when the patient was deemed as 'not getting better' this care was diffused without clear goals. As McClymont[15] writes, monotony and unremitting demand can lead to carer role fatigue and role disillusionment. Care givers may at times need more support than the patient. It is salutary to note that Barber and Kratz[16] remind us that 90% of all health care is given on a self-care or lay carer basis. It must also be remembered that patients and families may build up a wealth of knowledge about their condition, and the nurse needs to accept that the patient may have more detailed knowledge than she does.

Assessment for care

A full assessment of the chronically sick person may well take time to complete, as some of the more detailed and sensitive information may not be revealed until a trusting relationship has been developed. For example, the effects of a loss of sexuality in terms of role and being able to carry out sexually significant behaviours will not usually be raised at the first visit. A very important aspect of assessment is that of ascertaining an individual's particular strengths in terms of personality, motivation and emotions as well as physical ability. The nurse is invariably at a disadvantage, as rarely will she have known the patient before the illness developed. This may well be where the family and other carers are able to make a considerable contribution to the assessment. In making her assessment the nurse needs to bear in mind the likely effects of the disease and the reality of the prognosis. For example, in the instance of Mr Fisher with the progressive disease of multiple sclerosis it is important to be both positive and realistic.

The consideration of limitations on social interaction is important when assessing the needs of the chronically ill. It is marvellous that Mr Fisher can work from home, can continue to use his skills and can, therefore, experience a sense of achievement and contribution. One major problem is solved. The working from home means, however, that his normal activities are curtailed; gone are the pub lunches with colleagues and clients, gone is the membership of the work group and probably the sports or other recreational club; less easy is the trip to the theatre or the sports club dinner-dance with friends. Mr Fisher is actually one of the lucky ones because as a professional man he is able to continue earning and contributing to the household budget and can continue to satisfy his own and society's expectations in this respect. But what of the unskilled or skilled factory worker or the building-site craftsman? Their chances of continuing work from home are slight. They experience the loss not only of income but also of the social contact that the working group brings. Social interaction is important, and here a long-term patient's friends can be of tremendous value, if they are able to come to terms with and face his disability themselves.

Retraining is appropriate for some of the chronically ill, and should always be considered, as should membership of self-help and voluntary groups. Occupational and diversional therapy is essential and past skills should be used to advantage and should determine the type of therapy to be undertaken and promoted. An assessment of the financial situation and a knowledge of benefits available is also important (see Appendices 2 and 3). A reversal of roles is often seen when caring for the long-term ill; the husband cannot work so the wife goes out to work to supplement the family income while the husband stays at home. Role reversal is difficult for the average man to accept, and the psychological effects can lead to conflict within the marriage itself—in spite of the willingness of the wife to accept change. If such problems are evident, referral to a marriage guidance service might be useful, but the patient must be willing to accept help.

Planning care

One of the main objects of planning will be to communicate with others involved in the care to avoid the fragmentation described earlier. There is a paucity of services in the community such as therapists and home helps, and indeed a shortage of nursing time, so coordination of effort is required. It is also important to time visits to take account of the patient's social activities and as far as possible not to upset the normal family life.

Aids that enable and assist the chronically ill to continue occupational and diversional activities, together with necessary adaptations to the home, are of essential importance. Here the occupational therapist can offer advice if she undertakes home visiting. The Disabled Living Foundation has a wealth of knowledge and experience, and if their 'showrooms' cannot be visited they can supply leaflets and catalogues. It is often the charities and voluntary organisations that can be most useful because of their involvement in and experience of the needs of smaller, specific groups. Many of these organisations provide news-sheets and even newspapers to members, from which information about new aids can always be gleaned by the patient himself. A list of such organisations is included in Appendix 3. For nurses, all the nursing journals carry information about new aids and ideas and the local hospital's occupational therapy department could always be visited.

Care should also be planned to meet the needs of the family of the long-term sick. Mrs Fisher has a good job that will keep her away from the home most of the day but she will still need to do some housework. A common feeling of such spouses is guilt—guilt about leaving her husband and enjoying social and work contacts, guilt about needing more than he can give her. Common problems within such marriages concern the sexual life, or lack of it, the enforced role reversal, and financial pressures; and, of course, fear about the future. The family require support and, as participants in the caring plan, involvement in the decision-making, which must be dependent upon their knowledge of the diagnosis and the prognosis.

Any care plan for the long-term ill must focus upon prevention—prevention of unnecessary disability, the early detection and treatment of change and prevention of physical and mental strain in the caring relatives. One factor that is often forgotten because of the pressing nature of physical and psychological problems is the immediate environment in which the family live. Think of the family who have always prided themselves on the decoration of their house and their tidy, attractive garden; disability intervenes and the house cannot be redecorated or the spring bulbs planted. To see a previously cared-for garden become overgrown and ugly can be soul-destroying, especially when tidiness is a feature of the neighbourhood and 'keeping up with the Joneses' is important. Some people will be able to pay for help in the garden but many will not, and in this respect local volunteers can be invaluable, especially schoolchildren and Scout groups.

Another consideration in the planning of care is the provision of respite care for the carers. The problems of long-term caring have been increasingly acknowledged and will be discussed further in relation to the care of the elderly. A break from caring for the relatives can mean they can cope for longer periods and the district nurse should be aware of the facilities available in local hospitals or homes and by voluntary organisations to give this much-needed respite.

Intervention and evaluation

The nurse's role will be to carry out care as determined in the plan but also to teach the patient and carers how to cope during the remainder of the 24 hours when she is not available. Although the nurse should be reassessing the situation at every visit it is important to set dates for formal evaluation, as in the slow-moving situations of chronic illness perceptions of need may be blunted and cues may be missed. It may be useful periodically to ask a colleague to pass judgment on whether all that could be is being done. Another area of evaluation is that of observing all carers, including the nurse herself, for signs of 'burn-out'. Prevention of a situation where an individual cannot face caring for a particular person any longer is obviously preferable to a breakdown in relationships.

References

1. Dunnell K., Dobbs J. (1982) *Nurses Working in the Community*. London: HMSO.
2. Royal College of General Practitioners (1973). *Present State and Future Needs of General Practice*, 3rd edn. London: RCGP.
3. Hall C. (1982). Nurse with a stethoscope. *World Medicine*; **18** Part 1: 16 October 1982, 75–77.
4. Department of Health and Social Security (1986). *Neighbourhood Nursing—a focus of care* (Cumberlege report). London: HMSO.
5. Hockey L., Buttimore A. (1970). *Cooperation in Patient Care: Study of District Nurses Attached to Hospital and General Medical Practice*. London: Queen's Nursing Institute.
6. Skeet M. (1974). *Home from Hospital*, 4th edn. London: Macmillan Journals.

7. Gilmore M., Bruce N., Hunt M. (1974). *The Work of the Nursing Team in General Practice*. London: Council for the Education and Training of Health Visitors.
8. Kratz C. R. (1978). *Care of the Long-term Sick in the Community*. Edinburgh: Churchill Livingstone.
9. Werner-Beland J. A. (1980). *Grief Responses to Long-term Illness*. Virginia: Prentice-Hall.
10. McCarthy M., Millard P., eds. (1979). *Management of Chronic Illness*. London: King Edward's Hospital Fund.
11. Clarke M. (1979). Nursing care in chronic illness. In *Management of Chronic Illness* (McCarthy M., Millard P., eds). London: King Edward's Hospital Fund.
12. Bowlby J. (1969). *Attachment and Loss*; Volume 1: *Attachment*. New York: Basic Books.
13. Bowlby J. (1973). *Attachment and Loss*; Volume 2: *Separation, Anxiety and Anger*. New York: Basic Books.
14. Stockwell F. (1972). *The Unpopular Patient*. London: RCN Publications.
15. McClymont M. (1985). Intervention and care in long-term nursing of the adult. In *Long-term Care* (King K., ed.). London: Churchill Livingstone.
16. Barber J. H., Kratz C. R., eds. (1980). *Towards Team Care*. Edinburgh: Churchill Livingstone.

Further Reading

Baker G., Bevan J. M., MacDonnell L., Wall B. (1986). *Community Nursing: Research and Recent Development*. London: Croom Helm.
Griffiths V. E. (1970). *A Stroke in the Family*. Harmondsworth: Penguin.
King K., ed. (1985). *Long-term Care*. London: Churchill Livingstone.
O'Brian D., Alexander S., eds (1985). *High-dependency Nursing Care*. Edinburgh: Churchill Livingstone.
Roberts I. (1975). *Discharged from Hospital*. London: RCN Publications.
Strauss A. L., Glaser B. G. (1975). *Chronic Illness and the Quality of Life*. St Louis: C. V. Mosby.
Webb C. (1985). *Sexuality, Nursing and Health*. Chichester: John Wiley.

Chapter 15

Elderly People

The majority of elderly people fend for themselves or are looked after adequately by relatives, friends or the voluntary sector. It must be remembered that reaching the magical age of 60 or 65 does not mean that someone should be labelled 'elderly' and with this be stereotyped as sick, senile, old-fashioned, cantankerous or a nuisance, regardless of individual mental and physical abilities. For many the retirement period is one of the most active and fruitful times of their lives. Indeed, the French philosopher, Jean-Paul Sartre, when himself an octogenarian, said at an interview:

> 'I don't feel my age—so my old age is not something that in itself can teach me anything. What does teach me something is the attitude of others towards me. Old age is an aspect of me that others feel. They look at me and say "that old codger" and they make themselves pleasant because I will die soon and they are respectful. My old age is in other people'.[1]

However, the growth of the population over 65 years old has led to an increased demand for, and an expansion in, the health and social services. Of the district nurses' visits in 1985, 80% were to patients aged 65 years and over, and therefore these people have been identified as a special group. Figure 2.2 on p. 14 shows the use of the health services by the elderly.

The Audit Commission for Local Authorities in England and Wales[2] reports that by 1991 there will be 15% more people aged 75 and over than in 1981, and 35% more people aged 85 and over. These significant increases will obviously have implications for the health and social services including the work of the district nurse. Local authorities spend over one billion pounds a year on residential care and community services for the elderly, yet residential care is for only 2% of those over 65 and the support for a further 13%. This certainly does not meet the demand as the phenomenal growth of private residential care indicates; one of the resorts on the South Coast now has over 500 such establishments.

Some elderly people are inappropriately placed in residential care, and others are unable to get in and are left at risk in the community. Standard residential homes cannot accommodate the more severely handicapped, and a dilemma frequently occurs regarding the feasibility of keeping elderly residents in what has been home to them for several years when they require increasing amounts of nursing care. To help alleviate this problem and to consider alternative means of providing residential care the Department of Health and Social Security has supported three experimental NHS nursing homes manned by nurses; the evaluation completed in 1987 has shown these to be very successful and recommends that others should be developed.

As discussed in Chapter 5 the district nurse is increasingly involved in visiting patients in residential homes. One of the greatest problems in appropriately organising care for elderly people is inadequate coordination of health, housing and social services. Efforts to improve this have been made through joint financing.[3]

Allen[4] describes the growth in short-stay residential care for elderly people which has increased enormously over the past 15 years. This has risen from less than 30% of total admissions in 1967 to 59% in 1980. Short-stay residential care is defined as that providing holiday or temporary care whilst relatives or those who normally care for them are on holiday, in hospital or simply need a break. Short-stay usually implies 2 to 4 weeks but Allen poses the question whether it is a virtue to say 'our 40 beds for short-stay care have helped over 6000 people this year instead of 40 long-stay!'

The British Medical Association in 1986[5] considered the care of that large majority of elderly people living in their own homes. They found that families received little relief or support, only 11% of those over 75 being likely to have a visit from a district nurse or health visitor in the course of a month. They identified that the support provided by home helps is very variable from local authority to local authority, and needed to be increased by 40% in some and by as much as 400% in others. Only 3% of those over 65 have 'meals on wheels' and only 10% of carers have respite care—40% of those with confused elderly dependents have not had a break in 5 years.

The BMA report has three main messages:

1   Financial provision for elderly people should allow for leisure activities as well as for the necessities of keeping them warm, fed, clothed and housed. Economic self-sufficiency in old age should not be dependent upon employment history.
2   Far more resources should be allocated to community-based services in order to realise the official policy of maintaining people in their own houses.
3   Elderly people should not be treated as second-class citizens nor a race apart, and should have a right to participate fully in the life of the community. Their tastes, wishes and needs should be treated with the same consideration and respect as is offered to other groups.

The focus of nursing is to take action in a planned, organised and therapeutic manner in order to strengthen self-care capacities, to eliminate or minimise self-care limitations, and to provide care when self-care demands cannot be fulfilled.

Health education with elderly people

The district nurse must remember that she has a preventive role to play in helping people to adjust to change and to prepare for retirement and changed life styles. Unfortunately, although the value of preparation is well known and well documented, the attitudes of others to the elderly often colour the perceptions the elderly have of themselves. Phillipson and Strang[6] describe the district nurse as becoming 'quintessentially a nurse for the elderly'. The study considered how far the district nurse can carry out a preventive role with the elderly. Some questions raised were whether the work conditions were right, whether the district nurse had sufficient training and whether she had support from other professionals. They found that care of the elderly is very much a combination of practical and social care which is inextricably intertwined with the nurse clearly doing more 'educational' areas of work than identified in the earlier study of Dunnell and Dobbs.[7]

Turton[8] questions the use of social chatting, listening and unfocused general reassurance, and suggests whilst this is pleasant for the nurse and possibly for the patient, in terms of providing advice and health education it is totally ineffective. However, this does not support the finding of McIntosh and Richardson,[9] who in their study of district nursing staff in Scotland found that within the context of social support, valuable counselling and health education can be achieved. They state 'observation of, and conversation with, district nursing staff quickly dispels the view that their visits consist only of technical procedures and some social chat'. During nearly 600 visits the observer classified the main topics of conversation between patient and nurse as being history-taking, the progress and comfort of the patient, the nursing procedure and problems of daily living. This breadth of communication provides the nurse with a large amount of personal information about her patients. District nurses often find it difficult to identify the health education aspects of their role because it may be so closely incorporated into their routine activities.

Opportunities for health education with the sick elderly and their families visited by the district nurse are boundless, and with access to the home this should be realistic and appropriate to the situation. A group often neglected in terms of health education are the frail elderly. These people, who generally do not require nursing or supportive care, are an important group who could be enabled to avoid some of the problems of old age; but the role does not fall clearly into the province of any one worker. However, some health visitors and district nurses work either together or separately with groups or individuals in the promotion of health.

There are some specific problems associated with the elderly that invariably are preventable, such as hypothermia, misuse of drugs and falls; these are discussed below.

Hypothermia

It seems that in some elderly people the awareness of their ambient temperature becomes defective. The old person does not appreciate the coldness nor warmth in the room in which his daily activities are undertaken. If the room is too cold and the individual falls or becomes immobile for any reason there is an increased likelihood of hypothermia. The central core temperature of the body becomes too low and the individual thereafter feels tired, lethargic and is in danger of death. In fact in February 1986 over a thousand elderly people in the UK died as a result of hypothermia.

Anderson *et al.*[10] describe the predisposing factors of hypothermia as both exogenous and endogenous:

1 Ambient temperature
2 Impaired thermoregulatory response
3 Drugs—phenothiazines
　　　　alcohol
　　　　barbiturates
　　　　antidepressants
4 Hypothyroidism
5 Associated illness

A diagnosis of hypothermia is made with a temperature of 35 °C (95 °F) or below, and a low-reading thermometer must be standard equipment for the district nurse. Early diagnosis and treatment lessens the risk of severe complications, but prevention is better. Deep-body temperature does fall with age; around 60% of old people living at home in the UK are liable to develop a rectal temperature of 35 °C or less, and therefore constitute a group at risk. Some elderly people will understandably object to having a rectal temperature taken. An alternative means is to take the temperature of a fresh sample of urine, a temperature of 34.8 °C in this equates with a rectal temperature of 35 °C.

Many health authorities have hypothermia packs ready for crises, which contain soups, hot-water-bottles and possibly a foil wrap. It is important to restore the warmth of the person gradually, a rule of thumb being a rate of approximately 1 °C per hour.

Prevention may be by alerting the elderly to the dangers, but as described above this may be the very group not visited. Advice needs to be given regarding adequate heating and any relevant allowances for this; many would argue that the current allowances are far too low to be effective and their availability not generally understood. Advice regarding adequate clothing and nutrition is also important. This is an instance where an age/sex register helps a primary care team to identify those who may be at risk.

Drugs and the elderly

People over 65 years old receive a quarter of the total number of items issued on prescription, and it has been suggested that the elderly consume three times as many medicines (prescription and non-prescription) as the general population.[11]

Mathieson[12] cites the immense number of patients admitted to British geriatric units likely to suffer from drug reactions, the most commonly implicated drugs being hypotensive, anti-Parkinsonian, psychotropic or digoxin therapy. He suggests that the main causative factors can be considered under two broad headings: physiological changes associated with ageing, and the problems of patient compliance with drug regimes. Hamby[13] describes the many reasons for the physiological problems; although they may be seen to be more in the domain of the doctor than the nurse, the nurse does have a responsibility to check what drugs the patient is taking and be sure that all involved are aware of the regime.

In a review of the research into drug compliance, MacDonald and MacDonald[14] concluded that on long-term treatment courses patient compliance with prescribed drug regimes is about 50%. The district nurse has a responsibility not only to make sure that drugs are taken at the correct time but to ensure the elderly person is able to read what is written on the bottle label, understands the instructions and the reasons for taking the drugs. If the instructions are to 'take three times a day' the nurse needs to advise and possibly write out a chart of when these should be taken. Memory aids will need to be provided for many.

Another problem is that of the drug containers. Many elderly people have difficulties with child-proof containers and blister packs. A word with the chemist will be useful, and he may well put the drugs in new types of containers with 'butterfly' lids. One survey[15] showed that 87% of patients over 75 years of age taking tablets at home are responsible for supervising their own medications.

Falls in the elderly

The liability of falling increases with advancing age; the most common causes of home accidents are falls and the highest incidence is with the elderly.

A depressed body temperature increases the tendency to fall, which is another indication of the need to prevent hypothermia. Postural hypotension is relatively common in the elderly causing lightheadedness, and this creates a particular problem if the person gets up hurriedly in the night with urgency of micturition. Drugs may be a predisposing factor to falling, and as described in the previous paragraph the drug regime needs to be regularly checked.

The general process of ageing with a diminishing of the sensory functions, particularly that of failing vision, needs to be borne in mind. Once elderly people have had a fall they frequently develop a fear of falling and develop a reduction in moving around; a loss of confidence may also occur following illness or surgery. There are a range of appropriate aids and adaptations to the home that can be provided, usually through the local social services departments. In looking for the more complex reasons for falls in elderly people it is all too easy to overlook the simple hazards in the home such as loose rugs, frayed flexes and high cupboards. However, these seemingly easy-to-solve problems are often the hardest to deal with; the elderly person is not easily convinced of the need to remove such hazards, as 'they've always been like that'.

The district nurse, aware of the susceptibility to falls of an elderly person, has a dilemma in determining how often to visit. The nurse obviously cannot be expected to be there at the time of a fall; the important thing is to ascertain that someone takes responsibility for having seen the person at least once a day, noting if the milk has been taken in, the curtains drawn back and other such signs of activity or lack of it.

Psychogeriatric care

In October 1980 the Secretary of State for Health and Social Security said that there were some 70 000 psychogeriatric patients in the United Kingdom of whom only 13 500 were in hospitals or other institutions—the vast majority are therefore at home. Brocklehurst claims that the psychiatry of old age is now a speciality in its own right; he expects to see more psychiatrists with a responsibility for running psychogeriatric services within the next decade, and the recognition of dementia as a condition for care in its own right.[16] The need for such a service is demonstrated by recent studies which have shown that over a third of the people over 65 now receiving nursing care at home or elsewhere have psychiatric problems.[17]

There are now suggestions that a psychiatrist should be appointed to coordinate the services for psychogeriatric cases within a defined area, who would be able to plan hospital and community care and liaise with local authorities. However, the role of the primary health care team will remain of the greatest importance as a preventive service, especially in the detection and assessment of mental disease in old age. In the meantime experimentation continues into assessment based on the hospital, into small assessment units, and into home assessment.

In this area of work the district nurse will need to work closely with the community psychiatric nurse.

Assessment for care

When assessing patients and their families nurses are apt to concentrate on their recent social history and on social norms, but it must be remembered that to elderly people the past can be equally important. The age in which the patient grew up and the social conditions he experienced will have influenced his attitudes; for example, many elderly people are reluctant to divulge information about personal finances because of memories of 'means testing' and the treatment of the poor under the Poor Law system. This fact illustrates a principle of the application of the nursing process, namely that use must be made of knowledge derived from various fields including psychology, biology and other physical and social sciences when assessing the patient.

In making an assessment it is important to take into account the past working life of the patient; for example the carpenter who has no form of recreation and is depressed because he experiences no sense of accomplishment might well be persuaded to use his old skills to meet these needs. In order to promote communication skills in Mr Adams it will be important to introduce a subject immediately interesting to him, and something related to his past experience, such as what he did in the Second World War, is more likely to promote a response than trying to talk about the weather or the state of the economy. Knowledge of the patient's past occupation or wartime activity is sometimes essential when assessing his present financial situation and entitlements, as well as his physical condition. Examples of the importance of this are miners with lung disease or ex-service men with war wounds or disabilities.

When assessing an elderly patient the nurse must be aware of her own values and beware of imposing them. Mr Adams is old, handicapped, constantly wet and often difficult to manage because of his confusion. Being confused, he does not seem aware of his condition nor wish to seek improvement. Mrs Adams is not fit and there are no relatives to help; the house is old, facilities are poor—even squalid—and the environs are dangerous. The nurse who values modern living and who uses only her own preconceptions when making her observations might well want to remove the couple to a new house or even get Mr Adams into hospital. But, she should ask, is the house really dangerous? The 'clutter' constitutes a carefully built, cherished and familiar home environment. The paraffin heater is familiar, cheap and sensibly used, and although there are no relatives, villagers and friends abound and the couple have lived this way for over 50 years; they would hate separation and their attitude to it must be determined before any action is taken.

The observational skills of the nurse when dealing with the old are particularly important. For reasons of pride the elderly may not answer questions quite truthfully; for example they may deny incontinence out of shame or embarrassment, or they may claim their heating arrangements are adequate when in fact the fuel bills cannot be met and heat is only turned on when someone comes. The nurse's sense of smell and a suspiciously low room temperature may help her detect such problems. At the same time she must be alert to hazards in the home; accidents in the homes of the elderly are commonplace and the nurse must remember that hallways, bedrooms and bathrooms are as dangerous—or potentially dangerous—as are the kitchens and living areas.

As has been stressed in previous chapters the emotional needs of the patient and the family must not be overlooked. In Chapter 7 the need to discuss with John Davis his enforced lack of sexual activity was emphasised; this was not said of Mrs Adams even though the lack probably exists. There is now a great deal of literature about sex and the elderly and no better résumé can be found than that of Kastenbaum[18] who says 'the intimacy of two people who have shared years of joys and sorrows together is an excellent buffer against a world that looks at old men and women but does not really see them. In each other's arms they continue to be themselves rather than society's impoverished image of the aged. The small intimacies, the quiet conversation, the sense of togetherness, remain both precious and life-affirming'.

As stated previously the majority of sick elderly people are cared for at home, and it is important that the nurse determines the abilities of relatives to lift, fetch and carry, and that she is also aware of their attitudes to performing intimate tasks to patients. Some relatives feel they cannot give this intimate care and their feelings must be respected. All these factors need to be taken into account when planning care. Obtaining a complete nursing history with an elderly person will take time and information will be gathered over the period of many visits. It may be necessary because of the person's confusion or forgetfulness to verify facts with relatives, but this needs to be done in a sensitive way in order not to undermine the authority of the elderly person.

Planning care

The elderly have their needs as do all other individuals, and when the elderly person becomes dependent on care the nurse must always ask herself whether she is enhancing the quality of the patient's life. As an example, Mr Adams may find that eating fish and chips from a spoon is a degrading experience, yet be unable to communicate that feeling or express the desire to try to use his good hand to feed himself. The nurses and the family have taken over; individual need is not determined nor is independence promoted.

The problems of the elderly are frequently multiple and may embrace medical, social, psychological, financial and emotional needs. A multidisciplinary approach is therefore required but this has dangers in itself. The list of persons and agencies dealing with Mr and Mrs Adams could be lengthy, and without good liaison each worker could be aiming at a different goal and giving different advice. This could lead to confusion not to mention the sheer annoyance of having so many visitors in the home often asking repetitious and seemingly impertinent questions. The nursing care plan must take into account the number of agencies to be coordinated, and the nurse must be prepared for the role of coordinator to fall on her because of her continuous and intimate involvement in the household.

Problems often arise when an old person is brought into the younger generation's family home. Some difficulties can be anticipated in advance and the nurse should help and encourage families to discuss the problems and plan carefully. Agreement should be established from the outset about such things as money, the running of the house, the bringing up of the children and—the cause of many a family squabble—radio and television programmes. The old person should not be pressurised into moving in, nor the young family excluded from the preparations and discussions. The old require solitude as well as care, and if possible they should have their own room in which they should be encouraged to entertain friends and to continue with old interests. The life style of the family should change as little as possible; for example, if the mother works she should continue to do so, and family holidays should not be stopped but rather a holiday arranged for the elderly relative at the same time.

Planning diversional therapy is important for elderly patients if they are to avoid being lonely and to retain a sense of achievement, but 'filling time' is not sufficient; the occupation must have a recognisable purpose. A knowledge of the patient's past life is important. All too often it is practical therapy that is suggested but not all patients have practical skills; some have intellectual gifts and training which they should be encouraged to continue and possibly to share with the less fortunate; for example, retired schoolteachers are often invaluable in giving individual coaching.

Implementation

Whatever the reason for nursing intervention, and for however long the need for direct care continues, when caring for an elderly person the nurse must concentrate on preventive as well as active treatment. Elderly people become very reliant on routine and therefore it is important for the nurse to enable such a routine to be kept as far as is possible. Relatives and patients need to be educated that ill-health is not normal; far too readily, bodily deterioration, pain and other symptoms are accepted as part of the normal process of ageing. A positive attitude must be encouraged towards the vital ancillaries to health as people grow older: the provision of the correct spectacles, regular dental care, hearing aids if necessary, well-fitting shoes and chiropody services. As the Royal College of Nursing said in evidence to the Royal Commission on the Health Service, 'It is more important to keep the elderly on their feet, with their shoes on, than to provide geriatric beds'.

Evaluation

Evaluation is dependent upon continual assessment and the constant examination of the carer's own attitudes, prejudices and beliefs. Although nurses and social workers may express delight in the provision of such facilities as day centres, clubs and organisations for the so-called 'lonely and socially deprived', they are not necessarily a panacea for the problems many old people encounter. It has been suggested that people who have never had close friends at other stages of their lives, or single persons, are less likely to be unhappy or lonely in old age: what they have never had they do not miss. One study found that the elderly did not consider that communication with their own age group was of much value. One lady said 'it is not good to stay in one age group, but to make friends with younger people than yourself as well as people who are older'. Another study showed that enforced family gatherings such as at Christmas time could be conducive to mental trauma.

As we reach even higher survival ages with the likelihood of more patients over the age of 85 years, we must accept that we have not only pushed back the frontiers of death but also the wavy line that denotes old age.

A key area in evaluation with the care of the elderly person is the evaluation of the carers. A large proportion of the elderly require constant or supportive care from relatives, friends or other care givers. Non-accidental injury is usually associated with children, but there is an increasing manifestation of it in the elderly. This problem was first recognised in the 1970s and it is now more readily accepted by the nursing, medical and social professions; it is usually termed 'granny bashing', although it is certainly not confined to elderly females.

Hardie[19] identifies predisposing and associated problems that lead to an elderly person being at risk from violence. These include family violence between generations, children reared in violent environments, who batter and find themselves battered in later years; and resentment of son or daughter towards an ageing parent. This latter situation is found more commonly with the single daughter living with an elderly mother. A recently bereaved parent may have reluctantly been taken to live with a son and daughter rather than face widowhood alone. Such situations cause stress in the household and can result in violence. The nurse must be aware of the possibility of the occurrence of violence, and remember that both the abuser and the abused will require skilled help.

In her evaluation and reassessment the nurse will have to consider whether it is still appropriate for the person to be cared for at home or whether a break and the provision of respite care could be to the benefit of all. Sometimes relatives will feel guilty or a failure if this is suggested. A recent study[20] showed that 12% of patients admitted to a hospital in London for a holiday break die of bronchopneumonia (the normal for such a group would have been 8.9%).

Over recent years the plight of the carers has been recognised and there is a very active national Association of Carers (see Appendix 3). Oliver[21] reminds us that with the exception of theatre work there is probably no single nursing or paramedical task that is not carried out in this country every day of the week by a lay carer. Injections, manual evacuation of the bowels, physiotherapy, dietary control, occupational therapy, care of pressure areas, attention to spiritual and emotional needs—all these are done by carers. She pleads 'why are they treated so harshly by so many professionals?'; and continues by pointing out that if just 1% of carers of the elderly gave up, the health and social services would have to increase their spending by 20% overnight.

Rogerson[22] in a very perceptive article entitled 'Ignore them at your peril' examined the needs of people looking after elderly relatives. She discovered a demand for more services, particularly short-term inpatient care, and a plea for greater understanding of the stresses of the job.

Evaluation in the care of elderly people, as in every area of nursing, needs to include evaluation of the carers and may well need a reassessment of the situation and a change in plan. Early intervention and assistance for stressed, overloaded carers can pay dividends in the long run.

References

1. Nicholson J. (1980). *Seven Ages*. London: Fontana.
2. Audit Commission for Local Authorities in England and Wales (1985). *Managing the Social Services for the Elderly more Effectively*. London: HMSO.
3. *Care in the Community and Joint Finance*. DHSS Circular HC(83)6 and LAC(83)5.
4. Allen I. (1983). *Short-stay Residential Care for the Elderly*. London: Policy Studies Institute.
5. British Medical Association (1986). *All our Tomorrows: Growing Old in Britain*; Report of the BMA's Board of Science and Education. London: BMA.
6. Phillipson C., Strang P. (1984). *Health Education and Older People: The Role of Paid Carers*. Keele: Health Education Council/Dept of Adult Education, University of Keele.
7. Dunnell K., Dobbs J. (1982). *Nurses Working in the Community*. London: HMSO.
8. Turton P. (1983). Health education and the district nurse. *Nursing Times: Community Outlook*, 10 August; p. 228.
9. McIntosh J., Richardon I. M. (1976) *Work Study of District Nursing Staff*. Edinburgh: Scottish Home and Health Department.
10. Anderson W. F., Caird F. I., Kennedy R. D., Schwartz D. (1982). *Gerontology and Geriatric Nursing*. London: Hodder Stoughton.
11. Age Concern (1977), *Profiles of the Elderly 4: Their Health and the Health Service*. Surrey: Age Concern Publications.
12. Mathieson A. (1986). Old people and drugs. *Nursing Times*, 8 January 1986.

13. Hamby R. C. (1984). *Geriatric Medicine: A Problem-oriented Approach.* London: Ballière Tindall.
14. MacDonald E. T., MacDonald J. B. (1982). *Drug Treatment in the Elderly.* Chichester: John Wiley.
15. Law R., Chalmer C. (1976). Medicines and elderly people: a general practice survey. *British Medical Journal*; **1:**565–8.
16. Brocklehurst J. C., ed. (1978). *Textbook of Geriatric Medicine and Gerontology,* 2nd edn. Edinburgh: Churchill Livingstone.
17. Pasker P., Thomas J. P. R., Ashley J. S. A. (1976). The elderly mentally ill—whose responsibility? *British Medical Journal*; **3:**164–8.
18. Kastenbaum R. (1979). *Growing Old.* London: Harper Row.
19. Hardie J. (1986). Violence and the elderly. *Journal of District Nursing*; **4:** 10 April 1986.
20. Rai G. S., Beilawaska C., Murphy P. J., Wright G. (1986). Hazards for elderly people admitted for respite (holiday admissions) and social care (social admissions). *British Medical Journal*; **292:**240.
21. Oliver J. (1985). Eight days a week. *Nursing Times*, 16 January 1985.
22. Rogerson B. (1984). Ignore them at your peril. *Nursing Times: Community Outlook*, 12 December 1984.

Further Reading

Carver V., Liddard P., eds. (1978). *An Ageing Population.* Milton Keynes: Open University Press.
Clarke L. (1984). *Domiciliary Services for the Elderly.* London: Croom Helm.
Cormack D., ed. (1985). *Geriatric Nursing: A Conceptual Approach.* Oxford: Blackwell Scientific.
Muir Gray J. A., McKenzie H. (1980). *Take Care of Your Elderly Relative.* London: George Allen Unwin.*
Redfern S. J. (1986). *Nursing Elderly People.* Edinburgh: Churchill Livingstone.
Storrs A. M. (1985). *Geriatric Nursing: A Concise Text.* London: Ballière Tindall.
Tinker A. (1984). *Staying at Home: Helping Elderly People.* London: HMSO.

*Suitable reading for relatives and lay carers.

Chapter 16

Terminal Care

In a secular society few people contemplate death and few prepare for it. In the nineteenth century death was freely talked about, but sex was a taboo subject: now the topics have been reversed. Nurses are not immune to this; hospitals, particularly teaching hospitals, generally have an ethos of 'cure' and death somehow represents failure. The chances are that nurses witness death comparatively rarely. Moreover, the district nurse is unlikely to be present when death occurs, but will frequently have considerable involvement with the patient and family in the period leading up to the actual death.

Before a nurse can give support to families where a patient is terminally ill, she must come to terms with her own attitude to death and her own particular prejudices and convictions. A purely academic approach is not enough; the nurse must face up to her own acceptance of mortality. All too frequently the trainee nurse has been given little support in this sensitive and personal realm. Using the nursing process approach to care should help to improve this understanding. Effective terminal care involves not only looking after someone in his last illness but also helping his family in both the short-term conditions of bereavement and in their continuing problems.

A key question that arises is whether the patient and/or his family should be informed of his condition. The doctor may well be the person who thinks he should make the decision but ideally this should be made by the team and each member should be aware of the decision taken. The district nurse being closely involved with the patient and family may be the person asked and she needs to be prepared to answer questions honestly. The plan of care will be influenced by the knowledge held by the patient and family. For various reasons some patients are not told they are dying and the reasons why this is so should be analysed objectively; all too often the patient is aware that something is being withheld from him, and this can create a 'cruel absence of care' because the patient needs to be able to communicate his fears about pain, solitude and death itself. By not telling the patient, the carers may be protecting themselves from facing up to an embarrassment that they would rather deny. Moreover, it is increasingly realised that the separation of the terminally ill from their family and familiar surroundings is inhumane and that people deserve to die as they themselves choose. However, unless patients are given all the facts how can they choose? If they are fobbed off with being taken into hospital for the wrong reason there is no choice. The way people are told—or not told—often reflects the carer's own attitude to death. Kubler-Ross[1] comments that 'the manner in which the news is broken depends on the doctor's own ability to face terminal illness and death.'

It is one thing to cope with the patients who know their own prognosis, but it is even more difficult to deal with the patient with a terminal illness who does not know. Before entering the home the nurse should always ask the question, 'Who knows the diagnosis?' and then plan her care accordingly. If the continued assessment of the patient and his family lead the nurse to decide that the patient would benefit from knowing his condition, the doctor should be told and new care plans agreed on to meet with the situation, if and when the patient and his family are told the prognosis.

The majority of deaths still occur in some kind of institution and death is rarely witnessed by the family and friends. However, recognition of the inhumanity of removal to hospital for terminal care, the advocacy of the right of the individual to choose where to die, and the comparative decline of the number of hospital beds, mean that the primary care team, and especially district nurses, are more and more frequently meeting patients who will die at home.

During the 1970s there was an increase in the development of hospices in the voluntary sector together with further interest shown by health authorities. The aim of the hospice is to focus on maximum comfort and to control symptoms when health restoration is no longer possible. Only a small proportion of patients requiring terminal care will be able to take advantage of hospice care; many will still prefer to remain in their own homes but the essential principle is to attempt to include something of the philosophy of hospice care in the home.

Assessment for care

'Terminal' care implies that active attempts at cure have ceased. In some instances the course the disease will follow can be anticipated and care planned accordingly. Dying is unique to every individual, and besides the assessment of progress of the disease there are other factors to be taken into consideration such as the patient's religious beliefs (or absence of them), his age and previous health, his acceptance or not of mortality, and his family commitments and relationships. Nursing care must be unique for the individual and the assessment must take into account all these facts. Knowledge of the religious beliefs of the patient is essential for two reasons. The first is that the wishes of the patient for spiritual help and succour must be respected, and priests and clergymen will generally visit homes if they are told of the need. Such arrangements should only be made at the request of the patient, but it must be remembered that sometimes spiritual comfort is not sought because the patient is denying the possibility of death; once death is accepted such aid may be suddenly requested. This does not necessarily reflect on the essential faith of the patient but is part of the process of coming to terms with death. The second reason concerns the provisions of total care; it can be devastating to the nurse to find that following the death of a patient the rituals and customs of his religion have not been observed. For example, at the death of a Jew the body should not be touched and the Rabbi should be called. As was stressed in Chapter 4, in order to ensure that religious beliefs are respected the nurse herself must have some knowledge of the basic tenets of the main religions as well as knowing the beliefs and wishes of her particular patients, with a special emphasis on those who are terminally ill.

When death is accepted it is common for the patient to wish to settle his affairs and to put things in order for those who are left behind. Mrs Baker will undoubtedly be concerned about the future care of her children, and the need for Sarah to be able to lead as normal a life as possible. If patients wish to talk in this way they should be encouraged to do so and not be deceived with, 'Don't worry yourself about it, we shall sort it out and care for everyone'. This is to take all responsibility away when in fact the reverse should be encouraged; encouragement towards the maintenance of present standards as opposed to the immediate encouragement of false hope. The assessment should include an estimate of the normal standards, and the nursing plan should attempt to maintain them. A home help may be one answer (although, as always, with the agreement of the patient) and in this case the home help would work under the directions of the patient. The standards of 'self' are important too; Mrs Baker is anxious to wash and dress herself carefully every day, probably to put up a good front for her children but perhaps simply because she has always been neat and tidy. The nurse might well observe that there are cosmetics and perfumes in the bedroom or bathroom that suggest the lady is particular about her appearance and tactful questions might reveal that she has her hair set once a week. If Mrs Baker is determined to keep herself looking as she did before illness intervened, for whatever reason, a voluntary group could be asked to take her to the hairdressers or to arrange for a hairdresser to visit the home. For men, daily shaving may be very important to self-esteem.

Fear of pain is common among those who are terminally ill, especially when the diagnosis is known to be a cancer. The work of Cicely Saunders[2] and the hospice movement has shown that even severe pain can be controlled, especially if drug therapy is combined with psychological stability. However, care in the hospice is continuous and can hardly be emulated in the home. It is therefore necessary for the nurse to gain the fullest information about drug therapy and to determine methods of reviewing drug effectiveness from the beginning.

This detailed information may be gained from nurses with specialist knowledge of symptom control, invariably Macmillan nurses who work in close association with a hospice, continuing care unit or symptom control clinic. Macmillan nurses are generally district nurses funded by the National Society for Cancer Relief for the first three years, then funding is continued by the health authority. As explained in Chapter 5 such nurses should be used as a consultant for advice and referral. In this way, patient and nurse can discuss the fear of pain, and plan together to meet changing needs. Special attention needs to be paid to the assessment of pain and other symptoms. Contrary to popular belief Saunders[3] has identified that as many as 50% of those dying from all malignancies have no physical pain at all, 10% mild pain, and 40% severe or intractable pain. Other distressing symptoms are those such as coughing, nausea, constipation, vomiting and diarrhoea, all of which require careful assessment regarding degree and discomfort.

Assessment of the family and/or other carers is essential. Kubler-Ross[1] states that the family of a dying patient will experience similar emotions to those of a dying person himself, including denial, anger, depression and finally acceptance, but not necessarily at the same time as the patient is experiencing these emotions.

Munley,[4] however, argues with Kubler-Ross's series of stages culminating in acceptance and does not believe all patients or families reach this stage. She highlights the passage from life to death as being a complex process filled with contradictions and conflicting tensions, and praises the extraordinary capacity of ordinary persons to face with sensitivity, integrity and dignity their own deaths or the deaths of those they care about. Again, care must be on an individual basis and the nurse will need to understand the dying process and to accept that relatives may actually stay away from a dying relative. This may not signify any lack of love, but merely that the relative is denying the imminence of death. Assessment of the family response should be based on the knowledge of the defence mechanisms that may be used.

The acceptance of the death of a loved one is different from the acceptance of one's own death. What actually is death, and what is on the 'other side'? Where does the dead person go? These are questions relatives may ask, and some may actually say that their own fear of death makes the prospect of somebody dying in their home—the home in which they must afterwards continue to live—unwelcome, frightening and eerie. While the well-being of the dying patient is important, so is the future well-being of those who will be left behind, and they will need support in their preparations.

There is a tendency to strip the dying of individuality, but if the district nurse makes a sensitive assessment of the patient and carers it should be possible to create a context where it is possible for the patient to 'live while dying'.

Planning care

Assessment and planning are made difficult when patients and their family demonstrate contradictions in need, and scorn caring activities or are even abusive in their derision of them. Contradictions are common where there is denial of terminal illness or where the patient wavers between acceptance and renewed hope. The fact that defence mechanisms are being used to excess must be the basis for the assessment of need and planning of care, and not the contradictory messages themselves. Where anger is turned upon the nurse, she may respond with a feeling of resentment or personal affront, rather than accepting the right and need of the individual to verbalise his inner feelings. Uncertainty about the therapeutic value of her relationship is bound to occur and the nurse herself may then be in need of support from colleagues who can listen and give objective support.

These two points highlight the difficulties that exist in formulating a nursing care plan for the terminally ill. The nurse may be confident of achieving a caring situation one day, only to find herself unable to communicate or contribute the next. Plans should not be changed rapidly, however, as a greater knowledge and understanding of the dying process will make clear. What, then, should the nursing care plan include?

Physical care will include the maintenance of bodily functions. Constipation may cause unnecessary suffering; ill-fitting false teeth (a common occurrence as weight is lost) will cause mouth ulceration and feeding difficulties; pressure sores will also cause unnecessary suffering and should be prevented; and, finally, there is the need to control pain and assist in the maintenance of appearance.

Psychological care should not include unrealistic reassurance or encouragement. The amputee or the agoraphobic must indeed be encouraged to look on the 'sunny side', or 'round the corner', but with the dying such phrases are meaningless. Silence, presence and touch are more important. Being with the patient in silence is an important nursing contribution in itself, and the time available needs to be utilised appropriately. The accent in planning care for the dying must therefore be on flexibility;

routines will be difficult to adhere to anyway because of the fluctuating and contradictory nature of dying.

Fear of solitude is common in those who expect death, and at the same time relatives and friends may deny the realities and stay away. Nurses may gain support at such times from the clergy, or from local self-help groups such as Dorothy House (Bath) and national organisations such as the Marie Curie Memorial Foundation. The latter will also provide a night-nursing service for the terminally ill, and the Foundation's existence is invaluable. Liaison between all involved in the planning of care is essential, and especially in the careful recording of drugs administered and any reaction to them. For example, if nausea and vomiting are significant side-effects the drug may need to be changed, or its route of administration altered.

Terminal illness entails an increasing loss of function and strength, and therefore an increasing degree of dependence. The nurse must plan for this, perhaps by bringing in a commode to be placed in the bedroom rather than allowing the patient to struggle to the toilet, or by setting up a 'sick room' downstairs so that the patient does not feel isolated when bed-bound nor the family tired out by constant running up and down stairs. If the nurse is to organise things in this way she will need to use all her skills in communicating her proposed plans to the patient in order to gain total agreement. Mrs Baker might well prefer to struggle with stairs and toilet, and put up with the tiredness, until such time as the children are all aware that their mother is dying. Or she might feel that the children must have the downstairs room in which to play and watch television while she has a period of solitude and quiet.

A state of increasing dependence in itself is often feared, and a feeling of demoralisation often develops as independence is lost. Here the expertise of the professional is often welcomed, because professionalism is accepted where the attentions of relatives would be embarrassing. This applies especially to intimate acts such as bodily washing and toileting. For example, someone like Mrs Baker may not wish to ask her daughter to empty commodes, clean her after toileting or wash her vulva. The nursing plan will take this into account if the reasons for the patient's requests are understood. If the emotional aspect is not recognised, the nurse could decide that the needs of the patient are simply for unskilled care, for anyone can empty commodes and assist with washing.

It is interesting to note that much of the literature about death and dying is concerned with the discovery and documentation of psychopathology or with the course that individual diseases and ageing processes will follow. There is very little written about the possibility of the dying patient facing death positively and actually gaining from the experience, and yet it is known that the patient's initial fear and denial of death will often disappear or decrease with the passage of time. The fact is that impending death can be coped with and nursing staff have a crucial role in building up a relationship of trust with the dying person, within which all fears—past and future—can be openly discussed.[5] Death is inevitable, and patients should be helped to prepare for it. This may involve assistance with making a will, and nurses should seek the help of a solicitor if at all possible (Chapter 22). Dying patients may also need to discuss their wishes to give personal items away to friends and relatives, and their arrangements to ensure those left behind are cared for adequately.

Any nursing care plan will not end at the death, but will continue to provide support for relatives. Schoenberg *et al.*[6] have highlighted the phenomenon of 'anticipatory' grief, the growing sense of bereavement in relatives and friends who are anticipating the loss of a loved one. Whether it occurs before death or at the time of death, friends and family should be encouraged to express their grief—be it by crying, shouting or walking away. Nurses are no longer 'taught' to maintain composure on meeting death and if composure is not felt, emotion must be accepted. This can help relatives in expressing their own grief, for when the professional in attendance makes no attempt to suppress emotions the role model is shown to be human.

The nurse who is planning the care of relatives could well follow guidelines concisely laid down by Schneidman[7]:

1   Total care of the patient needs to include contact with survivors-to-be.
2   Begin as soon as possible.
3   Remember that there will be less resistance in talking to a professional person, especially one who has no axe to grind and no pitch to make (e.g. nurse, doctor).

4 The role of negative emotions towards the deceased—
   anger, envy, guilt—needs to be explored, but not at the very
   beginning.
5 The professional plays the important role of reality
   tester—the quiet voice of reason.
6 Medical evaluation of the survivors is crucial. One should
   be alert for possible decline in physical health and in overall
   well-being.

Implementation of care

As discussed in Chapter 9 it is only possible in a book such as this
to discuss some principles underlying the implementation of care.
Skills (other than those providing physical care) that are
obviously required by the district nurse are those of teaching,
health education particularly in the area of tertiary prevention,
and counselling. In the latter the art of listening is of paramount
importance in the picking up of clues.

Nursing skills required by the district nurse to relieve the many
distressing symptoms that may be incurred by the patient with
terminal illness are detailed by Copperman[8] and Hector and
Whitfield[9] and it is not intended to repeat them here. As
mentioned earlier in this chapter drug administration is of key
importance; as the district nurse cannot always be present when
drugs are required the use of a syringe driver to ensure a
continuous supply of a specific drug and to keep the patient
pain-free is increasingly being used.

Evaluation of care

Evaluation of care should be continuous because changes in
patient and family need, especially psychological need, are
continuous. Change requires reassessment, which in turn will
lead to further changes in the nursing care plan, and a constant
need for re-evaluation.

The ultimate evaluation will be a consideration of whether the
patient died peacefully and with dignity and that the family and
other carers were helpful to cope with the distressing situation.
Many people will say that in caring for a dying person they

reached a sense of 'serendipity'; a word coined by Horace Walpole that means the faculty for making happy and unexpected discoveries by accident.

Conclusion

The nurse working with a dying patient requires a great deal of support, including the availability of colleagues with whom her personal reaction to an individual death can be explored. Nurses have their own beliefs, experiences and feelings about death, which may limit their ability to support their patients and their families if, for example, they are denying death when the patient has accepted it. Nurses should be able to end a nurse–patient relationship if that relationship is no longer therapeutic, and here the support and understanding of colleagues is vital.

The involvement of the district nurse does not necessarily end with the death of the patient. The majority of people will cope adequately with their grief but are likely to feel helped and supported by visits from staff who were involved in the care of the patient.

During the process of the illness the district nurse should attempt to anticipate which people are likely to suffer from abnormal grief reactions and this may help to determine the need to seek advice from suitably skilled personnel.

Bereavement visiting is not the prerogative of any one worker and the team as a whole should determine who is the most appropriate person. This will usually depend on which worker has been most involved with the patient and the family. Some people will gain support from joining one of the self-help groups such as Compassionate Friends (bereaved parents); Cruse (widows, widowers and their children); or an organisation set up in 1985 called BACUP (British Association of Cancer United Patients and their families and friends). See Appendix 3 for details of these organisations.

Death should not be viewed as a nursing failure, but it remains for the patient a highly significant experience, and a uniquely individual one. Terminal care as Eliopoulous[10] observes, 'requires a fine blend of sensitivity, insight and knowledge of the vast topic of death'.

References

1. Kubler-Ross E. (1969). *On Death and Dying.* New York: Macmillan.
2. Saunders C. (1972). A therapeutic community—St Christopher's Hospice. In: *Psychosocial Aspects of Terminal Care,* pp. 3–15. New York: Columbia University Press.
3. Saunders C. (1976). Control of pain in terminal cancer. *Nursing Times;* **72,** 26:13.
4. Munley A. (1983). *The Hospice Alternative—a new context for death and dying.* New York: Basic Books.
5. Earle A., Argondizzo N., Kutscher A. H., Goldberg I. K. (1976). *The Role of the Nurse in the Care of the Dying Patient and Bereaved.* New York: Columbia University Press.
6. Schoenberg B., Carr C., Peretz D., Kutscher A., Goldberg K. (1974). *Anticipatory Grief.* New York: Columbia University Press.
7. Schneidman E. S. (1976). *Death: Current Perspectives.* New York: Aronson Jason.
8. Copperman H. (1983). *Dying at Home.* Chichester: John Wiley.
9. Hector W., Whitfield S. (1982). *Nursing Care for the Dying Patient and his Family.* London: Heinemann Medical.
10. Eliopoulous C. (1980). *Geriatric Nursing.* London: Harper & Row.

Further Reading

Archer Copp L., ed. (1985). *Perspectives on Pain.* Edinburgh: Churchill Livingstone.

Cartwright A., Hockey L., Anderson J. L. (1973). *Life Before Death.* London: Routledge & Kegan Paul.

Epstein C. (1975). *Nursing the Dying Patient.* Virginia: Reston Publishing.

Jury D., Jury M. (1976). *Gramps.* New York: Grossman.

Kastenbaum R., Aisenberg R. (1972). *The Psychology of Death.* Berlin: Springer.

Marris P. (1958). *Widows and Their Families.* London: Routledge & Kegan Paul.

Meinhart N., McCaffery M. (1983). *Pain: A Nursing Approach to Assessment and Analysis.* New York: Appleton-Century-Croft.

Neuberger J. (1987). *Caring for Dying People of Different Faiths.* London: Austen Cornish.

Parkes M. (1986). *Bereavement: Studies of Grief in Adult Life,* 2nd edn. London: Tavistock.

Robbins J., ed. (1983). *Caring for the Dying Patient and Family.* London: Harper & Row.

Sims R., Fitzgerald V. (1985). *Community Nursing Management of Patients with Ulcerating/Fungating Malignant Breast Disease.* London: RCN Publications.

Sofaer B. (1983). *Pain: A Handbook for Nurses.* London: Harper & Row.

'My view you know is that the ultimate destination of all nursing is the nursing of the sick in their own homes . . . I look to the abolition of all hospitals and workhouse infirmaries. But it is no use to talk about the year 2000.'

Florence Nightingale (1867)

'The district nurse is a generalist who must be prepared to cope with any condition in any setting and must have the professional competence and awareness to identify when and where specialist help, of any form, is required . . . she must have the knowledge and ability to contact and acquire help in the best interests of her patients.'

Panel of Assessors: *Report on the Education and Training of the District Nurse* (1978)

Since information about the various services contributing to the patient's health and welfare is often neglected in the basic nurse training this section is devoted to an attempt to remedy that omission.

District nurses are often in close and confidential contact with their patients. Sometimes they are the only people visiting the home on a regular basis and are therefore most likely to know about the unmet needs of the patient and his family. Helping the patients to meet their wider needs is part of total patient care, since ill-health and disability are generally caused by the inter-relationship of many factors. For this reason it is important that district nurses understand the work and the policies of other disciplines and how, and from where, the patients may obtain help. Some patients, like John Davis, will need a vast range of services, others, like Mrs Cray, will need to be persuaded to use the services that are available, while a number will be capable of organising any help they may need for themselves. Each patient presents an individual pattern.

The history of the development of the various services for care is complex and inconsistent. Although the Beveridge report of 1942 hoped to produce an integrated and coherent plan for all the social services, for the most part the different services, and the benefits they each offer, have, like Topsy, 'just growed'. Each service stems from a different tradition. Some have their roots in the voluntary organisations, most have been subjected to change due to political or ideological considerations and all have been influenced, and continue to be influenced, by the vagaries of the financial situation.

Because of this complexity it is impossible to deal with each service in detail, but if the district nurse understands the organisation of the services, the principles which guide them and the main controlling legislation, the day-to-day details can be filled in from up-to-date guides, leaflets and nursing journals to which every district nurse should have access.

Some services are universal, that is to say they arise from the assumption that the state has a responsibility to protect a minimum standard for all citizens in such areas as health, education and incomes. The philosophy behind universality was that being the concern of all, and not merely the poor and the powerless, there would be pressure to keep standards high. On the other hand, the Beveridge concept of a minimum standard for all immediately raised problems, because first, flat-rate benefits linked to flat-rate contributions were necessarily low, secondly, what is subsistence level varies with households depending on their special needs and how they organise their budgets, and thirdly, poverty is relative. The poverty line shifts with the expectations of society; not being able to afford the expenditure necessitated by custom, such as sending your grandchildren birthday cards, represents social deprivation. However, to raise the universal benefits to cover all exigencies would be immensely costly, and there has to be some element of selectivity to deal with special needs. It is this selectivity with its complicated variations from service to service that makes the benefits and their entitlement so confusing; they are apt to change with differing ideologies and the district nurse should acquaint herself with the main changes in benefits as they occur (see Appendix 2 for easy reference).

Since finance is the main controlling factor in all services, and as its provision is a minefield of misconception, a chapter has been devoted to this. Not only is the National Health Service the service that concerns the district nurse most, but also for historical reasons it belongs to a different tradition from the other services. It is, in fact, the 'joker in the pack', so for these reasons it merits a separate chapter. However, the other social services are even bigger spenders of public money than the Health Service and it must not be forgotten that they can affect the health of the patient as much, if not more, than the provisions of the Health Service.

Finally, because district nursing is about the provision of nursing care, a chapter has been devoted to the development of nursing policies, both in England and the countries of the European Community, with particular reference to the effects that these changes of policy have had on district nursing in the past 50 years.

Chapter 17

Financing the Health and Social Services

Across the spectrum of the developed world social and health services are financed in a variety of ways. Each country structures and pays for its services according to its own needs and resources, and its philosophy towards social and health care. The method of finding money for such services depends on inter-related, but at times apparently arbitrary factors, so that countries with the same health needs may deliver and pay for their services in strikingly different ways. Countries influenced by the Catholic religion continued to emphasise the role of the Church and institutions in health care, while the Protestant countries stressed the importance of individual and family responsibility, and fostered the concept of domiciliary care, the family doctor and the parish nurse. Whether countries use more nurses and fewer doctors can often be traced to the historical position of women in particular countries. A high ratio of doctors in countries such as Italy tells us more about the position of women in Italy than it does about the present Italian health needs.

How much a country spends on its social services depends not only on its total wealth but also on the priority it gives to social and health needs. Obviously countries with a high *per capita* income can afford programmes undreamed of by poor agrarian societies, but whether spending is effective depends on the state of knowledge and technology, how the services are delivered and whether they are meeting the real needs of the population. High spending on health care does not necessarily produce lower mortality and morbidity rates. In this respect it is of little avail for developing countries like the oil states to buy expensive hospital technology when their real needs are those of an agrarian population for better sanitation and food distribution.

Because of their success in overcoming the hazards of poor sanitation and their control of infectious and parasitic diseases the developed countries are in stage three of the demographic transition and have an ageing and slowly growing population

(Fig. 2.1, page 13). The health and social problems of these countries are now complicated and obdurate and it is this fact above all others that accounts for their cost. The conquest of bacterial infection by controlling animal and human waste, and through immunisation programmes and antibiotic therapy, was comparatively cheap. There will be no second bonus.

With the proviso that the comparison of international statistics is fraught with difficulty, it will be seen from Fig. 17.1 that in 1983 the health service expenditure in the United Kingdom as a proportion of the gross national product was the lowest in the western world. Until recently Great Britain had been well up in

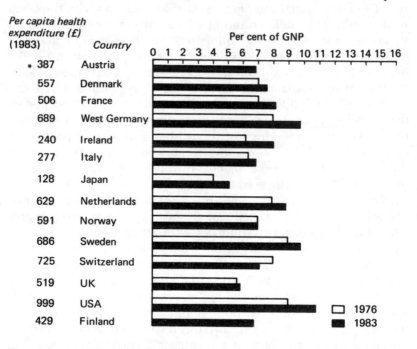

Note

* Public expenditure only
Average 1983 (excluding UK): 7.8 per cent of GNP
Average: per capita expenditure 533
Sources: IMF international financial statistics

Fig. 17.1. International comparisons of health care expenditure expressed as a proportion of GNP and per head of population, 1976 and 1983.

the perinatal and infant mortality rate league; now sadly it has fallen (Fig. 17.2) and it now has one of the highest infant mortality rates in the western world. Whether this high rate is due to low spending on health care is difficult to say; the United States, the highest spender on health care in the world, has a high infant mortality and perinatal rate and scores badly on other yardsticks by which the health of the nation is normally judged. On the other hand, Japan, apparently a low spender, has a low infant mortality rate.

Although the proportion of the GNP devoted to any service is important, other factors which are difficult to quantify are equally so, and these include barriers to the use of the services or the failure to deliver them to those whose needs are the greatest. In this respect it is worth considering the economy and the ideology of social services in the Scandinavian countries, whose performance in terms of health yardsticks has been universally good for medium expenditure expressed as a proportion of the GNP.

In 1974 Maxwell[1] analysed the health care systems in the developed world and placed them in a spectrum with those like the United States which rely heavily on private enterprise on the

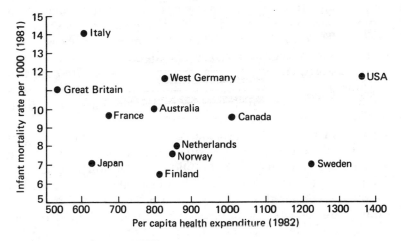

(Statistics provided by the DHSS)

Fig. 17.2. *Per capita* health expenditure (as a percentage of GNP) and infant mortality rate for Great Britain compared with other western countries, Australia and Japan (statistics provided by the DHSS).

right, and towards the left those like Britain whose services come mainly from taxation, with Russia, a fully collective society, at the extreme. In spite of these variations, the survey showed that no matter what the political philosophy, all systems were relying more and more on public finance; all were facing the ineluctable problems of soaring medical costs, higher wages and the fact that the main users of the service were the old, the disabled or the very young—in other words, those groups least able to pay charges or insurance premiums. In the United Kingdom the number of people over the age of 75 years has risen by 93% since 1951. In 1983 the amount spent in the hospital sector for each individual in that age group was £840 compared with the national average of £175.[2] The cost per week in a teaching hospital is now about £800 a week.

The British philosophy towards health care and the social services

Present health and social policies have their roots in the nineteenth century where the destitute were dealt with by the Poor Law and those above the pauper line, but in need and deserving, were often relieved by one of the charities so much a feature of Victorian England. This fact is important because the Poor Law system might have been the foundation of the welfare state, but unfortunately as it became more repressive after 1834 so it became more unpopular, and the twentieth century was concerned with finding an alternative to the Poor Law rather than an extension of it.[3]

Two important breaks with the Poor Law at the beginning of the century were crucial to the subsequent development of the social services. The first was the Old Age Pension Act of 1908 which provided a small pension to the low paid over the age of 70 years on a non-contributory basis; the other was the National Insurance Act of 1911, which, on the contrary, worked on the insurance principle and covered low-paid workers for unemployment benefit and medical treatment.

At the beginning of the Second World War the government set up a Reconstruction Committee under the chairmanship of Sir William Beveridge to prepare plans for the social services after the war. The Beveridge report, issued in 1942, was the foundation of all postwar social legislation and was built on the contributory scheme of 1911 to which various accretions had stuck like barnacles. There was a weekly contribution which provided for sickness, unemployment, old age, maternity, industrial injury and funeral benefits; both contributions and benefits were paid at a flat rate and it was envisaged that benefits would be sufficient to keep everyone above the subsistence level. But flat-rate contributions are hard on the low paid and therefore benefits had to be minimal. Beveridge, aware of this, argued that the scheme left scope for individual effort, thrift and voluntary endeavour. The scheme legislated for a pluralistic society, allowed for a certain freedom of choice and left room for that other traditional arm, the charitable organisation.

Imaginative though the plan was, it was soon in difficulty. The National Health Service interlocked with other social legislation, and budgets were prepared on the premise that once the backlog of illness was treated the nation would become healthier and demands for care would decrease. It was argued that the higher marriage rate would mean that fewer people were living alone and it was this group who were the high users of the service. It was not foreseen that earlier marriage meant a higher divorce rate, and also, that there would soon be an increasing discrepancy between the life expectancy of the sexes. Furthermore, it was not understood that good health care does not reduce the demand for care, it increases it. People live longer to have more incidents of ill-health, and good care of itself raises expectations.

The financial problems of the health service were exacerbated by inflation, the change in the demographic profile (Fig. 2.1, page 13) and the great increase in medical knowledge and technology.

As it was impossible to increase the flat-rate contributions steeply, the service was increasingly supplemented from general taxation. In 1948, to devote 3.5% of the GNP to the Health Service was considered exorbitant, and in 1953 the Guillebaud Committee was set up 'to find ways of avoiding a rising charge on the exchequer'. After 3 years, when the cost had risen by some £100 million, the Committee was unable to offer any alternative method of financing the service. The Royal Commission came to much the same conclusion 20 years later.

Financing the health and social services today

For half a century medical knowledge appears to have grown exponentially; more can be done for patients than there is money or manpower to achieve. Since not all needs can be met, choices must be made. But professional men and women pursue excellence and they do not like doing less than they know that they could if the resources were available, and this leads to conflict. Moreover, rationing the services and deciding who should receive organ transplants and who should be resuscitated usually falls on the professionals and this raises moral and ethical issues which create anxiety. On the other hand, if the government intervenes with guidelines, or consumer bodies offer advice, this is seen as 'interference with clinical freedom'.

The total budget for the National Health Service is now over £19 000 million, the steep rise in the past few years being mainly

Fig. 17.3. Comparisons of price indices in the NHS and the national economy: 1980 = 100 (by permission of HMSO).

attributable to rises in wages and salaries and the total wage bill (Fig. 17.3). After adjustment for inflation this is a *per capita* rise of 400% in 40 years. Nevertheless a slight drop in the proportion of the GNP spent on the health service in 1979 created an outcry because the Health Service needs at least another 1% on its budget each year to cope with the increasing numbers of elderly and to maintain existing services, with a further 1% increase to allow for advances in medical technology. Now the expenditure has crept up to 6.2% of the GNP but this is still woefully low and compares unfavourably with countries of a similar status in the European Economic Community. While other countries were spending more on health care, the proportion of the GNP spent in England actually fell in the period between 1983 and 1985, a fall that had considerable consequences for community care.

As there is no prospect of the total wealth of the country increasing, the next question is how the money should be divided between the competing services. Because of the fall in the number of schoolchildren it has been possible to reduce the amount of taxation allocated to education, but all the big spenders in the social services are in some way related to health. Health and welfare are intrinsically bound and although social security takes the biggest slice of government spending, pensions in England are lower than those in the leading EEC countries. It makes little sense to save the lives of pensioners in expensive intensive care units and return them to homes that they cannot afford to heat. Housing is fourth in the spending league, but to take money from that would mean more people suffering from ill health due to substandard housing, and more people like Mrs Adams continuing to cope with the inconvenience of an outside toilet. Even the smaller budgets for services like libraries impinge on health. Man does not live by bread alone.

Where the money comes from and where it goes

The 6.2% of the GNP now allocated to the National Health Service comes mainly from taxation, though there has been a slight fall in this proportion in recent years (Table 17.1). The contribution from the social security stamp has declined from 16% in 1962 to 10.8%, although in the past the proportion has been even lower than it is now. The 3% that comes from payments by patients includes about 0.5% from charges to private patients, while another small source of revenue comes from charges to insurance companies for road traffic accidents.

The total revenue from all sources is allocated by the Department of Health and Social Security on the basis of the Resource Allocation Working Party formulae which are currently under review by the government. The basic calculation for this uses population, mortality, socioeconomic statistics and the patient/bed ratio to obtain an index. The idea is to shift resources from rich regions such as Thames and Oxford to underfunded regions such as Northern and Merseyside.

Health authorities must spend their money within 'cash limits' which means that their allocation cannot be supplemented even when there are additional expenses such as large salary awards or changes in VAT; anticipated rises are allegedly accounted for in the original allocation. This is why government sources sometimes like to predict, or indeed threaten, that a rise in nurses' pay will mean a fall in services to the sick. Apart from keeping within their cash limits, health authorities have a statutory duty to spend within the broad guidelines and priorities laid down by the DHSS.

Table 17.1 Sources of NHS finance

Year	Taxation % NHS	NHS contribution % NHS	LHA % NHS	Patient payments % NHS	Total NHS £m
1951	82.3	8.3	8.2	1.2	503
1961	72.0	14.5	8.9	4.7	981
1971	80.2	10.0	6.6	3.2	2 323
1975	89.4	8.5	n/a	2.1	5 301
1981	87.6	9.8	n/a	2.7	13 729
1982	86.0	11.0	n/a	3.0	14 493
1983	86.5	10.7	n/a	2.9	16 375
1984	86.2	10.8	n/a	3.0	17 337
1986		breakdown not given			19 000

Notes: All figures relate to calendar year
Component items may not add up to totals because of rounding
LHA = former local health authority

Source: Statistics from the Office of Health Economics.

Alternative ways of financing health care

Many people argue that other countries can spend more on their health services because they are financed by insurance schemes or direct charges to patients, and that people are willing to pay more if they see a relationship between what they are paying and what they are receiving.

This argument ignores several facts. First, the high users of the health services are those least able to pay charges and it makes little difference whether they see a relationship between what they are paying and what they are receiving. In England over 60% of all patients are exempted from prescription charges, while in Germany it is calculated that if health charges continue rising at the present rate, and the years of retirement continue to lengthen, eventually workers will actually need to pay insurance contributions equal to their salaries. Secondly, ill-health strikes unevenly, and many of the long-term sick could not have made provision for such an eventuality however provident they might have been. Thirdly, as already mentioned, high spending does not necessarily produce better community health. Such yardsticks as we possess indicate no clear correlation between these variables. At times when England was one of the lowest spenders on health in the western world, she had also one of the lowest infant mortality rates and one of the best life expectancies. The USA, the highest spender shown in Fig. 17.2, has at present almost the highest perinatal rate, while Japan, the lowest spender, has one of the lowest perinatal rates and, incidentally, one of the best life expectancies. Finally, there is the problem of the what is the 'right' charge for an item of medical service, and there is evidence that fees and charges rise rapidly for the well insured.

Paradoxically, one reason why the British system apparently gives value for money is that, in spite of the fact that administration is the scapegoat for all its alleged ills, it is in fact comparatively simple, and the Royal Commission on the Health Service (1979) found no reason to believe that it was over-administered.

By no means everyone welcomed the National Health Service, and since 1948 a number of alternative methods of financing the service have been suggested—particularly by the medical profession. These range from state lotteries to the encouragement of private medicine and complex insurance schemes, or direct charges to patients at the point of delivery. Since the cost of the Health Service is an emotive issue all governments have tried to contain the costs, and most have explored the possibility of some charges, but even with the most determined 'market' approach, charges will only yield a fraction of the total cost. The Royal Commission came to the conclusion that even if patients were charged £20 a week for their stay in hospital (at 1978 prices) it would make little difference to the overall budget. Moreover, there is no concrete evidence to suggest that charges of themselves deter frivolous demands, and they might, as they did in the past, deter true needs. For example, would a charge of £5 for a visit to casualty be offset by a rise in long-term disability due to untreated wounds?

The strongest contender as an alternative system is that of a national, or seminational, insurance scheme on an actuarial basis like motor insurance. However, this is not as simple as it sounds; if the scheme were national and earnings-related it would be indistinguishable from income tax, and few people would see the relationship between the charge and the service provided. If, on the other hand, there were options for different premiums, like private insurance schemes at the moment, with the users reimbursed depending on their coverage, this would lead to higher administrative costs, hardship for the underinsured, a divisive service and different standards of care given to different patients, a prospect that most doctors and nurses find distasteful. Perhaps the most compelling argument against changing the system now is that most countries relying on such schemes are in difficulties and every European country is facing the fact that costs and claims are rising faster than either wages or the GNP.

Dividing the cake in the National Health Service

Since neither the GNP nor the proportion allocated to health care are likely to rise in the future, and there seems little hope of finding finance from elsewhere, we are left with the problem of making fairer and more efficient use of the £19 000 million we are currently spending. There are two main ways in which distribution might be changed; geographically, and between the different branches of the service.

Geographically

Historically the health services have always been unevenly distributed. In the voluntary system where honorary doctors gave their services free to the hospitals, but made their money out of private patients, they tended to concentrate in London and the south-east where more private patients lived. This tendency was aggravated by the depression of the late 1920s when there was a southern drift of the population; but for climatic, occupational and socioeconomic reasons the greatest health needs were in Wales and the north. In 1842, Edwin Chadwick (1800–90) noted that the labourer in Liverpool had half the life expectancy of the labourer in the rural south; this discrepancy, although less marked, has continued. The north still has an infant mortality rate higher by five per thousand than the most favoured region, and one-third more deaths among children under 14 years. However, to suggest that a redistribution of the health services would of itself change the position is to misunderstand the relationship of the curative health services to prevention. 'There are many reasons why chronic sickness or days lost from work are higher in the north than in the south; lack of provision of hospital beds is not one of them.'[4] In 1980 the working group chaired by Professor Sir Douglas Black reported concern about continuing inequalities in the health of the nation; the chances of pregnancy ending in a dead baby are twice as high for the wife of a manual worker as for the wife of a doctor, lawyer or university professor, and this discrepancy, and others like it, have continued unchanged for the past fifty years. This has been confirmed since by the report *The Health Divide* (1987).[5]

In 1976 the Resource Allocation Working Party (RAWP) produced formulae by which populations, weighted by the indicator of mortality experience, received more according to their need, the favoured areas marking time. When the Health Service budget was increasing, such plans, though crude, were acceptable, but in a period of retrenchment it means that the 'giving' areas actually suffer cuts and the 'receiving' areas merely mark time. Now the rough justice of the RAWP formulae are questioned; poor health is due to more things than are controlled by the National Health Service.

Distribution of money between the branches of the service

The acute general hospitals have always attracted more money; the interesting and the dramatic afforded prestige, and prestige brought in donations and medical students. On the other hand, the medical services that grew up under the shadow of the Poor Law were poorly provided and housed. The first budget in 1948 was allocated according to the current costs of the service at that time. The poor remained poor.

The reorganisation of 1974 did nothing to alter the allocation of resources, but the Family Practitioner Service remained outside the control of the health authorities as an open-ended service, and as this service does not operate with cash limits it gets proportionately more during a time of retrenchment. Although it is agreed that an increase of resources for primary care is desirable, this is a haphazard method of distribution and does nothing to encourage planning.

From time to time the health departments issue guidelines about the need to move capital and revenue resource to the underprivileged branches of the service. However redistribution is slow because over 70% of hospital costs goes on salaries and wages, and short of dismissing staff there is little that can be done about this. Moreover, because medical training is expensive it is axiomatic that all who train as doctors must be found posts and the number of medical students qualifying has increased by one-third in 10 years. All consultant posts have a revenue consequence and many have nursing manpower consequence. However, as hospital costs rise the greater is the need to return the patient to the community quickly. The beds are then filled by more patients needing expensive care and so hospital costs spiral; the quick turnover creates a vicious circle, generating as it does ever more work for the community.

In the past 10 years the number of district nurses has risen by about 30%, but their official working week has been reduced and their holidays increased. In spite of this district nurses have treated just over twice as many people and made half a million more home visits, the majority of which were to people over 65 years.[6] Although visits are not separately given for the over-85s, these must have increased and are likely to be time consuming.

Apart from this, district nurses are treating twice the number of physically handicapped and otherwise disabled people under 65 years old than they were doing 10 years ago. The policy of community services for the disabled is praiseworthy, but it founders on lack of manpower and resource. In this respect it is a matter for concern that there has been a fall in the number of student nurses qualifying in recent years. Even more alarming, in the light of proposals for increased community care, is the fact that the number of nurses entering district nurse training in 1986 was virtually unchanged from the previous 4 years.[7]

The future of the health services

Resources for health care are finite and must be used effectively. The government has set up 'cost-effect' studies under the chairmanship of Lord Rayner. However, obsession with cost-effectiveness can have dangers and ethical consequences; can we, for example, balance the cost-effect to the community of so many more years of working life for a patient by giving him a transplant, against the diversion of money from such things as long-term or preventive medicine? It may be cheaper not to overlap nursing shifts in hospital, but this ignores the fact that hospitals should also be places of nurses' education.

One way of employing resources more effectively, although in the long run it will not be cheaper, is to make people aware of their personal responsibility for their own health. Much current ill-health is due to unwise habits and behaviour, which include the effects of alcohol, inappropriate (if expensive) diets, smoking, addiction to drugs (whether prescribed or otherwise), and the effects of air and water pollution by a society on the make. It makes little economic sense to push up tobacco sales in order to garner tax and at the same time spend millions on thoracic surgery—and, equally perversely, fail to use the media for health education because it is 'too expensive'. Nor does it seem logical to plan more drug-addiction centres and not spend money on prevention and education, or to pour money into research for AIDS but fail to educate the public on its means of transmission.

The district nurse, so often in a long and close relationship with her patients, is in a position to influence them by example and advice. This was the chief role of the early district nurses. Miss Nightingale, writing about the aim of district nursing in 1887, said it was

'putting the home in good healthy order, teaching the family to keep it in good order, how to help nurse, knowing how to teach Sanitary Authorities to do what individuals cannot do for themselves. . . . Above all by teaching them self-help and healthy ways and habits, besides, of course, the best skilled sick nursing at the poor people's homes.'

References

1. Maxwell R. (1974), *Health Care: The Growing Dilemma*. McKinsey Survey.
2. Office of Health Economics (1985). *Health Service Statistics: The Cost of the National Health Service*. London: OHE.
3. Fraser D. (1973). *The Evolution of the British Welfare State*, p. 50. London: Macmillan.
4. Royal College of Nursing (1977). *Evidence to the Royal Commission on the National Health Service*. London: RCN Publications.
5. The Health Education Council (1987). *The Health Divide: Inequalities in health in the 1980s*. Health Education Authorities. London: HMSO.
6. *Social Trends* (1985). London: HMSO.
7. United Kingdom Central Council for Nursing, Midwifery and Health Visiting (1985). *Annual Report 1984–85*. London: UKCC.

Further Reading

Brown R. G. S. (1978). *The Changing National Health Service*. London: Routledge & Kegan Paul.

Garner L. (1979). *The NHS—Your Money or Your Life*. Harmondsworth: Penguin.

Institute of Health Services Management/British Medical Association/Royal College of Nursing (1985). *Public Expenditure on the NHS: Recent Trends*. London: IHSM/BMA/RCN.

Office of Health Economics (1984). *Understanding the NHS in the 1980s*. London: OHE.

Open University (1985). *Caring for Health: Dilemmas and Prospects*. Milton Keynes: Open University Press.

Royal College of Nursing (1984). *Nurse Alert*. London: RCN Publications.

Townsend P., Davidson N. (1982). *Inequalities in Health: the Black Report*. Harmondsworth: Penguin.

Chapter 18

The Development of the National Health Service

The hospital services of the nineteenth century developed along three main lines: the voluntary system with its roots in the charity hospitals; the provisions of the Poor Law, which eventually came under the aegis of local government and at the end of the century extended hospital services to non-paupers; and the mental hospitals, which were first under the Lunacy Commission, then in 1913, under the Board of Control.

There were also lines of health care in the community: some, like the Queen's District Nurses or the 'Lady Health Missioners', had their origins in voluntary societies; others, like the school health service, came into being because of legislation and were statutory. For the sake of convenience the statutory community services, and often their associated welfare services, were placed under the control of the local authority public health department and the medical officer of health.

The health services evolved piecemeal to meet changing needs, with the voluntary services often showing the way; but although this rich variety provided adaptability and flexibility the services were confused, unevenly distributed and full of anomalies. More importantly, by the 1930s many health services were almost bankrupt and all the strategems of 'popular' insurance schemes, charges to patients, national and local appeals and flag days were merely the rearranging of the deckchairs on the *Titanic*; the new possibilities of medicine and the expectations of patients were about to overwhelm the ship.

The structure of the national health service

In spite of the fact that plans for a comprehensive health service had been discussed since 1909, when the Beveridge proposals were put forward in 1942 the various vested interests could not agree, and the 1944 White Paper aroused deep passions and positive hostility from the British Medical Association. In order to break the deadlock Aneurin Bevan, Minister of Health in the new Atlee administration, produced a compromise solution which largely gave the services back to the people who had run them before and was particularly generous to the medical interest. The National Health Service Act of 1948 took the services as they had developed so far and fixed them by legislation; it was, as it were, a snapshot of the services as they had evolved by 1948 (Fig. 18.1).

The structure exhibited many of the old historical divisions. The main change was that all types of hospitals were brought together within the Hospitals and Specialist Services division; but even here some of the old dichotomies remained, with the mental hospitals having separate management committees and the teaching hospitals remaining outside the control of the regional hospital boards. The service was tripartite, with each division funded from a different source. The administration of the hospitals was delegated to regional hospital boards consisting of members appointed by the Minister; the boards devolved responsibility to hospital management committees, who were accountable for the day-to-day running of the hospitals in their group, but the teaching hospitals had separate boards of governors and were directly responsible to the Minister. The general practitioners, who had been particularly vociferous in opposition to the service, managed to retain their independent status and had a contract *for* service, not *of* service, and were remunerated through executive councils by *per capita* payments and a complicated system of reimbursement for practice expenses. The general practitioners retained their independence but the price they paid was their isolation from other branches of the service. The local authorities lost control of their municipal hospitals but retained responsibility for the community health services which now included the domiciliary nursing services, preventive medicine and most of the personal social services. A divorce had been made between preventive and curative medicine and between the institution and the home, but at least the community health and the social services remained in wedded partnership in spite of matrimonial quarrels.

Fig. 18.1. The NHS in England and Wales in 1948 (from *Understanding the NHS in the 1980s*. London: Office of Health Economics).

Criticism of the national health service—Green and White Papers

The National Health Service achieved its broad objective. A reasonable standard of health care became available to all citizens whatever their financial position and when charges were made there were usually exemptions. Furthermore, as Chapter 17 has shown, by such crude measuring rods as we have, it gave value for money. Nevertheless there was much to criticise. First, because the service was a compromise it inherited the old—and often outdated—priorities and it was primarily an 'Ill-health Service' with the prestige, money and manpower going to acute general medicine. Secondly, the services, including the ancillary services like dentistry, were geographically unevenly distributed, and branches of health care like mental health and long-term care received proportionally far less than general medicine. Thirdly, because of their divisions the services were poorly coordinated and communication between the different parts was poor or non-existent, and in addition their complicated structure made them bewildering to the average citizen. As late as 1966 the survey *Feeling the Pulse*[1] showed that district nurses were often working in isolation and that general practitioners were ignorant of their nursing qualifications, frequently sending their patients to hospital for treatment that was well within the scope of the district nurse. Moreover, hospital staff, lacking understanding of the patient's home conditions and having little contact with the community health services, often sent patients like Mr Adams home to unsuitable conditions with no proper provision for further care. In fact the Dan Mason research study *Home from Hospital*[2] is full of such examples. Surveys like this and *Care in the Balance*[3] brought home to the health professions that the barriers in the service were being paid for in terms of unnecessary suffering; and it was these reports, as much as anything, that made people take a more urgent look at the need to unify the services.

Meanwhile, as professional conferences discussed 'unification' those working in the community health services embarked on experiments to make the delivery of care better coordinated and more effective. District nurses and health visitors in some areas were 'attached' to specially selected groups of general practition-ers, and by 1963, these experiments provided an impetus for the Committee on the Future Scope of General Practice.[4] This committee, under the chairmanship of Dr Annis Gillie, found that many elderly patients needed a variety of services but they were often unaware that these services existed or of their entitlement to them—a finding of both *Home from Hospital* and *Care in the Balance*. To overcome these problems the committee recommended that district nurses, health visitors, midwives and social workers should be attached to group medical practices to form a *primary care team*. Within the next 10 years 60% of all health visitors and most district nurses were attached to group practices, and while there were losses as well as gains, most participants would agree that communication has improved even if in some cases the 'team' concept is more honoured in the breach than in the observance (Chapter 5).

The reform of the social services

While the Minister of Health, Kenneth Robinson, was preparing the first Green Paper on the unification of the health services in 1968, the social workers were looking at their future. The personal social services, like the health services, had developed from voluntary organisations and the Poor Law; some were offshoots of other services like education, and some had come from the public assistance committees of the 1930s. But poverty and ill-health are linked, as Edwin Chadwick showed in 1842[5] and the Black committee demonstrated in 1980[6] and the health and social services frequently dealt with the same users. Therefore, when the local authorities, set up after the 1888 Act, took more responsibil-ity for the personal social services they found it simple to group them under the Medical Officer of Health. However, there is no denying that the services were confused, with different authorities trying different administrative patterns. By the 1960s the social workers themselves were anxious to improve their training and career structure; indeed, many of their problems were analogous with those of the nursing profession in the nineteenth century when they tried to establish themselves as a profession.

Because of these factors, and new attitudes towards social

problems, in 1966 a committee was set up under the chairmanship of Sir Frederic Seebohm, 'to review the organisation and responsibilities of the local authority personal social services in England and Wales and to consider what changes are desirable to secure an effective family service'.

The report, which was published in 1968, concluded that the only solution to the present confusion was the establishment of an independent social services department in each local authority under the control of a Director of Social Services. The report was welcomed by the social services, and in spite of warnings from the Central Health Services Advisory Committee about the need to keep health and welfare integrated, the Local Authority Social Services Act came into force in May 1970.

The reform of the health service

Ever since a 'health service' was first considered in 1909 many people thought that the logical structure would be within the framework of local government, and the first plan for the National Health Service in 1944 was based on this concept. However, although this was a tidy solution it had become increasingly impractical. First, the cost of the health service was now so great that it would destroy the delicate balance between the rates and the exchequer grant and, secondly, the medical profession thought such a plan would interfere with their clinical freedom and they would not cooperate with such a scheme. However, since health depends largely on other social services and factors outside medicine it is important that the administration of the health and social services be viewed as a whole and concurrently. Once the social services were placed firmly within local government the reform of the health services had to be linked with the reform of local government.

The Royal Commission on Local Government, set up in 1966, reported in 1969 and recommended that outside the metropolitan areas there should be about 61 'unitary' authorities, which it was thought, would be large enough to deal with the demands of the modern services and small enough to have a local identity. The Royal Commission's report (Redcliffe-Maud) was accepted in principle and new plans for a reformed health service were put out based on the unitary authorities, that is to say a single-tier health authority covering an area much the same as the 'single district' areas. In May 1970 the Labour administration fell from office.

The reorganisation of the health service

The incoming administration rejected the plans for a reformed health service and much of the report of the Royal Commission on Local Government, and prepared a new White Paper on local government reform which was in fact the basis of the Local Government Act of 1972. This act provided for a two-tier system with 44 county councils covering the old traditional boundaries and 6 new ones like Avon and Teesside carved out of old counties. Below the county council tier there was the district council which was to be responsible for services like housing and slum clearance, refuse collection and amenities such as parks, although some services, confusingly, involved both types of authority. The structure of the local authority service and the fact that the social services were now under the aegis of the new county councils, determined the shape and structure of the reorganised health services. The Secretary of State for the Department of Health and Social Security consulted with the Brunel Institute of Organisation and Social Studies whose advice was reflected in the policy of consensus management with 'maximum decentralisation and delegation of decision-making downwards matched by accountability upwards'.

The structure

In order to unify the services, which was the *raison d'être* of the exercise, the personal health services, including of course the district nurses, were brought under the control of regional health authorities (which covered the same areas as the old Hospital Boards). Scotland, Wales and Northern Ireland had their own health departments and organised their services on similar lines except they had no 'regional' tier.

Below the regions there were area health authorities (Fig. 18.2) based on the 44 units of local government outside London. The areas were intended to be conterminous with the local authorities,

Fig. 18.2. The NHS in England in 1974 (by permission of HMSO).

with which they were to set up liaison committees, while the special needs of the teaching hospitals were met by designating certain areas as 'teaching'. Because they were based on the old counties the area health authorities were uneven in size; some were so large that they had to be divided into six districts, while others were 'single-district areas'. The other outstanding anomaly was the fact that in England the area health authorities were not given responsibility for the family practitioner services; the area health authority was responsible for the administrative costs of the family practitioner committees but the real costs of the services—the money which was paid to the general practitioners who provided the services as independent contractors—was paid directly from centrally held funds.

Criticism of the reorganised health service

Although it was agreed that the health services must be unified and reorganised the proposals when they came met with much criticism and hardly any journal on health matters expressed approval. First, the health services were divorced from the social services, and no papering over the cracks could disguise this; secondly, there was concern about the loss of the Medical Officer of Health with his distinctive role; thirdly, there were still anomalies—for example, the teaching hospitals were still set apart and the family health services were outside the main structure. Now this lack of coordination affected district nurses in a way that it had not done in 1948, for now most district nurses were attached to family practices.

The loudest complaints, however, were about the structure of the service. It was alleged that the number of tiers of management would delay decision-making and would be expensive of resources. Moreover, it soon became clear that consensus management and worker participation without sensible discrimination would mean a vast increase in the number of committees, and one authority reported having to consult with 26 committees before any decision could be taken. In 1976, the government having changed again, the Wilson administration appointed a Royal Commission, whose job was 'to consider in the interests of both the patient and those who work in the National Health Service the best use and management of the financial and manpower resources of the National Health Service'.

The Commission's report of 1979 made it clear that by no means all the problems of the National Health Service stemmed from reorganisation and that many were there before 1974. However, they pointed out that inasmuch as managerial problems arise from the structure of the service itself, these problems were due to the fact that each 'tier' of management had a team of officers and each member of the team was responsible to the appointing authority for the services in his or her control. This meant that an authority with six districts had to deal with seven teams and some 31 chief officers, but area officers were only advisory, and although they had a duty to 'monitor' they were not empowered to instruct if they did not like what they monitored. In this situation, matters that were once dealt with by the head of a department were now passed up and down the management chain.

The Commission agreed that the management arrangements of the service were cumbersome, but it recommended that the regions should be retained and given more power and a positive financial role. Below the region there should only be one management tier carrying operational responsibility for supplying services and cooperating with local government. The Commission advised that 'these authorities should be formed from existing single district areas and by merging districts or by dividing areas'. It was stressed that the new pattern should be flexible and should take into account geographical, historical and demographic considerations.

The Commission saw the community health councils as having the two-fold task of representing the public to the health authority and of informing the public about the health services. The councils had been more successful with the former task largely because they lacked resources and were not sufficiently involved by the authorities, and of course, because they had been excluded from anything to do with the family practitioner services. The Commission recommended that the community health councils should be strengthened.

Reorganising the reorganisation

In the life cycle of confrontation politics, the incoming Conservative administration did not accept all the findings of the Royal
Commission. It did, however, agree that criticisms of the 1974
structure were well founded, and it therefore, in 1982, issued a
document entitled *Patients First*, which in spite of its title was about
management structure rather than patient care. In particular it
sought to devolve decision-making within districts to a point
nearer the level at which the services were actually delivered, by
the creation of 'management units'. How services were divided
into units was left for the districts to decide; the definition of a
large hospital or group of hospitals as a unit was a relatively
obvious choice, but units were also based on services for particular
client groups (e.g. psychiatric services) and community nurses up
and down the country lobbied hard to ensure that in most places
community health services were managed by a community unit.
The management arrangements at the new unit level mirrored
those at district and regional level—a consensus team consisting
of a nurse (the director of nursing services), an administrator, and
(depending on the type of unit) one or more doctors.

The Griffiths reorganisation

As far as health services are concerned, politicians are like
children with a kitten—they cannot leave it alone. Before the 1982
reorganisation was complete and before the new unit teams were
fully established, another enquiry into NHS management
arrangements was set up under the chairmanship of Roy Griffiths,
the managing director of Sainsbury's. The Griffiths enquiry
directly reflected the current government's policy in other fields,
namely that managerial decision-making needed to be speeded up
and strengthened and that there should be much stricter financial
control.[7] The concept of consensus management (by a multidisciplinary team of equals) was replaced by the concept of general
management (a single individual who would be responsible and
accountable for the whole enterprise, in particular the control of
the budget). The Griffiths recommendations were accepted by the
government for immediate implementation in England. The

arrangements for Scotland and Wales were slightly delayed and have been implemented rather differently.

At central government level a new Health Services Supervisory Board chaired by the Secretary of State was established to be responsible for the determination of the broad direction of the services and strategic decisions. To plan and ensure the implementation of the Supervisory Board's broad policies the NHS Management Board was established under the chairmanship of a general manager and included directors of finance, personnel, and procurement (supplies) drawn from the highest echelons of industry. However, when the first chairman resigned, the reality of the political as opposed to the purely managerial functions to be performed at this level was recognised by his replacement by a government minister.

At health authority level (regions and districts) each chairman was required to appoint a general manager whose first task was to review the management structure within the regions and districts, in particular to use the concept of general management to devolve decision-making as near as possible to the level of services to the patients, and to abolish separate functional management structures (e.g. nursing). It was anticipated that many of the new appointments would come from outside the NHS, for example from industry, but managers of any discipline within the NHS could also apply; the Secretary of State hoped that doctors in particular would by this means be drawn into management. In the event relatively few 'outsiders' and a very few nurses were appointed general managers at regional and district level (Fig. 18.3).

Unlike previous reorganisations, guidance from the centre (e.g. DHSS circulars) about how the changes were to be implemented was deliberately avoided, and structures below the level of the district general manager (DGM) vary widely across the country. In many areas the units established in 1982 were changed, and this in some places has led to the breaking up of community units into units based on 'programmes' such as 'services for the elderly' or 'child health and women's services', or the amalgamation with other units, for example psychiatric and mental handicap services. In the pursuit of the concept of general management, as opposed to consensus management, a unit general manager was

Fig. 18.3. The NHS in England in 1984 (by permission of HMSO).

appointed to each unit and the consensus team (the unit management team) was abolished. At unit level about 10% of general manager's posts were filled by nurses.

Although the Griffiths report explicitly stated that its proposals would not necessitate any major reorganisation of services, the management arrangements that have emerged constitute—especially for nursing—a reorganisation far more fundamental than either the 1974 or the 1982 reorganisations. The concept of general management, and in particular the general manager's personal accountability for managerial and financial control, has meant that nursing services are no longer managed or financially controlled by nurses. At health authority level the chief nursing officer no longer manages the nursing service or holds the nursing budget; the post is now advisory only, and is often combined with other functions such as quality assurance. Similarly, at unit level, the director of nursing services may also be merely advisory; in some places, the post has disappeared altogether.

It is important that district nurses working at field level recognise and fully understand the implications of these changes for their day-to-day work. In areas where a community unit is retained and proper authority is delegated by the unit general manager to a director of nursing services, the district nurse may continue to be able to look for support to more senior and experienced nurses; in other areas she may be much more vulnerable. In these circumstances the nurse must fully understand the implications of her professional and legal accountability as a nurse. The UKCC has stated that

> 'In implementing the general management concept, due account should be taken of the professional responsibilities of nurses, midwives and health visitors and nothing should be done which would undermine their ability to fulfil their professional responsibilities and so place them at risk in the context of the Code of Professional Conduct of the UKCC.'[8]

These issues are discussed in Chapter 22.

Family practitioner committees

Meanwhile changes were also taking place in the family practitioner services. Under the Health and Social Security Act

1984, family practitioner committees were reconstituted as independent health authorities alongside the regional and district authorities. Their statutory responsibilities now include, in addition to administering the family practitioners' contracts, responsibility for joint planning of services with other health authorities and the control of their own administrative costs and the staffing arrangements. Membership of the revised committees must include a community nurse. Unfortunately, however, the boundaries of the FPCs remain as they were established at the time of the 1974 reorganisation, so they are not conterminous with district health authorities; one FPC may relate to four or five district health authorities, or one district authority may relate to one or two FPCs.

The primary health team

From the point of view of the individual patient, however, the organisational complexities of the National Health Service are at best an irrelevance, at worst a nuisance. It is part of the responsibility of the district nurse to ensure that the organisational systems, however complex or unsatisfactory, do not impede or reduce the standards of nursing care the patient is entitled to expect and to receive. The district nurse continues to act professionally within the context of a multi-disciplinary primary health care team who, even though they may be individually employed by different agencies or within different management units, must communicate and cooperate to provide an integrated and comprehensive service to the patient.

The choices about how money is spent are made mainly by professionals and clearly their opinion is of importance, especially about the possibilities (or dangers) of a particular course of care. But in a service which is mainly about non-curable complaints where what is being provided by the service is mostly intervention and support, it seems sensible that the general public should have the opportunity to express a view on whether they want more home helps and 'meals on wheels', or whether they wish to see more hospital beds and transplant surgery. Mrs Cray might well prefer a ground-floor flat to anything the health service can offer, an indoor toilet might be more beneficial to Mrs Adams than drugs for her arthritis, while cuts in school meals could devastate the Johnson family.

The medical profession decides who in society is 'ill'; as a corollary it plays an important part in making the decisions as to how the money should be allocated to those labelled 'ill'. The time has come to modify this concept.[9]

Health for all by the year 2000

A WHO Expert Committee in 1985[10] suggested that within the context of the development of health care in the western world three broad and overlapping historical periods can be identified:

1   The individual care era (up to the 1950s): in which emphasis is placed on curative medicine, services are provided for as many people as can reach them or seek them out, and the doctor is the key health-care provider with the nurse acting as his assistant.

2   The community care era (the 1960s and 1970s): in which curative care is still the key service, but the role of social factors in health and the importance of preventive medicine are increasingly recognised; the health-care system differentiates between a high-technology hospital system and a system of local facilities which depend less on medical interventions.

3   The health for all/population care era (the 1980s and 1990s).

The history of the National Health Service described in this chapter shows that the United Kingdom's health services, like those of most of Europe, is currently in the second phase. Until recently few countries in Europe had formulated broad health policies designed to make health care universally accessible or to improve the health of the population as a whole. During the 1970s countries with highly developed health-care systems began to be concerned at the rapidly escalating demands of their populations for increasingly sophisticated and expensive services which nevertheless seemed to have no impact on general mortality and morbidity levels.

The year 1977 marked the turning point towards the third phase. In that year at the World Health Assembly the member states of WHO (including the UK) resolved that 'the main social target of governments and WHO in the coming decades should be the attainment by all citizens of the world by the year 2000 of a level of health that will permit them to lead a socially and economically productive life.' The following year at Alma Ata all countries signed a declaration which identified the development of primary health care as the means of achieving this goal and committed themselves to a global strategy. In 1984 the European region (including the UK) expressed its strategy in the form of 38 targets to be achieved, 65 statistical indicators that would continuously measure the progress—or lack of it—made by each country, and agreed to report back to WHO the result of their monitoring every 2 years.

Since 1978 many European countries have begun to reorientate their health policies and their health services towards the concept of primary health care. In the UK the process has begun slowly but is gathering momentum. The implications for community nursing are momentous. As Dr Halfden Mahler, the Director General of WHO, has pointed out:

> 'If the millions of nurses in a thousand different places come together and articulate the same ideas about primary health care they could act as a power-house for change. I believe that such a change is coming and that nurses will greatly help to bring it about.'

References

1. Hockey L. (1966). *Feeling the Pulse*. London: Queen's Nursing Institute.
2. Skeet M. (1968). *Home from Hospital*, 4th edn. London: Macmillan.
3. Hockey L. (1968). *Care in the Balance*. London: Queen's Nursing Institute.
4. *The Future Scope of General Practice* (Gillie report, 1963). London: HMSO.
5. Chadwick E. (1842, reprinted 1965). *Sanitary Conditions of the Labouring Population of Great Britain*. London: Longman.
6. *Inequalities in Health: Report of a Research Working Group* (Black Report, 1980). London: HMSO.
7. Department of Health and Social Security (1983). *NHS Management Enquiry*; HC 84/13. London: HMSO.
8. UKCC Annual Report. (1984–5). Objective 2: *To Promote Heightened Awareness Among Student Nurses, Midwives and Health Visitors*.
9. Kennedy I. (1981). *Unmasking Medicine*. London: Allen & Unwin.
10. WHO (1985). *Targets for Health for All*. Geneva: WHO.

Further Reading

Allsop J. (1984). *Health Policy and the National Health Service*. London: Longman.
Bruce M. (1968). *The Coming of the Welfare State*, 4th edn. London: Batsford.
Fraser D. (1973). *The Evolution of the Welfare State*. London: Macmillan.
Klein R. (1983). *The Politics of the NHS*. London: Longman.
Levitt R., Wall A. (1984). *The Reorganised National Health Service*, 3rd edn. Beckenham: Croom Helm.
Office of Health Economics (1984). *Understanding the NHS in the 1980s*. London: OHE.

Chapter 19

The Social Services

Social services may be statutory or voluntary; they deal with personal services such as social security, or with non-personal services like education, housing and employment. Many of our present statutory services have their origins in voluntary action as does district nursing itself and most of the child care services. Often they were formed in response to a special need; for example a Royal Commission in 1861 found that the majority of school leavers could not read a newspaper, and the report led to the idea of cheap elementary education. Similarly in 1885 the Commission on Housing gave rise to the revolutionary idea of 'council houses'. The solutions were usually pragmatic, uncoordinated and were in fact often merely attempts by society to accept some responsibility for the industrial revolution and for what Professor Titmuss later described as 'socially generated dis-service and socially caused dis-welfare'[1].

After the Local Government Act of 1888 the new authorities assumed responsibility for some of these services with varying degrees of accountability to central government, with each authority adopting its own pattern. At first these services were concerned with the administration of the Poor Law through Boards of Guardians, but soon other duties became statutory such as the setting up of Local Education Authorities after the Education Act 1902 (Fig. 19.1). On the other hand, some duties were merely permissive; after 1850 municipal councils were allowed to provide public libraries and by the end of the century civic pride and new wealth had produced a rash of museums, galleries, parks and those other cultural facilities that were so much the hallmark of the late Victorian city. Generally speaking, by the end of the century the sanitation and personal health services were grouped in the Public Health Department under the Medical Officer of Health, who was the most important officer in the sanitary movement. However, many health services were in fact outside his control and these included the new-style 'hospitals' that had

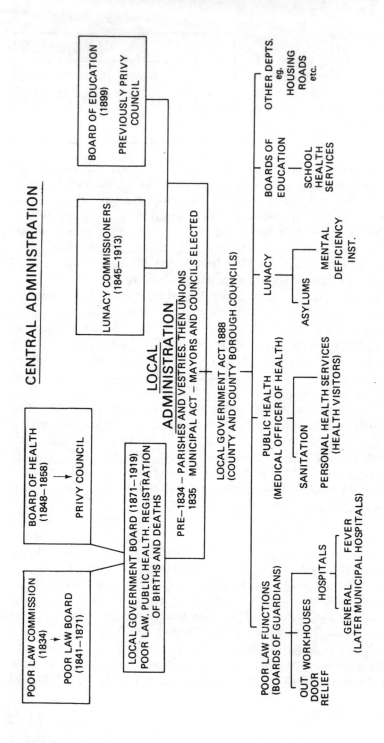

Fig. 19.1. Health services in the nineteenth century.

been built under the Poor Law after 1867. Meanwhile the social and welfare services developed *ad hoc* and were spread through all the departments of the local authority.

All social and welfare services impinge on health and, with the possible exception of Mr Evans—provided he returns to his old job—all the cases in Chapter 1 will require a number of different services. However, it is probably the personal social services with whom the district nurse will have the most contact.

The personal social services

In the past, social work was usually associated with philanthropic and charitable organisations, although some welfare work was done by officials of local government departments. For example, the School Board Attendance Officer often found hardship in the homes he visited—perhaps children were not attending school because they had no shoes; the housing departments began to employ Welfare Officers, and perhaps best known of all was the Relieving Officer who assessed people for 'parish relief'. However, both the state and the voluntary system operated within the economic philosophy of *laissez faire* and differentiated between the 'deserving' and the 'undeserving' poor, justifying their intervention with the former on the grounds that if people could be 'got back on their feet' they would return to work, which helped the market economy. Morally, of course, the work ethic was all-important.

Since the Second World War, attitudes have changed because of the greater understanding of social problems and their causes, and as a reaction to the massive misery caused by inter-war unemployment. Nearly a quarter of the population on the dole made a mockery of the concept of the 'work ethic'. After the Beveridge report in 1942 there were new ideas about what was meant by a 'welfare state' and with a change of emphasis from utilitarianism (Chapter 22) to humanitarianism it was regarded as reasonable that the state should intervene to ward off the worst effects of stress in all classes.

For these reasons, and others, the social services changed their ideas about the organisation of communal services to meet social needs, but while the social services were fragmented through different departments there was little chance of developing these ideas, nor of improving the training of social workers themselves. Discussion of this problem led to the setting up of the committee under the chairmanship of Sir Frederic Seebohm[2] which reported in 1968 and, although not all the philosophy of the report was put into practice, this was the basis for the Local Authority Social Services Act 1970. The Act set up a social services department which carved out an empire from other departments; home helps, services for the disabled and mentally handicapped were taken from health departments; other services, such as the responsibility for children in care, from the children's department, and other social responsibilities were hived off from education and housing. The original concept was for a community service for groups of 50 000 to 100 000 people, but the Local Government Act 1972 made this impossible because most of the country areas were too large. In order to overcome the problem social service departments were set up in each of the metropolitan and non-metropolitan counties and in the 33 London boroughs: they therefore often covered areas unequal in size, and also areas that had no matching health authorities. Now that metropolitan counties and the Greater London Council are being abolished, social services departments will be located in non-metropolitan counties and boroughs.

The social services, many of which have their roots in voluntary organisations, are trying to establish a fully professional service; they cover a wide range of problems which often involve the whole family and its environment, and for this reason they try to offer a 'family orientated service'. However, although the training of social workers is now comprehensive and generic, certain aspects of the work can be divided into different skills which for convenience can be grouped into: services for children, the physically handicapped, the mentally handicapped, the elderly and services dealing specifically with income need.

Services for children

In 1946 the Care of Children Committee (the Curtis report) recommended the setting up of Children's Departments under the aegis of the Home Office and the appointment of Children's

Officers who, incidentally, took over some tasks from the health visitor and unwittingly hastened the divorce between health and welfare. Although the new Children's Department tended to concentrate on what had already happened it did eventually lead to a more preventive approach, and in 1963 the Children and Young Persons Act required authorities to take steps to diminish the need to take children into care. Since then there have been a number of experiments including the idea of cash payments to relatives or friends, or for payments for someone to live in with the children. Although this was hailed as a new idea it was in fact a device often used by the Overseers of the Poor in the eighteenth century.

Children may come into care either through a court order or because the authority is fulfilling its duty under the Children Act 1975. Court cases usually arise from matrimonial, wardship or criminal proceedings, and in matrimonial cases where it seems that neither parent should be given custody, the child or children may be committed to the care of the local authority. Court cases may also arise from offences committed by children, and although children under the age of 10 cannot be charged they may be taken into care. Apart from court cases, children may come into care because they have been abandoned or because for some reason the parents or guardians are incapable of providing for the child. It must, however, be emphasised that a local authority has no power to keep a child against the wishes of the parents although it does have a duty to ensure, as far as possible, that the child will have proper care. Only on rare occasions, after stringent conditions have been fulfilled, will an authority over-rule the wishes of the parents.

In this area come the problems arising from suspected non-accidental injury to children. The battering of children is not new and literature is full of reference to it, but recent reports such as that of the National Society for the Prevention of Cruelty to Children[3] must come as a shock to a society that is both affluent and better educated than previous generations. Identifying children at risk is difficult but the latest surveys show that the families at greatest risk are those where the parents are young and immature and lack the ability to respond to the needs of a demanding child. In nearly half the cases of child abuse marital discord is a factor, and the lower income groups (particularly when unemployed) are heavily represented.

In 1974 the Department of Health and Social Security (England) issued a memorandum on the subject[4] and health authorities were urged to set up Review Committees. Since then there has been much discussion and research centred on non-accidental injury, and particularly on the question of sexual abuse of children and of incest. In July 1985 the DHSS issued a consultative document on Child Abuse Inquiries;[5] health authorities were asked to review their practices in relation to this problem, and principles were laid down. Again it was reiterated that one of the most frequently occurring problems was the exchange of information between professional workers. Although the district nurse is less likely to be involved with cases of child abuse than her health visitor colleague, she should, nevertheless, be aware of the directives laid down by her authority and the guidelines for dealing with suspected cases, and she must not shirk the issue when it comes her way. As press reports show, these cases need sensitive handling and a calm, non-judgmental approach. Advice on the professional handling of suspected cases of child abuse is well set out in *Health at School*.[6]

Services for the physically handicapped

Because of increased longevity the number of handicapped people in the community is increasing. In 1944 the Education Act laid down that handicapped children should receive appropriate education and the Disabled Persons (Employment) Act provided for a disabled persons register, the appointment of Disablement Resettlement Officers and for the setting up of industrial rehabilitation units, work which was eventually extended by the Chronically Sick and Disabled Persons Act of 1970, the provisions of which are all important to someone like John Davis.

The aim of all work with disabled persons is to assist them to independence within their limitations, help them to come to terms with their disability and to give help and support to their families. Disabled persons are defined as 'those who are blind, deaf or dumb, or who are substantially and permanently handicapped by illness, congenital deformity or old age'. Local authorities have a duty to make known to such persons the services they offer. The needs of the severely disabled like John Davis are complicated and require the coordination of many services which in his case have already included the health and housing services and the social services department, and may well soon involve others. For some patients the employment services will be vital, and for others the educational services may be important.

It is useful to remember that the Open University has a special service for handicapped persons, has made a study of meeting their particular educational needs, and manages to cope with the severely disabled in summer schools.

Services for the mentally ill and the mentally handicapped

The services for the mentally handicapped have passed through many vicissitudes, with needs and attitudes changing.[7] Some mental illness has declined, particularly that which was the sequela of acute infections, but there is evidence, difficult to measure, that anxiety and depression are less well tolerated than they were formerly. Furthermore, in a technical society with a rigid notion of the 'rate for the job' it is more difficult to find work for, or to fit in, the mentally handicapped. The electronic age favours the quick and slick.

About 5 million people a year consult their doctors about mental health problems. Few are admitted to hospitals and even then their stay is likely to be short, which means that all problems have to be dealt with in the community. Before the Social Services Act of 1970 the psychiatric social workers, who worked from the department of the Medical Officer of Health, often had a close relationship with the local mental hospital, the psychiatrists, the qualified mental nurses and, if they existed, the community psychiatric nurses. Now the psychiatric social worker has disappeared and this, together with the divorce between the hospitals and local authorities occasioned by the 1974 reorganisation of the health services, means that there was a lack of coordination in the services dealing with mental ill-health. Since then there has been a marked increase in the number of training courses for community psychiatric nurses and in their numbers, and there is now Community Psychiatric Nurses Association. It is the policy of the government to return psychiatric patients to the community as quickly as possible and where possible to avoid their admission to hospital. This, however, means that increased resources and more trained workers are required in the community, and while there are a number of notable experiments the general impression is that these services remain underfunded.

In particular there has been disquiet about the cooperation of the services dealing with mental handicap. The social services are responsible for mentally handicapped persons in the community; if they are in hospital or residential care the health service is responsible, while under the Education Act of 1975 the education department has a duty to provide suitable education. In order to try to resolve some of the problems a Committee on Residential Care for the Mentally Handicapped was set up under the chairmanship of Mrs Peggy Jay. The committee came to the conclusion that a new caring profession should be created with all workers trained in a course designed to qualify students for a Certificate of Social Service.

This suggestion did not find much favour with the nursing professional although to some extent it was similar to the long-term solution proposed by the Committee on Nursing in 1970 (the Briggs report). However, whatever its merits or demerits the proposal is likely to founder because of the lack of money to pay for the extra staff it would require. There are, however, a number of schemes to build a bridge for the mentally handicapped patient between the hospital and full independence, using small houses to create a homely atmosphere with trained staff being redeployed; this is not a cheap option but it does provide a better and more humane service.

Services for the elderly

There are now some 16% of the population past the age of retirement compared with 6% in 1911, and the percentage in the higher age groups is increasing. It is the over 85s, of which Mr Adams is a typical representative, who will make the greatest demands on the health service (Fig. 19.2). Fortunately the problem is partly offset by the fact that the younger retirement groups are fitter, more independent, have greater expectations of

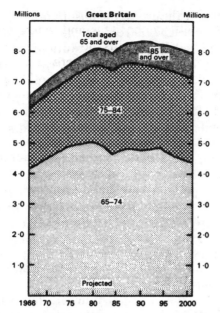

Fig. 19.2. Elderly persons in Great Britain 1966 to 2001 (by permission of HMSO).

continued activity, and with better pensions and facilities, they are able to continue to play a role in the community. Indeed they themselves often make a significant contribution to the voluntary services. On the other hand, this very independence and the tendency to move to 'retirement areas' often cuts them off from the younger generation. Moreover, smaller families and smaller houses, the mobility of much employment, and the fact that daughters and daughters-in-law often work outside the home, all militate against older people living with their children even if they wished to do so, which they usually do not. All these factors make family support in times of crisis that much more difficult.

Ageing is a variable process; Mrs Cray at 68 has aged early whereas Mrs Adams seems to have coped into her 80s, but the document *A Happier Old Age*[8] points out that the proportion of people who are bedfast and housebound rises steeply with age, with mental infirmity becoming an increasing problem. The Almshouse, that legacy of the Elizabethan Poor Law, was the traditional way of dealing with the unsupported 'aged infirm', and in 1960 there were still 37 000 old people in Part III Accommodation in old converted Poor Law institutions, and in some cases 'conversion' was more apparent than real. Since then, with a greater understanding of the needs of old people, and the fact that residential care is becoming increasingly expensive, there has been a reversal of policy and there is more emphasis on keeping the elderly mobile and at home, which of course has enormous implications for district nursing.

When it is clear that an infirm person can no longer cope alone it is always worth finding out if any particular service is available to them; for example, do they belong to any particular church or denomination, for most have homes for old people and some of the old 'dissenting' groups like the Quakers offer a number of services. It is worth finding out whether patients have served in the armed services and if they belong to the British Legion, or whether they are members of a professional organisation, occupational group or trade union which offers facilities. Most people have a touchstone somewhere. In dealing with elderly nurses, help may be had from the Counselling, Help and Advice Together (CHAT) of the RCN which has a directory of funds and trusts. The more usual services offered by local authorities and voluntary societies are listed in Appendices 2 and 3.

Services dealing with poverty

At the end of the nineteenth century Charles Booth (1840–1916) pointed out that for most people income and need followed a cyclic pattern. Young couples with no children were comparatively well-off but when children arrived and the wife stopped working the needs rose and the income fell. When the children were grown up and working (probably at the age of 13 years) there was another period of comparative ease, only to be followed by hard times again when the breadwinner stopped working because of age. Basically, the provision of benefits in the twentieth century has aimed at restoring income at least to subsistence level during the troughs of childbearing, sickness, unemployment and old age.

Different countries and ideologies have met these needs in different ways. In France, when the birth rate fell sharply, generous child allowances were introduced; in England when it was feared that the unfit school children would not be suitable as recruits to the army, there was the provision of a school health service and school meals. In both countries, be it noted, welfare provisions were related to the defence needs of the country.

In England, for historical reasons, we have dealt with the main needs of Booth's cycle through a pragmatic variety of contributory and non-contributory benefits. Contributory benefits are as of right, that is to say they are universal and paid to all people who qualify regardless of income or class, although it must be stressed that payments do not derive from actuarial calculations and are supplemented from taxation. On the other hand, non-contributory payments are usually (though not always) subject to a means test; that is, they are selective and paid to those whose needs are the greatest. Usually these are families whose total income is below the official 'subsistence' level. This level varies with inflation and the district nurse should have some idea of the current rate. Benefits can be complicated and may take the form of cash or kind, such as school milk, clothing grants, and rebates on rent or rates (see Appendix 4).

Other statutory services

Apart from the personal social services, the work of the district nurse may be affected by the operation of other statutory services, including education, employment, housing and a range of legal services.

The education service

At the end of the nineteenth century, England was at least 60 years behind her neighbours in the field of general education, and to try to remedy this Parliament created a Board of Education followed by the great Education Act of 1902 which made elementary education to the age of 14 years compulsory. The Fisher Act of 1918 empowered authorities to raise the school leaving age and also made provision for more medical services and the greater care of defective children. However, the main educational services of today stem from the Education Act of 1944 introduced by R. A.

Butler as part of the overall Beveridge report. All fees for maintained schools were abolished, the system of primary, secondary modern and grammar schools established, and provisions for dental and other services strengthened. In the past 20 years there has been a continuing move towards the comprehensive system and in 1972 the school leaving age was raised to 16 years.

As a response to the Warnock Committee which in 1978 looked at the educational provision for young people handicapped by disabilities of body and mind, the Education Act of 1981 was passed. The Act required local education authorities to review their educational provision for the disabled, and placed a duty on them to identify educational needs and to provide assessment on a multi-professional basis. The Act defined special educational need as a learning difficulty which calls for special educational provision. It is the duty of the authority to enable a child to engage in as many of the school activities as possible. This definition of special educational need and the way in which provision is made highlights the responsibilities of health authorities for the delivery of services to parents and to education departments.

The school health service

This service is of particular concern to district nurses because patients are often concerned about the health of their children, or (as in the case of Mrs Baker) the health of the parents reacts on the children, and for this reason the school nurse must be seen as part of the primary care team.

The school health services have their origins in the revelations of the Committee on Physical Deterioration of 1904 which showed that 40% of Army recruits were physically unfit—and the Army's standards were hardly high. In 1907 the Education (Administrative Provisions) Act required authorities to provide for the medical inspection of children, thus making the Board of Education a health authority; and in spite of protests from the British Medical Association, the services were extended to give treatment for minor ailments. At the same time, authorities were empowered to provide school meals and milk, a move that provoked much protest and outraged letters to *The Times*. After the

Notification of Births Act of 1907 and 1915 more authorities began to employ health visitors and to attach them to the Medical Officer of Health; consequently they often assumed responsibility for the health of school children. Some authorities, however, especially in the large towns, preferred to employ specially recruited school nurses and, if necessary, to give them an in-service training.

After the setting up of the National Health Service it was questioned whether the school medical service was still necessary, since now children had the right to free medical treatment. The debate, which was not unrelated to the desire to cut costs, meant that the position of the school nurse was not clarified and the service took on the mantle of Cinderella. But hopes that the service would be redundant soon faded. Children now stayed at school longer, they matured earlier, they had psychological and emotional problems about examination pressure and competition which were unknown in earlier years. Old problems like malnutrition have largely disappeared, although they may still be met in immigrant groups, but their place has been taken by the complicated problems arising from an affluent society such as obesity, smoking, drinking and drug-taking, to say nothing of the fact that in 1978 there were 4600 pregnancies in girls under 16 of which 3000 ended in abortion.[9]

While the district nurse may not be much involved with the question of teenage pregnancies, the arguments about contraception without the parents' consent and the guidelines emerging from the Gillick appeal, she should be aware of the current legislation, the advice of the BMA and the RCN, and be able to make the appropriate referral or give the right advice if asked.

Today the school health service tries to fulfil three main aims: to be a health education service, an occupational health service and to provide liaison with other services. Since 1974 the school health service have been the responsibility of the NHS and health authorities have appointed Child Health Nursing Officers who have been responsible for coordinating all the health services for children. The Education Act of 1981 and changes in the health problems and habits of school children have greatly extended the work of the school nurse who should be a valued colleague of the district nurse; for instance, she might well liaise with her over the problems of Mrs Baker's children and Rose Johnson.

In 1976 the Court Committee[10] recommended that there should be an integrated child health service, with each group medical practice having one doctor with paediatric training and a similarly qualified health visitor who would oversee other child visitors and school nurses. The committee also recommended that each school should have its own nominated doctor and nurse, trained in educational medicine, who would act as general mentors to the children. The report has not been implemented, partly because it goes against the philosophy of the primary care team where workers are 'all purpose', and also because of cost and because health workers have already undergone enough upheaval. Nevertheless, the report is a salutary reminder that child health care in England is now falling behind other western countries and there is no room for complacency.

Special schools

The 1981 Education Act has changed the whole basis of the education of handicapped children. As far as possible handicapped children will in future be integrated with other children in ordinary schools, although some special schools (including boarding schools) will continue to be necessary for the most severely handicapped. Rose Johnson attends an ordinary primary school where she receives the special support of the school nurse during a normal education.

Nursery schools

Although these have existed since the Education Act 1944 they have always been in short supply and in 1967 the Plowden Committee recommended that children in deprived areas should be given better than average schooling to compensate for their social and environmental deprivation. For this reason there has been a tendency to concentrate such schools in deprived areas, but for families relying on the mother as the breadwinner, or even partial breadwinner, the lack of nursery schools can mean real difficulty and can lead to unsatisfactory child minding.

Housing services

The Housing Acts of 1885 and 1890 allowed local authorities to provide working-class houses, but as this was seen as interference with the market system with a vengeance, little was done, and the provision of cheap houses came mainly from charitable trusts like Peabody or Guinness. The First World War saw the beginning of rent control, and although in the inter-war period there was some council house building it was often of poor quality and design. However, as the country recovered from the economic slump there was a burst of suburban building, and owner occupation spread down the social scale.

During the Second World War a Ministry of Town and Country Planning was created with the hope of avoiding the mistakes of the past unplanned development, but the overall shortage was so great that the aim was only partially met. Since then much attention has been paid to the way in which cities grow. Originally the city centre was the high point of prestige but in the late nineteenth century it became increasingly fashionable to move away from the scene of work.

Different classes, however, have different abilities to compete with one another in terms of housing and of transport, and those with no cash tend to get trapped in areas of high-density living. The once desirable becomes undesirable; working-class families move to the next zone with white-collar workers moving further away. Cities therefore develop in concentric circles with the ripples spreading outward. It will be noticed that Mr Fisher commutes from a dormitory town to the city. Post-war speculation, assisted by convenient bomb damage, has tended to concentrate on office blocks and luxury flats in the centre of cities and now it is the outer ring of the centre, once so fashionable, that has become the twilight zone. Because of planning blight these areas tend to be poorly served with health and education services and for this reason they become even less desirable. The Johnson family are likely to be trapped for some time.

Post-war planning emphasised the need to tie housing schemes in with road networks and to avoid the evils of ribbon development. People like Mrs Cray were rehoused in tower blocks which, it was thought, would break down barriers and give social cohesion. What was not foreseen was the high maintenance costs and the invitation to vandalism. These flats have been particularly unpopular with mothers of young children and with elderly people, and since the partial collapse of Ronan Point in 1968 few authorities have continued with this type of building. Recently there has been a move to rehabilitate old buildings but unfortunately not before whole neighbourhood communities have been obliterated beyond recall.

The pattern of housing

The Department of Housing is responsible for housing policy but the actual administration is devolved onto local authorities, with functions divided between the county councils and the districts. Basically there are four types of housing: owner-occupied, local authority, voluntary housing association and private rented accommodation. In the past 25 years owner occupation has doubled but local authorities still supply one-third of the total stock. Local authority housing is usually allocated on a points system and it is estimated that there are over a million people like the Johnsons waiting for a council house.

Rights of tenants

Most tenancies are protected by the Rent Act, but rents are not now controlled; instead they are fixed by the Rent Officer who works within a local authority area, but who is not a servant of that authority and who is in fact employed by the central government. Objections to rents will be heard by the rent assessment committee, where the appellant can be represented by a solicitor or some other authorised person if he so wishes.

Since housing conditions may well affect the health of the occupants the district nurse should know something of the many improvement, repair and special grants for which householders and landlords may apply to bring a house up to a reasonable standard. Sometimes the nurse may find a patient suffering hardship, or even being in danger of injury, because of disrepair; in such cases the local authority may issue an order requiring that the repairs be done and the danger removed. The authority also has the power to act in the case of deficient sanitation and to recover the costs later; similarly, they can take steps to insure that property, and sometimes people, are cleansed of vermin and that rats and mice are eradicated.

The employment services

These services are most important to the district nurse when she is dealing with disabled people and in this respect they are discussed elsewhere. It is important to remember, however, that the Department of Employment has directly employed Nursing Officers who give help and advice on nursing matters.

Voluntary organisations

Probably half the population of Victorian England was poor. The lowest tenth, the 'perishing classes' found relief from the Poor Law; for those who managed to keep above the pauper line but who were distressed because of illness, accident, unemployment or some other disaster, there was a wide range of charities.

Victorian charity was a response to the growing disparity between rich and poor in an increasingly affluent society, and was largely prompted by the Christian belief in good works, and the notion that it is 'more blessed to give than to receive'. The Victorians firmly believed that the personal connection was more valuable than the cold hand of the state. There was also a growing concern about law and order; the powerless, impoverished masses were a focal point for criminal activity and political agitation. Finally, there was the evangelical point of view; as General Booth of the Salvation Army put it 'you can't save a man's soul when he is hungry'.

In 1861 there were 640 charities in London alone, and to bring some order to the chaos of overlapping and competition the Charity Organisation Society was formed. Some of these charities were the forerunners of later statutory services such as the National Society for the Prevention of Cruelty to Children, which pioneered much of the Child Life Protection legislation, or St Dunstan's which demonstrated the need for the services to the blind.

Many branches of social work have a similar lineage. However, after the Second World War as the statutory services took over more and more of the social services and as social workers put their work on a client basis, the role of the voluntary societies began to look ambiguous. In this atmosphere the voluntary societies tended to experiment and to pioneer new forms of service (for example, the aftercare of prisoners, hostels for unmarried mothers, support for drug addicts) while, at the same time, supplementing the statutory services with such things as 'meals on wheels'. However, the Seebohm Committee, while fully accepting the need for a professional service, saw the voluntary societies, not as a secondary source, but as a positive force for 'developing citizen participation in revealing new needs and shortcomings'.

In recent years there has been a burgeoning of voluntary societies, many of which receive government subsidies. The expectation of help with social needs, like expectations for health care, rises faster than professional manpower and official resource can keep pace, and social workers, like professional health workers, need to rationalise their skills and promote community self-help.

There are about 77 000 organisations registered with the Charity Commission of which over 10 000 were formed between 1960 and 1970—a figure which gives the lie to the idea that modern society is lost to self-help and voluntary endeavour. Furthermore, it must be remembered that the needs for social help are much more complicated than in previous generations. At the beginning of this century anyone of reasonable intelligence could comprehend the services to which they were entitled—which were pretty few. Now, with the best will in the world, this is manifestly untrue. Who, for example, understands exactly who is entitled to a rate rebate?

However, the great rise has been in the number of self-help groups, particularly where sufferers of a disease or disability, such as ileostomy patients, spastics or alcoholics, form a group to help one another; the afflicted have an empathy with the afflicted and often form not only a society for mutual aid but also a pressure group. Mr Fisher, John Davis and Rose's parents can all be helped by such groups.

The greatest difference between the Victorian charity and the present-day voluntary organisations is not the current emphasis on 'self-help' (the Victorians tutored by Samuel Smiles were strong on that), but the fact that Victorian society saw charity as an *alternative* to state aid whereas today it is a supplement and a spur to state welfare. But perhaps, more significantly, voluntary organisations are supported by all classes of society instead of merely being seen as a duty of the rich towards the poor; the builder's wife may well be delivering meals to the retired judge who is housebound because of his arthritis and arteriosclerosis; money does not buy service and the days of housekeepers are over.

Professor Ralph Dahrendorf in the Reith lectures of 1975 suggested that there was an urgent need for society to get away from the work ethic that has been so much the basis of the Protestant capitalistic society, where 'work' is seen as something that a person is paid to do for so many hours a day, then at a certain age is 'put out to grass to the world of non-work'.[11] He went on to point out that there is a need to adopt a more flexible notion about work and retirement, and to ask why, provided that in our affluent society we have enough for reasonable subsistence, the early retired or the redundant cannot undertake some useful work according to their various abilities without being penalised or accused of undercutting? This might well prove more interesting and rewarding than participating in those 'retirement hobbies' which are sometimes merely filling in time.

References

1. Titmuss R. (1968). *Commitment to Welfare.* London: Allen & Unwin.
2. *Report of the Committee on Local Authority and Allied Social Services* (Seebohm report, 1968). London: HMSO.
3. National Society for the Prevention of Cruelty to Children (1979). *Annual Report.* London: NSPCC.
   Also (1976) *Child Victims of Physical Abuse.*
4. Department of Health and Social Security (1974). *Memorandum on Non-accidental Injury to Children.* London: HMSO.
5. Department of Health and Social Security (1985). *Consultative Paper on Child Abuse Inquiries.* London: HMSO.
6. Nash W., Thruston M., Baly M. (1985). *Health at School*, p. 252 ff. London: Heinemann Medical.

7. Baly M. E. (1980). *Nursing and Social Change*, 2nd edn, Chapters 7, 20. London: Heinemann Medical.
8. Department of Health and Social Security (1978). *A Happier Old Age—a discussion document*. London: HMSO.
9. Davies S. (1980). Comment on the report of the Joint Working Party (1979). *Pregnant at School and Schoolgirl Mothers*. What every child should know. *The Times*, 21 February 1980.
10. *The Future of the Child Health Services* (Court report, 1976). London: HMSO.
11. Dahrendorf R. (1976). *The New Liberty*. London: BBC Publications.

Further Reading

Family Welfare Association (1986). *Guide to the Social Services*. London: Family Welfare Association. (Updated annually.)

Nash W., Thruston M., Baly M. (1985). *Health at School* London: Heinemann Medical.

Townsend P. (1979). *Poverty in the United Kingdom*. Harmondsworth: Penguin.

Chapter 20

Policies for Nursing

Until the nineteenth century nursing tasks had been carried out by a variety of people ranging from aristocratic ladies and devoted Augustinian nuns to village nurses, medical students and paid attendants. No one asked what was the 'proper task of the nurse'; people were cared for by the person on hand and care varied according to the changing mores, the knowledge available and the expectations of the community. By no means all care was bad, indeed some of it was devoted beyond praise, and nursing care often gave more comfort than the medical treatment of the time. However, Miss Nightingale was right when she pointed out that nursing, even if devoted, was for the most part untrained. In spite of the general belief that 'every woman makes a good nurse', Miss Nightingale insisted that 'the elements of what constitutes good nursing are as little understood for the sick as for the well'.[1] When she said that she used 'the word nursing for want of a better' Miss Nightingale clearly meant that nursing should apply to something more than 'the application of poultices and the administration of medicines', and her concept embraced a whole range of social and environmental factors that cause ill-health and which the nurse must be trained to prevent, or advise and treat when prevention has failed. The cryptic comment that 'the causes of the enormous child mortality are perfectly well known . . . the remedies are just as well known and among them is not the establishment of a Child's Hospital',[2] shows that she considered an understanding of the causes of illness to be essential to nurse training—it was for this reason that nurses needed to be educated.

The Nightingale reforms

During the Crimean War the Nightingale Fund was set up to enable Miss Nightingale to start an institution for the training of nurses when she returned to England.[3] Miss Nightingale was not enthusiastic about the idea because she had more pressing work:

her first priority was the reform of the Army Medical Service and if necessary the army itself. After much procrastination and many delays St Thomas's hospital offered to accommodate nurses supplied by the Fund Council and in 1860 a small school was started under the aegis of the matron, Mrs Wardroper. The probationers, as they were called, were assistant nurses; they received little instruction because there was no one to give it, and the standard of candidate was not high. However, the Nightingale Fund Council was prestigious and its propaganda effective; it coincided with the introduction of Listerian surgery, the greater use of anaesthetics and the changed use of the voluntary hospitals which impelled hospitals to seek a better class of nurse. At the same time many women were receiving a better education and there was a general move for their emancipation. However, opportunities for work for educated women outside the home were limited, and the new style of nurse as advertised by the Fund became what Miss Nightingale later somewhat scathingly described as 'fashionable'.

By the 1870s the Fund Council was able to advertise—and get—what they called 'special probationers' who were better educated and who, it was intended, should be groomed for superintendence. By no means all such recruits were successful, but some, backed by Miss Nightingale herself, went forth as matrons to start schools elsewhere. By this time other voluntary hospitals had started similar systems and by the late 1880s there were numbers of the new-style nurses being appointed as matrons and carving out empires. The important change made by the Nightingale reforms was not so much that they offered a training for nurses (this, as the records show, was often haphazard) but that in nursing matters it made nurses accountable to a trained nurse.

The administration of the voluntary hospitals became tripartite with the matron having direct access to the Board of Governors. When this access was lost after the inception of the National Health Service nurses reacted sharply and the restoration of this right was one of the reasons for setting up of the Committee on Senior Nursing Structure (the Salmon committee) in 1966. The structure proposed by the committee may now seem hierarchical, but the health service structure was itself hierarchical (see Fig.

18.1, p. 275). This line of accountability has again been lost; this is important, not because nursing posts have been lost, but because, if the reform of nursing demonstrated anything, it was that nursing matters are best dealt with by trained nurses. The improvement in nursing in the late nineteenth century came not because nurses were better trained, but because they were better managed.

The idea of reformed nursing spread to the Poor Law infirmaries especially those new hospitals erected after the Metropolitan Poor Act of 1867, and two training schools were started by the Nightingale Fund Council. In 1881 a Royal Commission recommended the general accessibility of these hospitals, and by 1891 the citizens of London had the right to use the hospitals for infectious fevers that were being erected by the new Metropolitan Asylums Board. As time went by these too began to train for 'fever nursing' which, owing to the new knowledge about bacteria was becoming an art in itself. Generally speaking, however, the hospitals administered by the Boards of Guardians attracted fewer candidates for nurse training and the standard of selection was less rigorous. Thus began the great divide between nurses trained in the voluntary hospitals and those in the municipal system. To some extent this was also a reflection of the differing priorities given to the acutely ill and the chronic sick 'not suitable for general hospitals'.

As well as nurses trained in the voluntary and Poor Law systems, in general and later in specialist hospitals, there were nurses specially trained for nursing in the community (Chapter 21) although, as with their colleagues in hospital, for many years the untrained outnumbered the trained.

Miss Nightingale never ceased writing and talking about the need for the prevention of illness by health education, and she realised that the 'health missioners' attached to the various visiting societies also needed a definite training. The great 'sanitary movement' which followed the publication of the report of Edwin Chadwick and the Health of Towns Commission in 1845 had produced a spate of sanitary societies, and some, like the Salford Ladies Health Society, actually employed women to visit and instruct mothers in domestic hygiene. Miss Nightingale's contribution to this movement was that she designed a training scheme for such visitors who were not nurses but who would form a back-up service to the new trained district nurses. Her plan for a course of lectures in 1890 classed as technical education, is important because it established the idea of health visitor training within general education and also the fact that hospital training was not a necessary prerequisite for such work. Health visitors, who had a variety of backgrounds, including medicine, continued on this basis, with Bedford College and Battersea Polytechnic offering training schemes by 1907.

The campaign for state registration

The rise of a large middle class in the nineteenth century produced an increased demand for services of all kinds which led to the growth of 'professional' occupations, and, as each tried to enhance its status by examinations and diplomas, so there was a demand for 'registration' and the denial of practice to the unregistered. Doctors had been registered since the Medical Act of 1858 and it was not long before the new-style matrons were clamouring for registration for nurses. However, there were difficulties, not least of which was the problem of defining the limits of nursing practice. It is comparatively easy to say what is the law—and therefore what is the lawyer's province—but it is less easy to define nursing care. Furthermore, was it to be a 2- or even 3-year training, what standards were to be set, and did the mere length of training guarantee safe practice? If the standards were high then what about the livelihood of all the others who practised nursing? Above all, there were Miss Nightingale's wise reflections on the nature of nursing which, as she pointed out, needed not only the acquisition of knowledge but had another aspect, the vocational, which could not be tested by an examination. The nurse has 'to nurse living bodies and spirits'.[4]

Undaunted by the difficulties, the registrationists led by Mrs Bedford Fenwick, the erstwhile matron of St Bartholomew's Hospital, founded a variety of organisations to further the policy of registration for nurses, the best known of which was the Royal British Nurses' Association. The movement was to some extent associated with the suffragette campaign which at the beginning of the twentieth century was at its height. Nursing, except in the mental hospitals, was almost entirely feminine and, not without reason, attributed its difficulties in advancing as a profession to the general position of women in society. Partly because of the association with the militant wing of the suffragette movement, but mainly because of dissension in the profession itself and the conflicting advice given to the Committee on Registration (1904), the early Registration Bill of 1908 came to nothing, and soon the general expectation of war obscured its claim on the attention of the government.

Nursing organisations and their policies

The Royal British Nurses' Association, the National Council of Nurses and the Matrons' Council all had as their main aim the registration of nurses, a 3-year year training and a high registration fee. These early associations tended to be exclusive and there was much dual membership. On the other hand, at the beginning of the century the rapidly growing trade union movement was expanding into hospitals, especially in the county asylums and the Poor Law hospitals. The trade union movement was essentially male-dominated and linked to the new Labour party; if women were recruited at all they either had their own underfunded association or a separate, and often powerless, section. Most nurses remained unorganised.

The First World War highlighted the lack of organisation in nursing and the fact that there were no national criteria to judge what was meant by a 'trained nurse'. To overcome some of these problems the leaders of the Joint War Organisation of the British Red Cross and the Order of St John put forward the idea of a new College of Nursing, unattached to any political movement and not associated with either the registrationists or the suffragettes, with a constitution in line with the other professional Royal Colleges and with power in the hands of the members themselves.

The policy of the College of Nursing, which was set up in April 1916, was to promote the better education of nurses and uniformity of the curriculum; to recognise 'approved' schools of nursing and to maintain its own register of persons who had certificates from such schools; and generally to pursue such objectives as 'would advance the art and science of nursing'. By the end of the war the College had about 15 000 members and as it increased in strength it too pursued the cause of registration but in a somewhat more accommodating manner.

When the new Ministry of Health was set up in 1919 it was clear that some form of registration would have to come, not to protect or enhance the status of the nursing profession as the early campaigners had intended, but to protect the public from the vast numbers of women who had had nursing experience in the war and called themselves 'trained'. Many thought that the College of Nursing would be the registering body, but the Royal British Nurses' Association was still campaigning for its own rigid Bill and in the internecine warfare that followed, the exasperated Ministry eventually set up its own statutory body, the General Nursing Councils under the Nurses' Registration Act of 1919 which allowed for a separate Council for Scotland and another for Ireland (to be the Northern Ireland Council after 1922). Thus, the profession lost the right to control its own basic education.

The General Nursing Council was controlled by the Ministry who also had the responsibility for the oversight of the health services. Because impoverished hospitals before the war had been quick to see the advantages of biddable, educated probationers, and because of the lack of opportunity for a career for women elsewhere, there seemed a never-ending stream of devoted young women coming forward to nurse. As about one-third of these recruits left fairly quickly the main labour force of many hospitals had come to be made up of probationers, a fact that would have made Miss Nightingale turn in her grave.

The Ministry of Health was in no position to help the finances of either the voluntary hospitals or the municipal system and therefore it could do no more than accept the status quo; the new Council was designed to accommodate nurse training *as it was at that time*. Accordingly, the Council recognised most hospitals giving a training and divided the register into five, and later six, parts. There was a part for nurses trained in general hospitals and, because they had a different training, a part for male nurses; then there were also supplementary parts for the nursing of fevers, children, mental diseases, and finally, a part for the care of mental defectives.

This fragmentation of the basic training was against the educational policy of the College of Nursing who had been looking at developments in America and who favoured a 'comprehensive training' with specialisation to follow as in medicine. However, this was an issue on which the profession has always been split. Miss Lückes, the matron of the London Hospital, giving evidence to the Select Committee on Registration in 1904, had argued that it was 'a waste to train all for everything'.[5] The mental nurses saw little advantage in would-be psychiatric nurses doing a training in a general hospital, and the health visitors have always been sceptical about the value of a spell in an acute general hospital as the foundation to a career in health education.

The new Nursing Council brought some order, eventually only approving schemes that met its standards, and set up machinery for removing the names of unsuitable practitioners, but because it fixed with legislation a training and education that ought to be evolving to meet new needs, its contribution to the advancement of the art and science of nursing was hardly revolutionary.

The inter-war years

Policies for nursing remained pragmatic and disparate. The different branches had come from different traditions; not only was the register divided into six parts, there was also that other division between those trained in the voluntary and the municipal systems where not only the social status of the patients, but often their diseases, and certainly the structure of the administration, were different. A 'trained nurse' compassed a much wider range than say, a trained doctor or solicitor. Furthermore, mental nursing had come from the county asylums, first under the Lunacy Commission and then under the Board of Control, and mental nurses had taken examinations under the aegis of the Medico-Psychological Association since 1891; many regarded its certificate as of more value than that offered by the General Nursing Council. Also, mental nurses tended to organise through trade unions so there was practically no point of contact between general and mental nursing.

Midwives had always been a separate profession. Miss Nightingale had tried to found a School of Midwives at King's College Hospital but it had closed because of puerperal sepsis; nevertheless the College of Midwives was formed in 1881 and was influential in getting the Midwives Act of 1902 passed which set up the Central Midwives Board as an independent examining body with the College of Midwives responsible for the postcertificate courses.

Health visitors, as already pointed out, were originally not necessarily nurses but often had another qualification such as sanitary inspector or medical practitioner, and usually did a special course such as the one organised by Bedford College. As time went by, with more emphasis on maternity and child welfare, nurses tended to predominate and particularly nurses with more than one certificate.[6] In 1925 health visitor training became the responsibility of the Ministry of Health and more full-time courses were set up in technical and other colleges, including the College of Nursing, with the Royal Sanitary Institute becoming the examining body. In 1946 all health visitors were required to be state registered nurses and to hold the first part of the certificate of the Central Midwives Board, and, in 1962, the Royal Sanitary Institute handed over to the Council for the Training of Health Visitors.

Apart from the Queen's Institute for District Nurses (dealt with more fully in Chapter 21) which was another training and examining body, the Royal College of Nursing, as it became after 1928, was offering its own certificates for post-basic courses which in 1932 included the Certificate of Industrial Nursing (later called occupational health nursing) and a Ward Sisters' Certificate. At the same time the sister tutors were usually qualified through a diploma of the London University and later registered as 'tutors' with the General Nursing Council, while the Diploma in Nursing of the London and Leeds Universities offered registered nurses a more demanding course in the basic sciences and the philosophy relating to nursing. To complicate matters even further there were a number of 'national certificates' which might be taken before or after training in such fields as orthopaedics, ophthalmics and tuberculosis (later thoracic nursing) or in tropical diseases.

Policies for nursing since the establishment of the National Health Service

Unlike the First World War, the 1939–45 war did not attract large numbers of nursing recruits and in 1946 30 000 beds had to be closed because of the nursing shortage. The government tried to make good the deficit by any means and these included short, 'crash' courses for ex-service auxiliaries, not reintroducing the educational entry test, the introduction of a variety of cadet schemes, often without safeguards, and relying on the work of 15-year-olds. The results of these measures were to affect nursing for the next 20 years.

Meanwhile the nursing profession itself was looking for ways to meet the new demands on nursing, and partly as the result of the Horder Report the Nurses Act of 1943 was passed which established a Roll for 'assistant nurses' with the General Nursing Council. However, the new grade was not universally welcomed and for a long time only marginally affected the shortage. In the early years assistant nurses (later known as enrolled nurses) were confined to work in the long-stay hospitals but eventually they were accepted as a valuable component of the nursing team in all hospitals, including the mental hospitals in 1967 and also in 1970 in the district nursing service.

The new demands of the National Health Service highlighted two main problems for nursing: firstly the need to change the system of training and education to meet the new health needs and expectations of patients, and to meet the aspirations of nurses themselves; and secondly to improve the economic status that nursing had inherited largely as the result of being a women's profession. The two problems were related and were, to some extent, a vicious circle.

Nursing education

There were three major reports on nurse training within the first 18 years, the *Report of the Nursing Reconstruction Committee* (Horder), the *Report of the Working Party on the Recruitment and Training of Nurses* (Wood), and *A Reform of Nursing Education* (Platt), all of which, if accepted, would have placed more emphasis on community nursing.[7] It is now a matter of history that these reports, although widely debated, failed to bring about the necessary legislation to bring about a change in the status of the student nurse and the educational programme. Finally in 1970 as the result of pressure from the profession itself, which was brought to a head by a fall in recruitment due to low pay and dissatisfaction with the standards of training, the government set up the Committee on Nursing under the chairmanship of Professor Asa Briggs (later Lord Briggs). The recommendations of this committee were important for district nurses because it was the first committee to plan for nursing within an integrated health service, and the first to offer a plan based on the total health needs of the community rather than the service needs of hospitals.

The committee's recommendations in 1972 were generally well received although the various training councils were unable to agree on the structure of the new council and this subsequently raised problems for district nursing (Chapter 21). The committee saw nursing education as a continuum in much the same way as had earlier committees, but whereas the Platt and Horder reports had thought that the range of people attracted to nursing was so wide that it was necessary to have two basic courses, the Committee on Nursing recommended a single portal of entry. The committee's plan was that all students should take five modules in a foundation course which would lead to a Certificate in Nursing, but contrary to the advice given by the Royal College of Nursing and other professional bodies, the learner was to remain a health service employee. Some students would stop there but others would take modules in greater depth leading to registration, with the student free to build in a variety of patterns. Finally, the Certificate of Higher Education would replace the various special trainings and the separate examination bodies and there would be further links with universities. This last certificate would take the place of the various post-basic nursing certificates including the present certificate for district nursing.

Although the recommendations of the Committee on Nursing were accepted in principle, it was not until April 1979 that the Nurses, Midwives and Health Visitors Act reached the statute book. Reasons for the delay were the various vested interests that had developed during the long and complicated history of nursing and midwifery, and the fissiparous nature of the nursing profession. In 1981 the United Kingdom Central Council for Nurses, Midwives and Health Visiting was set up with National Boards for each country. In 1983 these new bodies took over the functions of the General Nursing Council for England and Wales, the General Nursing Council for Scotland, the Council for Northern Ireland, the Central Midwives Board, the Council for the Education and Training of Health Visitors, the Panel of Assessors for District Nurse Training, the Joint Board of Clinical Nursing Studies and the Committee for Clinical Nursing Studies (Scotland). The UKCC, in conjunction with the National Boards, is now responsible for 'making statutory rules governing entry to training and the criteria for registration and improving standards of training.' The four National Boards approve 'institutions to provide all training and education courses for nurses, midwives and health visitors and control examinations.' The Boards provide a direct point of contact for schools and other institutions running courses for nurse training or those contemplating training.

Within the new structure a District Nursing Joint Committee was set up to serve the interests of district nursing throughout the UK. This is a statutory committee of the UKCC and the four National Boards and its advice has to be sought on all matters relating to district nursing.

The Committee on Nursing advised on a reform of nursing education and since then much work has been done in formulating new plans and schemes. In 1984, the Royal College of Nursing set up its Commission under the chairmanship of Dr Harry Judge, director of the Department of Educational Studies, Oxford University, which reported in 1985.[8] The Commission reviewed the position of nursing education as it was then with 391 820 nursing and midwifery staff employed in the NHS. Of these only 38.4% were registered and over 20% were trainees who had a wastage rate of 21%. This meant there were comparatively few qualified staff to supervise the trainees and that most nursing tasks were performed by unqualified staff. Having considered the possible options the Commission came to the conclusion that a radical solution was necessary and that nursing education should take place outside the NHS, within or linked to establishments of higher education. The Committee advocated a progressive educational programme built up in modules with the final year embracing choices in mental handicap nursing, mental illness nursing, general and community nursing, paediatric nursing, health visiting and midwifery. Such a course would be the foundation for further study which should be seen as a continuum. The revolutionary feature of the Judge report was that it suggested the complete transfer of nursing education into higher education and advocated a system of bursaries rather than allowances or grants.

In the meantime, in 1984, the UKCC inaugurated Project 2000:[9]

> 'To determine the education and training required in the preparation for the professional practice of nursing and midwifery and health visiting in relation to the needs of the 1990s and beyond and to make recommendations.'

The Committee has now reported and its recommendations have been largely accepted by the profession. They are a variation on the theme of the Committee on Nursing and the Judge report, with certain innovations. The recommendations include a common foundation programme lasting up to 2 years and the preparation for a new registered practitioner to be completed in 3 years. The course would prepare the candidate to work both in the institutional and non-institutional setting. There would be branch programmes in mental illness, mental handicap, nursing of adults and the nursing of children, with experimentation in a branch of midwifery. All future practitioners would register with the Council and their area of practice would be indicated on the register. Health visiting, occupational health nursing and school nursing would be specialist qualifications in health promotion, and district nursing, community psychiatric nursing and community mental handicap nursing would also be specialist qualifications, all recordable on the Council's register.

The most controversial recommendation, however, is that 'students should be supernumerary to the NHS staffing establishments throughout the whole period of preparation and they should receive training grants which are primarily NHS controlled but administered by the National Boards from a separate budget and education costs clearly identified'. Other proposals include the introduction of a new grade of helper under the supervision of a registered nurse practitioner and the provision of opportunities for enrolled nurses (who would be phased out) to undertake conversion courses to become registered nurses.

Project 2000 differs from the Judge report in that the student, although supernumerary, remains within the NHS, and the suggested specialities are slightly different. It differs from the Committee on Nursing in that there is only one course, that leading to registration, whereas the Committee on Nursing suggested a course leading to certification and a further course for registration.

The nursing profession has pressed for students to be made supernumerary to the workforce for 40 years. The difficulty in the government acceptance lies in the cost and the implications for manpower as we move into a period when there are fewer young people in the population. If these proposals are accepted they will have consequences for the future education of district nurses.

However, of perhaps greater immediate consequence to district nurses are the recommendations of the Review Team on Community Nursing in England, under the chairmanship of Mrs Julia Cumberlege, contained in the report *Neighbourhood Nursing: A Focus for Care*.[10] This report could be implemented without heavy implications for cost and without undue disturbance. The report suggests that each district health authority should identify neighbourhoods with populations of between 10 000 and 20 000, and that each should have a neighbourhood nursing service with the work of the community midwives, community psychiatric nurses, nurses for the mentally handicapped and other specialist nurses fully coordinated into the service.

The report's proposals for training are revolutionary, for it advocates that

'Within two years the English National Board should introduce a common training and education programme for all district nurses, health visitors and school nurses.'

Students would then study their speciality in greater depth, with all trainings having equal value.

Another important proposal is the suggestion that the principle of the nurse practitioner should be introduced into the primary health care team. Here the term 'nurse practitioner' has a different connotation from the use of the term in Project 2000. This idea is not new but is now being more actively canvassed.

Such designated practitioners would be able to prescribe from a limited list set out by the DHSS, they would be highly trained and could be consulted by patients if they so wished, and this, it was hoped, would cut down the burden on the general practitioner's time. Allied to this proposal is the controversial recommendation that the 70% subsidy to general practitioners for the employment of practice nurses should be phased out. This does not mean there would be no practice nurses, but they would be employed by the district authority.

Although the Cumberlege report has been favourably received by most nurse members of the primary care team, and if implemented it would go a long way to resolving the differences that have grown up in the historical past concerning the training and status of the different members of the nursing team, there are many hurdles to overcome. Not least of these will be the attitude of the general practitioners who over the years have become used to the idea of nurses being employed exclusively by them. Another problem is that some practice nurses lack the further training for the tasks they undertake. However, a quarter of a century ago group attachment was a novelty, now it has become an accepted fact. If the family practitioner service and the primary health care team are not to be overwhelmed by the growing needs of the population, then some rationalisation of tasks and duties will have to be made. The district nurse in the past was often underused; the Cumberlege proposals could lead the way, not only to utilising her potential more fully, but also providing a better service to the patients. It will be interesting to learn the results of the consultation on this document and the one on primary health care.

Nurse management

Apart from education and pay the other great concern of the nursing profession after the setting up of the Health Service was the structure of nursing administration, and related to it, the career structure. The old style did not fit the tripartite structure of the hospital service nor yet the new pattern for the local authority services. The Committee on Senior Nursing Structure under the chairmanship of Sir Brian Salmon (1966) attempted to rationalise and simplify the position by proposing three bands of administration, top, middle and first line, with only two grades in each. Unfortunately in some cases the report was hastily implemented and without sufficient preparation, and some of the fundamental philosophy was often ignored. Nevertheless, the implementation did restore the nursing voice to the decision-making levels, and, contrary to popular myth, it actually reduced the ratio of nursing administrative posts to ward posts.

A similar report was introduced for the community nursing services under the chairmanship of Mr E. Mayston and was important for district nurses because it merged the three arms of community nursing, midwifery, 'home nursing' and health visiting. The report recommended that the structure should be based on geography and not on function, and that at the top, the policy-making level, a chief nursing officer should be appointed to coordinate the nursing services and to provide a single line of communication on nursing matters to the Medical Officer of Health. In middle management only one grade was recommended, which equated with the Senior Nursing Officer in the Salmon structure. However, when dealing with first-line management there was a fundamental difference between the community and the hospital services; nurses in the community had an additional training and functioned as independent practitioners, and it was difficult to make a valid comparison because the community nurse had to organise her own priorities and workload without other nursing support. The committee considered, therefore, that all grades in the community services should receive management training.

The implementation of the Mayston report was over-shadowed by the reorganisation of the health services (Chapter 18) but the fact that there was a clear 'line' structure for services that were integrated made it comparatively easy to dovetail with the hospital services. But for the Salmon and Mayston reports, the reorganisation of the health services would have proved even more traumatic for nursing than was the case.

The changes which followed these reports were, however, strongly opposed by the medical profession and by some nurses. In particular, in the community services general practitioners saw nurse managers as remote bureaucrats who 'interfered' with the work of the primary health care team. Some community nurses, resenting the restrictions that some nurse managers (whether because of health authority policies, rigid attitudes, or financial constraints) placed upon their expanding clinical role, chose direct employment by general practitioners as practice nurses. The number of nurse managers was constantly criticised, and in response to this and other political pressures (Chapter 18) was gradually reduced. By 1986, however, the Cumberlege team, which included a management consultant among its members, suggested that community nursing was, on the contrary, suffering from inadequate management, especially in respect of objective setting, planning and monitoring. It therefore recommended a strong role for the managers of neighbourhood nursing services, with proper training for the role and an appropriate level of remuneration. These recommendations, which mirror similar developments in hospitals, are a reflection of new management theories in general and a changing approach to nursing management in particular, in which the function of the manager is seen not as the wielding of supervisory control implied by a Salmon-type hierarchy, but as facilitating clinical practice by providing appropriate resources, organisational frameworks and professional support systems.

Developing new roles

The clinical career structure in nursing which many have advocated has not yet been achieved, but the clinical role of nurses, including district nurses, is developing rapidly. Nurses are demanding (and in many cases achieving) greater autonomy and accountability. One indication of this change in community nursing is the development of the nurse practitioner in primary health care. This concept, which began in North America but is now being developed in several countries as part of the Health for All strategy, was commended to the Cumberlege review team by many of those who gave evidence, including the Royal College of Nursing. The review team's public opinion poll found that two-thirds of those interviewed were prepared to talk to a nurse instead of a doctor, and 60% would actually prefer to see a nurse for certain purposes. There is now sound research evidence to support the effectiveness of the nurse in this role both in this country and elsewhere. They therefore recommended that the nurse practitioner role should be introduced into primary health care and also that nurses should be allowed to prescribe from a limited list of medications which are currently restricted to medical prescription; this recommendation has been widely supported within community nursing, but needs further debate on definition and detail.

The European Community regulations

These regulations are important to nursing. Article 57 of the Treaty of Rome requires mutual recognition of diplomas and qualifying certificates and the coordination of conditions of practice. The directives issued by the Commission are only concerned with broad parameters regarding the quantitative aspects, and they point out that emphasis should be on the quality of training. Each country has to have a 'competent authority' responsible for implementing the directives and in the case of Britain this is now the United Kingdom Central Council. Representatives of the Council take part in appropriate European Community discussions, and Officers of the Council serve on advisory committees for training in nursing and midwifery.

The directives for general nurses

The requirements are broad and flexible: all nursing recruits must have 10 years' general education, and the quantitive requirements are that the training should be 4600 hours or 3 years, although it is recognised that mere duration is meaningless and it is likely that in the future training will be measured in terms of hours. However, it seems clear that only the registration of course of the Committee on Nursing would be acceptable, but the main problem arises in ensuring that students of nursing have theoretical knowledge and experience in the seven areas laid down by the directive, which include: general and specialist medicine, general and specialist surgery, child care and paediatrics, maternity care, mental health and psychiatry, care of the old and geriatrics, and home nursing. Although these can be accommodated in the proposed 'modular' system, if they are to be anything but perfunctory then there is little chance of the student giving much service to the wards and this must raise the question as to whether she should be on the payroll and counted as 'ward staff'.

These directives are of course important for district nurses since *all* students must now have experience and teaching in home nursing and this can only reasonably be done on a one-to-one basis. It will be time-consuming and it implies that all district nurses must be able to teach students, which requires a different skill from that exercised when teaching patients. There are at present 49 000 students in training in England alone.

Conclusion

Policies for nursing have undergone a change in the past 30 years. In many ways the wheel has gone full circle because having cured the curable and prevented, or intervened with, much that is now preventable, we are left with the inescapable fact that we must all age and eventually die, and before we leave this world what we are most likely to need is care. Therefore, more and more the nurse must take on the role of the prescriber and organiser of care, and administrative support services and nursing education must now be directed to this end. For six of the cases described at the beginning of this book medicine can now do little, but good nursing care can still do much; for two at least the best hope is that good care will see the patients 'comfortably out of this world' and it will support and comfort the relatives, and other carers, to the end and beyond.

References

1. Nightingale F. (1859, facsimile ed. 1970). *Notes on Nursing*, p. 16. London: Duckworth.
2. Ibid; p. 17.
3. Baly M. E. (1986). *Florence Nightingale and the Nursing Legacy*. London: Croom Helm.
4. Ibid; p. 571.
5. *The Select Committee on the Registration of Nurse*, p. 15, (1904). London: HMSO.
6. Ministry of Health (1919). *The Training of Health Visitors* (Circulars 4 M and C W). London: HMSO.

7. Baly M. E. (1980). *Nursing and Social Change*, 2nd edn, Chapters 14 and 23. London: Heinemann Medical.
8. Commission on Nursing Education (1985). *The Education of Nurses: A new dispensation*. London: RCN Publications.
9. *Project 2000* (report of the United Kingdom Central Council, 1986). London: UKCC.
10. Department of Health and Social Security (1986). *Neighbourhood Nursing: a focus for care* (Cumberlege report). London: HMSO.

Further Reading

Abel-Smith B. (1960). *A History of the Nursing Profession*. London: Heinemann Medical.

Baly M. E. (1980). *Nursing and Social Change*. London: Heinemann Medical.

Clay T. (1987). *Nurses Power and Politics*. London: Heinemann Medical.

Maggs C. J. (1983). *The Origins of General Nursing*. London: Croom Helm.

Royal College of Nursing (1986). *What the Rcn Stands for*. London: RCN Publications.

Salvage J. (1985). *The Politics of Nursing*. London: Heinemann Medical.

WHO (1986). *Targets for Health for All by the Year 2000: Implications for nursing and midwifery*. Geneva: WHO.

SECTION V

The Professional District Nurse

'A district nurse, competent to undertake duties in the community, will be held individually accountable for the professional standards of her own performance and must understand the legal and professional implications of caring for patients in their own homes.'

Panel of Assessors: *Report on the Education and Training of the District Nurse* (1978)

In their evidence to the Briggs Coordinating Committee the Panel of Assessors stressed the fact that the district nurse has unsupervised access to the homes of people who are ill, frail and at risk, and that there was therefore a need for a high standard of professional conduct and practice to safeguard both the patient and the nurse.

Although this need is common to all nursing, because the district nurse works alone and is isolated from her medical and nursing colleagues, questions about professional responsibility, accountability and ethical considerations have an even greater urgency.

This urgency is now exacerbated by the fact that the nurse may be dealing with patients with a wide variety of religious beliefs (or none at all) and that advances in medical knowledge and technology have produced ethical problems undreamed of by earlier generations. For these reasons, and because in the past there has been much confusion about the professional responsibility of the nurse, and in the present there is much concern about her extended role, two chapters have been devoted to the basic questions that must guide and influence nursing practice, and to the way district nursing itself developed as a profession.

Chapter 21

The Development of District Nursing

Although it is commonplace to think of professional nursing beginning with the Nightingale reforms of 1860, from time immemorial men and women with a vocation have cared for the sick in their own homes. Some, like the Vincentian sisters in the seventeenth century, belonged to orders that gave a training and had rules about bedside care that few would quarrel with today. Moreover, there have been periods when nurses attending patients in their own homes were trained in extended duties such as lancing, blood-letting and, later, vaccination. The performance of such tasks largely depended on who was on hand to do them.

Nursing in the community in the nineteenth century

The old Poor Law committees usually employed parish nurses to care for their pauper sick in their own homes and, even after the Amendment Act of 1834 (the New Poor Law) it was often found to be cheaper to care for the poor sick at home rather than put them in the workhouse. The standard of care offered to paupers varied widely—as did the nursing duties which at times embraced everything from administering dangerous drugs and applying leeches to minding the baby. However, by the standards of the times, and the general expectations for care, by no means all parish nursing was bad and records suggest that many earned their patients' gratitude.

The pauper sick were cared for by the employed 'parish' nurses and doctors, while the non-pauper 'poor sick' were often cared for by one of the many charities or visiting societies. In the middle of the nineteenth century efforts were made by charities to employ a more elevated cadre of women with some training in nursing, a notable experiment being that of Mrs Elizabeth Fry who, in 1840, founded a nursing institution in Devonshire Square, London. Although the scheme was inspired by the deaconess movement of Kaiserswerth it was not particularly successful because the objectives were muddled and the nurses lacked systematic training; indeed it was this confusion of spiritual proselytising with physical nursing that made Miss Nightingale vow that she would rather found a 'highly paid profession of nursing than a religious order'.

In 1859, William Rathbone, a wealthy shipowner in Liverpool, employed Mrs Robinson from St Thomas's Hospital to nurse his wife in the final stages of her consumption; Mrs Robinson so impressed her employer—a proof if one were needed that not all nursing before 1860 was bad—that he retained her to look after the 'poor sick' in the surrounding area. William Rathbone was of Quaker stock and came from a family with radical political views and a history of philanthropy, and he realised that good nursing not only alleviated suffering but it prevented pauperism by restoring the breadwinner to work; a nice example of charity going hand in hand with nineteenth-century utilitarianism. Since Mrs Robinson could do little on her own, Rathbone consulted Miss Nightingale who was just starting her School of Nursing at St Thomas's hospital, about the possibility of supplying trained nurses to look after the sick in their own homes. Miss Nightingale gave the matter much consideration and eventually suggested that the Liverpool Infirmary may be persuaded to train its own nurses for hospital work and home nursing in a joint training scheme. The Liverpool Infirmary cooperated—no doubt spurred on by the fact that Mr Rathbone promised a new training school built at his own expense—and the first 'trained' nurses were allocated to the districts of Liverpool in 1863.

The Liverpool scheme is important because it was the model for other provincial schemes and was at times at odds with the views and objectives of the later Queen's Institute of District Nursing. Each 'district' was run by a Ladies' Voluntary Committee which was responsible for collecting money and dispensing welfare, and each committee had a Lady Superintendent who was not a nurse but who supervised the work of nurses. Such superintendence was contrary to Miss Nightingale's dictum that 'only those who have undergone the training should rise to the position of Superintendent.' This is the heart of the conflict about 'amateur' and 'professional' that dominated so much of the correspondence about district nursing in the later part of the nineteenth century.

In 1868 Mr Rathbone became a member of parliament for a district of Liverpool, and as he then spent much time in London he was soon involved in a venture of the Order of St John of Jerusalem to promote district nursing in London. Miss Nightingale was again consulted, and although she was now out of London managing the complicated affairs of the Nightingale family and their two houses, she found time to write *Suggestions for Improving the Nursing Service for the Sick Poor*. These suggestions formed the basis of The Metropolitan Nursing Association which was founded in 1874 with Miss Florence Lees, one of Miss Nightingale's ablest pupils, as superintendent. Disciplined and well educated, Miss Lees converted Miss Nightingale to the view that 'district nursing should be a profession for educated women rather than a craft for the lower orders',[1] which was contrary to the opinion held by the ladies of Liverpool.

It is clear from the content of the lectures given by Miss Lees that she herself was adept at a number of skilled tchniques, which is no doubt why the doctors of the day were not enthusiastic about the idea of the new-style district nursing as 'an occupation for educated ladies'. The doctors argued that the new nurses would take the bread out of their mouths; but it must be remembered that many of the sick poor could not afford a doctor and for many poor families the district nurse *was* the substitute doctor; well might Miss Nightingale say 'the district nurse would carry more responsibility than her hospital colleague because there would be no doctor to call on.'

The candidates for the Metropolitan Association were carefully selected and spent 9 months training in the Home in Bloomsbury, followed by a year's training in a hospital operating the reformed nurse training system and, finally, a further 6 months studying district nursing. Apart from the theoretical knowledge required, the standard of conduct and ethics was strict. Nurses were not to interfere with the religious beliefs of the patients or influence them in any way, which was the antithesis to the philosophy of Mrs Fry's Institute and the Ranyard Bible Nurses. Furthermore, nurses must be prepared to do everything necessary to put even the most degraded dwellings in 'nursing order', and on no account were they to accept gifts. An interesting injunction was that a patient's hair should never be cut off unless it was hopelessly infected since it was better to take any trouble rather than lessen the patient's self-respect; a maxim that might stand at the heart of the nursing process.[2]

Queen Victoria's Jubilee Institute for Nurses

In 1887 after much diplomacy and counter-diplomacy, the greater part of the Women's Jubilee Offering to Queen Victoria amounting to £70 000 was given by the Queen for an extension of the work of district nursing. A provisional committee was set up under the chairmanship of the Duke of Westminster with Mr Rathbone, Sir James Paget and Miss Lees (now Mrs Dacre Craven) among the moving spirits. Thanks to Mr Rathbone, supported by Miss Nightingale, who now shared Miss Lees's view that district nurses must be well educated, the Bloomsbury centre for the Metropolitan and National Nursing Association became the central training home and its principles and ideals were accepted. Similar homes were set up in Dublin and Scotland and later elsewhere. Rosalind Paget, a niece of Mr Rathbone who had trained as a nurse at the London hospital, was appointed the first Superintendent General. Existing district nursing associations were invited to affiliate with the Queen's Jubilee Institute provided they conformed with the conditions laid down by the Institute and were duly inspected by them. Only nurses that had the requisite training and whose names were on the Roll were accepted as Queen's nurses and allowed to wear the specially designed uniform, the brassard and Queen's badge worn as a pendant.

In 1890 the Rural District Nursing association which had been founded earlier by a Mrs Malleson affiliated with the Queen's Institute, and County Nursing Associations were formed with Queen's nurses as superintendents. By no means all districts employing nurses could afford a Queen's nurse, and some were run by religious organisations while the Queen's Institute was strictly non-sectarian. By 1898 there were 639 Queen's nurses on the Roll but they were, of course, a minority. One difficulty was midwifery; associations often employed village midwives, who were at times under-employed and were often expected to give general nursing care and advice. After much discussion it was decided to offer village nurses a special training at Plaistow and, when the district was affiliated, to take them under the wing of the Queen's nurse and the inspection of the Queen's superintendent.

After the Midwives Act of 1902 midwives were required to be certified with the Central Midwives Board, and this applied to the village nurses. By now the Queen's Institute had introduced examinations and the training embraced principles of health teaching, infant care and feeding, and school nursing, not to mention assisting with operations in the home. The district nurse in the early part of the century was an all-purpose community worker dealing with all age groups and very conscious of her sanitary mission. With new social and health legislation and the National Insurance Act of 1911 the work of the district nurse expanded, and there was discussion as to whether one type of professional worker could encompass so many aspects of care. Already some authorities, including the London County Council, were employing nurses solely for school nursing, and with the Notification of Births Act more authorities were recruiting specially selected health visitors to work with the Medical Officer of Health and to be direct employees.

In 1919 state registration became a reality. Although the register was divided into parts and the standard was not high, it was at least now possible to differentiate between the trained and the untrained. Registration with the new General Nursing Council now became a prerequisite for starting district nurse training for which the Queen's Institute retained responsibility. In 1928 the charter of the Institute was revised and the name changed to the Queen's Institute of District Nursing. Throughout the inter-war period a large proportion of district nurses were employed through the agency of the Queen's Institute. Each association was responsible for raising money to pay for the salary of the district nurse, although by now this was supplemented by certain statutory payments. The Midwives Act of 1936 required all local authorities to employ salaried midwives, and this some did by employing midwives directly through their public health department. Each authority was a law unto itself, but there was a tendency in rural areas to use Queen's nurses for combined duties, using nurses who were often triply trained and who were, like their early counterparts, all-purpose workers and very much part of their community.

Like so many other voluntary services the Queen's Institute pioneered the way for a statutory service, for in 1948 the National Health Service Act required what the Act described as 'home nurses' to be provided by all authorities. A working party set up in 1955 to consider the training required for such nurses noted that out of the 9203 district nurses then in employment less than half were Queen's trained, and because of the increased demand for such nurses it was decided that other arrangements should be made for this training. In 1959 the Panel of Assessors for District Nurse Training was set up to advise the Ministry of Health, which reduced the length of training from 6 months to 4. The Panel took over the organisation of training as an interim measure, but although the granting of a National Certificate had the effect of increasing the number of nurses with a 'certificate', it was a retrograde step because the district nurses now had no independent educational body, and the emphasis was on numbers rather than preparation to meet the future health needs of the community. In 1968 the Queen's Institute finally surrendered its training responsibility.

District nurses, having lost the prestige once offered by being 'Queen's nurses' with a distinctive uniform and the attention it attracted, now felt their position as the Cinderella of the primary care team, more acutely because since 1962 their colleagues in the team, the health visitors, had had an independent Council for Training and Education of Health Visitors which provided a longer, more heuristic and prestigious educational programme. The Committee on Nursing (Briggs) which reported in 1972 recommended that nurse training should be seen as a continuum and that more emphasis should be placed on community care, and the district nurses looked to the implementation of the committee's recommendations to put their anomaly right. However, some training bodies that were to be replaced by a Council for nurses and midwives and the health visitors were fearful that the new training to be offered for *their* speciality would be lower than they had already achieved; they therefore demanded, and eventually received, a separate committee within the proposed new structure. This left the district nurses in the same anomalous position, and still a far cry from the days of the superior standard of education demanded by Dame Rosalind Paget which had made them the envy of the nursing world. In 1979 the Panel of Assessors was reconstituted and its membership enlarged, which together with professional organisations lobbied for recognition. By dint of determination district nurses obtained their own committee under the aegis of the Central Council and National Boards. A new curriculum was approved and introduced in 1981 and the new training was mandatory before anyone could use the title and practise as a district nurse.

District nursing as a profession

Much of the debate about district nursing at the end of the nineteenth century turned on the question of whether or not it could be regarded as a profession. Discussion centred on the fact that the district nurse was required to do many non-nursing tasks and was involved in social questions beyond her competence. Therefore, the argument ran, district nurses should be honest working women, supervised by Lady Superintendents who could deal with the social and welfare problems. Usually these superintendents were from a class much involved in charitable work and they were, as Mary Stock points out in all fairness, 'not only well educated but experienced in social work'.[3]

Miss Nightingale and Miss Lees had other ideas. Miss Nightingale always insisted that a nurse must be educated because she had to be what she called 'a sanitary missioner' and teach people. This wider concept required educated women and a system in which nurses were accountable to a trained nurse for nursing matters. Paradoxically, the Nightingale experiment proved its worth as medicine became more scientific, and the younger doctors soon found that the educated nurse—originally trained to organise and give care—was a valuable assistant in the new technical medicine, and could be trusted to do much of the measuring and recording. It is therefore slightly ironic that nursing was hailed as becoming a profession at a time when, in hospitals at least, it became to a large extent an adjunct to another profession. In this respect the district nurse, concerned with giving care and unsupported by doctors, had a greater claim to be considered as an independent professional.

It was this coincidence of the rise of the Nurse Superintendent, to whom the nurse was supposed to be responsible for nursing matters, and the use of the nurse as the doctor's assistant, to whom she was responsible for clinical matters, that led to confusion about her professional responsibility and her accountability. Not only were the public and administration often misled, but nurses themselves had a muddled perception of their own role.

The hallmarks of a profession

Many writers have tried to describe the distinguishing marks of a profession but setting aside Plato's immortal phrase, 'the pursuit of excellence', perhaps the most succinct is that given by Sir Harold Himsworth because he manages to reduce to two main hallmarks most of the characteristics given by other writers.[4] These are set out more fully in *The Professional Ethic* especially written for nurses by Norah Mackenzie.[5]

Sir Harold argues that for a profession to exist at all there has to be a 'social contract' between society and the professional body. Society has a special need, and in order that this need can be met it allows the professional person 'the status, authority and privilege necessary for him to discharge his duty,' and it tacitly agrees to this person being above the law in certain respects. For example, the doctor and nurse are allowed to handle dangerous drugs and to do certain things to patients that in other circumstances would be an offence, lawyers are allowed to possess incriminating information and not be made to disclose it. In return for these privileges society requires that the professional person has a special competence and skill to meet the needs that brought the profession into being. If doctors can order their patients to take dangerous drugs or make incisions into their bodies, then society wants a positive assurance that the training and skill is of the best. Therefore, the first hallmark of a profession is that it embodies a *competence and skill that is more than ordinary*. This skill must always be improving, and for this reason requires the continual prosecution of research which is the essential criterion of professional endeavour.

However, it is not just 'competence' that distinguishes the professional person, and the second hallmark relates to the fact that professions deal with people and there is a special relationship between the practitioner and his client. As knowledge advances and science becomes more esoteric so medicine (and other professions) become less intelligible to the man in the street, and with every step towards more specialisation he becomes more vulnerable. How then can the patient or the client be sure that his professional adviser will act for his particular good? Of course he cannot be sure, but the bridge across this doubt is trust, and for this reason the professional person 'must act always so as to increase trust'. This is the reason why professions not only have registers of qualified practitioners, but why they also remove the name of anyone who is deemed not to be a fit and proper person. What constitutes improper conduct may vary from profession to profession, but the outstanding reason is always the betrayal of the special trust; in the case of doctors and nurses it is the misuse of drugs and the abuse of a relationship with a patient, whereas in law and accountancy it is the misuse of information or the client's money. Any conduct, however, on duty or off, which destroys trust in the profession may be cause for disciplinary action. Therefore, the second hallmark of a profession is that it adheres to a *standard of conduct and a code of ethics more exacting than that expected of the public in general.* It is for this reason that taking industrial action that inflicts harm on one's patients cannot be reconciled with professional status. Harm destroys trust and without trust the professions are helpless.

Is nursing a profession?

It is generally agreed that Miss Nightingale's aims to raise nursing to the status of a profession was realised inasmuch as nurses were trained and had 'competence and skill'. Later, the General Nursing Council ensured that no one could practise as a 'nurse' who was not, by the Council's standard, a safe practitioner. In 1921 the Council set up a Disciplinary and Penal Committee to deal with those nurses whose conduct, on or off duty, had in some ways destroyed trust. Broadly speaking Sir Harold's two main hallmarks were met, but there were large areas of doubt.

Firstly, while many nurses did possess a high degree of competence, the standard for registration was not high and it might only be in one branch of nursing. The reason was that because of the squabbles within the profession in 1919, nursing allowed the control of its basic education and training to pass to the Ministry of Health who was also responsible for the staffing levels. An important hallmark of a profession was surrendered—that it controls its own educational programme. On the credit side the profession did keep control of its post-basic education and although this was consistently higher it was to some extent dictated by the level of the foundation course.

In addition, the nursing profession did not possess a 'body of knowledge extended by united effort'. Much nursing, including district nursing, was concerned with how things were done and not why they were done, and a great deal of nursing practice was based on folklore rather than scientific findings. The position is now changing; the demographic profile and the changed health needs set out in Section I are placing a fresh emphasis on nursing care. Medicine can do little for Mr Adams, but planned nursing and cooperation with other agencies can do much, and thanks to this realisation there are nurses who, by virtue of research, practice, education and experience, are extending the body of knowledge about nursing practice. For example, sheer longevity, if nothing else, highlights the importance of a scientific approach to the care of pressure areas.

There has also been confusion about professional responsibility, as was mentioned earlier. Not only have nurses not had a clear perception of their own responsibility, but the confusion has been compounded by other and conflicting ideas about their role including those of the doctors and of official administration.[6] If the nurse is merely an assistant to someone else 'who takes responsibility' then there is little obligation to provide further training, refresher courses, libraries, journals, textbooks and all the other essentials for professional growth. Failure to meet the true needs of a profession means that eventually, cut off from the necessary tools, we become the way we are perceived.

Remaining a safe practitioner

If district nurses are to fulfil the first hallmark of a profession, 'to possess skill and competence above the average extended by united effort and continual research', then certain obligations are laid upon them. This implies a pooling of knowledge and experience which can only be achieved by meetings and conferences at various levels, or by the written word. One thing is certain, in a time of rapid professional change, excellence cannot be pursued in isolation. In this respect group practice offers an opportunity for inter-change of knowledge, experience, opinion and new developments as reported in professional journals, and although there has not been much favour for the Court Committee's idea of a 'designated specialist paediatric nurse and doctor', nevertheless, members of the team will have different interests, which can be used as a source of sapiential authority on an informal basis. Apart from this, each member of the team has a duty to participate in meetings, designed to advance the practice of his or her particular branch of health care, held outside the practice locality. If people do not do this the ideas of the team will become conservative and inbred.

The pursuit of excellence can only be carried out by regarding qualification as a first step in continuing education. There must be a commitment to regular professional reading through journals, and every practitioner should possess his basic reference books. Also, as will be seen from Chapter 22, ignorance of new knowledge is no excuse in law if a patient has suffered avoidable harm. The aphorism, 'half that you teach your students today will be out of date in 5 years; the trouble is you do not know which half', must now be speeded up, and even recently qualified nurses can no longer rely on what they learned in training.

The philosophy behind the Committee on Nursing was that nursing education should be seen as a continuum, with a progression towards specialist qualification for those who have the ability and motivation. Even then, however, some abilities will not be fully developed, and it is important that district nurses who have the motivation and ability to do so take opportunities for further study, not necessarily because it 'will make them better nurses' but because it makes life richer and more satisfying.

The commitment to continuing nursing education is ever changing. As opportunities for specialisation in community care develop, so new opportunities for further study and specialisation occur. It is the policy of professional organisations to cater for new groups as they arrive and some groups like the community psychiatric nurses feel the need to have their own association. As the health needs of the community changes, and medicine and care techniques advance, so nurses must regroup to study and meet those needs.

Nursing as a research-based profession

One of the most cogent reasons for denying that nursing has a professional status is that its practice is based on tradition modified by trial and error and not on scientific understanding. Some have argued that nursing is primarily a practical matter and to such arcane and pretentious flights nurses should not aspire. But, if nursing has been defined as 'assisting the patient, sick or well, in the performance of those activities contributing to health or its recovery that he would perform unaided had he the necessary strength, will and knowledge'—if this is the case, then it follows that the nurse must understand what is involved, and the inter-personal relationships that occur when she assists with these activities. Practice must be based on proper understanding and the results of professional action must be seen and evaluated.

In the past nursing has not had that group of research workers that are the usual concomitant of a profession, and research has not been the basis of the foundation training nor yet of post-basic education. However, in the last two decades strides have been made; Nurse Research Officers were appointed to the Department of Health, to the General Nursing Council, to the Royal College of Nursing, the Queen's Institute and to health authorities. A number of universities involved in nursing education supervise research into nursing practice and train nurse researchers, while the Royal College of Nursing has a Research Society and there are a number of opportunities for research appreciation.

For district nursing to become research-based there is a need for some district nurses with special aptitude to be trained as research workers and to identify nursing problems on the district that are either specially obdurate, or are now changing and in need of further study. Although comparatively few will be so trained, and not all research yields valuable results, all professional nurses should be aware of the main tenets of the research approach and the different types of methodology, and all should be able to read a research report with understanding. Moreover, they should know and act on such research as has been validated, such as the Norton Pressure Sore Scale, and they should continually question their own practices. It is the duty of every district nurse to those she trains not to hand on blind obedience to standard practice, but to advocate a questioning of what we do, why we do it, and even whether it needs to be done at all.

Research should not be seen as a thing apart but should inform all practice. For this reason the authors of this book decided against a separate chapter on research, and also because, like Miss Nightingale's 'handicraft of nursing', it cannot be taught in a manual.

References

1. Stocks M. (1960). *A Hundred Years of District Nursing*, p. 44. London: Allen & Unwin.
2. Dacre Craven F. (1889). *A Guide to District Nurses and Home Nursing*. London: Macmillan. (Quoted by Stocks, 1960[1])
3. Stocks M. (1960) *op. cit.*; p. 30.
4. Himsworth H. (1953). Change and permanence in education for medicine. *The Lancet*, Oct. 17; p. 789.
5. Mackenzie N. (1971). *The Professional Ethic*. London: English University Press.
6. Anderson E. R. (1973). *The Role of the Nurse*. London: RCN Publications.

Further Reading

Baly M. E. (1980). *Nursing and Social Change,* 2nd edn Chapter 24, Appendix 8. London: Heinemann Medical.
Baly M. E. (1987) *A History of the Queen's Nursing Institute*. Beckenham: Croom Helm.
Hockey L., Macleod Clark J. (1979). *Research for Nursing*. Aylesbury: HM & M.

Chapter 22

Ethical and Legal Considerations

When Stephen Undershaft in Shaw's *Major Barbara* told his father that he had the qualifications for becoming a politician because he 'knew the difference between right and wrong', his father regarded this as a joke because, as he said, it was a subject that had always puzzled philosophers and baffled lawyers. We by no means always know 'what things we ought to do' as recent debates on medical ethics demonstrate all too clearly.

Nurses, if they claim to be professional people, cannot stand aside from ethical issues; indeed being closest to the patients they should be their advocates. Apart from a duty to speak up in public debate or in the professional press about the use of scarce resources or questions of an abuse, for example, the failure to get proper consent for a transplant, nurses are confronted with their own ethical problems for which the answer is by no means always clear.

The professional ethic

The fact that professions lay down ethical codes is indicative of how important this subject is to professional people. The UKCC issues a Code of Professional Conduct[1] which every nurse should know. The code stresses that every registered nurse, midwife and health visitor is accountable for her practice, and, in the exercise of professional accountability must take into account the 14 points laid down in the code (see Appendix 1).

The International Council of Nurses also issues its own code but this is only a general statement endorsing the fact that nurses believe in essential freedoms and the preservation of human life, and that their activities will be 'unrestricted by considerations of race, colour, politics or social status'.[2] However, as the RCN discussion document on ethics points out, 'codes are never a substitute for individual moral integrity'.[3] If we are left relying on individual integrity, what guides can practitioners find to help them make the right decisions in controversial matters?

Some people will say that there is no dilemma, and that their own religious beliefs or personal philosophy provide all the answers. Stephen Undershaft belonged to that group. But religious creeds are usually in archaic language, and in a time of rapid change even the most devout and learned can draw different conclusions from the same basic teaching, as the terrible conflict at the time of Reformation serves to testify. Moreover, although religious teaching lays down guidance about living it is usually couched in general terms or through parables and can be interpreted equivocally. Nor have the great moral philosophers been more explicit, but at least they have shown the questions that ought to be asked. This is the value of including some moral philosophy in all professional education.

Nearly 2500 years ago Socrates (469–399 BC) asked the abiding question, 'How ought men to live?' and tried to find the answer through dialectical logic, working out by question and answer, what contributes to virtue and what makes a good citizen. Socratic teaching was written down by his disciple Plato (427–348 BC) who fused it with his own philosophy and the concept of the 'idea' or 'ideal', the eternally existing pattern of which individual things are but imperfect copies. Plato held that right behaviour stemmed from a proper balance of the elements within us and that correct harmony led to goodness; therefore, balanced actions were just actions, that is to say, they were disinterested actions, and hence, the figure of Justice is often depicted holding a pair of scales. The Socratic tradition emphasised that if man was wicked it was due to his ignorance, therefore virtue must be pursued through the pursuit of knowledge. Aristotle (348–322 BC) whose ethics were the lodestar of mediaeval philosophy, stressed that good could only be achieved through contemplation and the rational principle, which is why his works on politics and ethics were closely related. Stephen Undershaft, brought up in the nineteenth-century public school classical tradition, thought the same. The Greek system of thought dovetailed with the Christian ethic with which it was largely in tune, and this fusion gave the moral philosophy which governed western civilisation until the coming of modern science. Even after that it was commonplace to describe subsequent philosophy as a 'footnote to Plato'.

A new attempt at laying down principles of behaviour came in the eighteenth century with the philosophers of the so-called 'Enlightenment' who challenged the idea of an innate conscience and whose work gave rise to the principle of 'the greatest good for the greatest number' and Bentham's idea of 'utilitarianism' which was the underlying force of so much nineteenth-century legislation.

The greatest influence on modern moral philosophy, however, has undoubtedly been Immanuel Kant (1724–1804) who maintained that 'goodness' was not an inborn characteristic and that 'good feelings' such as sympathy could lead to wrong actions. For Kant a human action is only morally good when it is done for the sake of 'duty', that is to say it is done for a disinterested reason; Kant places much emphasis on the right motivation. To find a governing principle Kant posited two imperatives, the second of which is generally known as the 'categorical imperative' and states '*Act only on that maxim through which, at the same time you can will it, will become a universal law*', sometimes rendered as 'am I willing that everyone should act the way I am acting now'. Although much Kantian philosophy is difficult and convoluted, nevertheless Kant does provide a useful working guide in dealing with patients and colleagues. It is always well worth questioning our motivation. Kant, like Plato, is explicit about the danger of inflicting harm for our own ends, which of course would include harming patients to achieve a salary award, but he offers no golden key about the problem of disinterested harm to avert a greater harm. For example, are war, civil disobedience or revolution ever justified?

Philosophers such as Bertrand Russell have looked at 'the right action' in terms of contemporary values and mores; others have tried to rethink moral philosophy in terms of current problems, for example, over-population and finite resources. Still others, especially since the first explosion of the nuclear bomb, have been concerned whether in fact all knowledge *is* good and whether truth *should* be followed wherever it leads, even if it leads to genetic engineering and to the abyss.

Meantime, as life becomes increasingly complex the practical problems for the district nurse multiply. Records on the computer and the ever-increasing size of the team change the old concept of confidentiality; there are new questions about the 'pill' and who should have it; and the possibility of prolonging life artificially raises terrible dilemmas about 'saving life at all cost'.

Some ethical problems for nurses

Confidentiality

In recent years a number of inquiries, particularly into the deaths of children in care, have highlighted the strain that the commitment to confidentiality can place on the professional worker. Nurses have, quite rightly, taken from the doctors that part of the Hippocratic oath which says 'whatever I see of the lives of men which ought not to be spoken of abroad, I will not divulge, deeming that on such matters we should be silent.' But what should a nurse do if she suspects that a child, or an old or disabled person, is being cruelly treated and abused? Such suspicions can place the nurse in a difficult position, and she has to weigh up whether the danger is immediate and whether reporting her suspicions would risk having the door closed against all workers and thus making the last state worse than the first.

The district nurse is less likely to come across child abuse than her health visitor colleague, but she may well suspect abuse or gross neglect of an old person, and the guidelines laid down by the Department of Health dealing with suspected child abuse could be adapted. In the case of an emergency, if the person in question is already apparently injured, there should be prompt consultation with the doctor and possibly the social worker with a view to getting the patient removed to hospital for an assessment. However, if suspicions are not strong enough to warrant this the nurse should discuss the case with the family doctor and at least one senior colleague, or a colleague in a different profession. The risks should be weighed and a case conference called. Senior nursing staff should ensure that nurses know what to do when faced with such a dilemma. In the end the nurse herself must decide when to seek advice and her judgement will be based on her knowledge and experience, an inexperienced nurse may well have over-estimated the ability of a family to cope when faced with the burden of giving continual care to someone like John Davis, and have given the family more responsibility than they can stand. Sometimes we hear what we want to hear and all too often we listen to what people are saying rather than grasp what they are trying to tell us.

However, in the event of a tragedy such as a patient being injured, or even killed, by relatives, it must be remembered that no one involved is above the law. Professional workers have been severely criticised in court for failing to report suspicions about neglect, and it was of little avail when they told the judge that they were 'trying to establish a client/worker relationship based on confidence.'

There may be cases where a nurse is subpoenaed; if so she must appear in court and give evidence on oath, and to refuse to do so is contempt of court. If a nurse is called as a witness she should take care to confine her answers to factual, truthful statements and never allow herself to be drawn into giving an opinion. This is something which must be left to the 'expert witness'. If the nurse feels uneasy about the prospect of cross-examination she should seek advice from her organisation. Fortunately, in actual practice conflicts concerning confidentiality and the requirements of the law are comparatively rare, but there have been cases where doctors have been prepared to be prosecuted rather than betray a confidence and journalists have gone to prison rather than reveal their sources. Each professional must judge for himself whether a principle is at stake, act accordingly and be prepared to take the consequences. It must be borne in mind that there is a special question of confidentiality concerning patients with AIDS. This comes within the Sexually Transmitted Diseases Act, when to reveal confidences is against the law and not really an ethical and moral dilemma.

There may be other problems concerning confidentiality. Sometimes the nurse through her own perspicacity learns something that the patient wishes to be secret, or the patient or relatives, in a moment of stress, may reveal something and then beg the nurse to say nothing. Such confidences must be respected and are best forgotten and certainly not recorded. However, if it impinges on the health of the patient, then the nurse should try to get the patient to accept help voluntarily. Such situations can be delicate and time-consuming, they may involve such problems as wife-battering, an unwanted pregnancy, fear of violence due to mental disorder or alcoholism, suspicions of drug addiction or worries about AIDS. On these occasions the nurse must give such lonely support as she can until those concerned are ready to accept help; but there may be rare occasions when the matter seems so serious that in the interest of the greater good, and perhaps the safety of other people, confidence has to be broken. This is a big decision, but if it has to be taken the person concerned should be warned that in their own interests and possibly someone else's, another person must be consulted; this of course could very well in the first instance be the doctor or the social worker. Never act behind the patient's back. Once the step has been taken, provided it is done honestly, the patient may well be relieved that the decision to act has been taken from them. In fact this is something the nurse needs to be quick at discerning: the occasion when 'Don't tell anyone' means 'Please help me'.

Saving patients from themselves

It has been pointed out in Chapter 13 that an order for compulsory removal will only be made in exceptional circumstances, but nurses sometimes come across people who are elderly, confused and apparently unable to cope with their hygiene and nutritional needs, but who refuse help and are determined 'to keep their independence'. This is a problem likely to get worse as the age group over 80 years increases. Because of the discrepancy between male and female life expectancies many of these will be women living alone, and as they get older, some will be eccentric and some confused. But who is to say that they should not be allowed to finish their lives among the unwashed dishes if they are determined to do so? 'Is life a boon?' asked W. S. Gilbert in *The Yeomen of the Guard*, but not everyone worries about staying alive until July when 'perchance they might have died in June'. If we start coercing those we regard as unfit to live alone, what criteria do we use, and who will watch the watchers?

No one can be forced to accept help against their will; but the district nurse who may have been the friend of the family for a long time is often in a good position to give advice early and to apply gentle persuasion when things begin to go astray, and she may be able to ease patients into the idea that sheltered accommodation is not necessarily the end of all independence. The secret lies in getting people to make the decision before they become confused, but this is advice more easily given than taken.

Suspicions of criminal activities

Sometimes it comes to the nurse's notice that the family she is visiting is engaged on some illegal activity and she may wonder if she has a duty to the law. It is not the job of the nurse to play policeman; if those plants in the front garden could possibly be cannabis, so be it; or if she becomes aware that Mr Evans is conducting a rewarding side-line while off sick, that is not her concern. However, as in the case of confidence, there may be rare occasions when she has to consider the greater good. Rarely are district nurses going to stumble on a cache of home-made bombs, but there may be other instances, such as the much-discussed dilemma about the patient who arrives at surgery with an apparent bullet wound of the shoulder after the news of a bank robbery. There can be no rules in such cases, except that a patient's confidence should only be betrayed if some greater issue is at stake, and this calls for personal judgement, wisdom and, above all, the ability to see a situation from several perspectives.

Terminal care and the wishes of the patient

The Victorians accepted death and talked about it, largely because theirs was, at least superficially, a religious society, but also because, with a high death rate and a high birth rate, both were frequent occurrences. Now, in a secular society and with death a less frequent visitor, it has tended to become a taboo subject, and this failure to be able to talk about death is at the root of some of the current problems concerning the wishes of the patients themselves, and their adviser's ideas about what is best for them. However, it must be remembered that a person is not obliged to accept medical treatment, even if refusal may result in an earlier death, and there is no legal, moral or ethical obligation to use drugs, or apply treatments if they can at best be described as prolonging the process or distress of dying.

The nurse may well be troubled about patients dying alone with perhaps only intermittent care, but sad though this is, and however much it is an indictment of modern society, is it worse than being moved into hospital for the last few days of life? Although hospices like St Christopher's have provided centres of excellence and research and have to a large extent revolutionised the medical care of the dying, it is now important that, as far as is humanly possible, these principles be applied in the domiciliary setting. Of the cases outlined at the beginning of this book, three are 'terminal' in the sense that they will not recover, and for two at least death is not far away. It is hoped that they will both be able to die at home, with dignity and as free from pain as possible, and that 'their nurse' will support them to the last.

Research ethics

The RCN discussion document on ethics says that although 'the initiation of clinical research is usually a medical responsibility nurses have the right and duty to express opinions about the effect of such procedures on the patients under their care.' Miss Norton has suggested paraphrasing Miss Nightingale with 'it is the first duty of the researcher to do the patient no harm.' To which wise counsel it should be added, that if avoidable harm occurs the patient may seek legal redress through the law of damages. Advising district nurses to be research-minded is not an invitation to rush into unsupervised studies which may do more harm than good; researchers must be trained and there must be sound reasons for the study. It must be remembered that patients have a right to withdraw and any duress put on a vulnerable group such as the old or the mentally handicapped is an abuse of professional power and can only bring research, and the profession itself, into disrepute. Whatever the purpose of a research study, it must be designed in such a way that the dignity of those participating is protected.

Communications about colleagues

In the hierarchical structure of a hospital there are exact procedures for staff appraisal and counselling but this is less easy within the primary care team, for to a large extent the members are independent practitioners. Difficulties may arise when colleagues know that a member of the team is failing in a way that is not obvious to the Nursing Officer. Failure may be due to domestic anxiety, poor health or incipient mental ill-health; it is no kindness to cover up until something does happen. Tragedies have occurred this way. Probably the best person to take action is the colleague who is nearest at work, maybe the one with whom the nurse in question works in harness, or in the case of an enrolled nurse, the district nurse who supervises. Sometimes a sympathetic approach is enough to persuade the nurse to become amenable to help, but occasionally, particularly in the case of mental illness, the nurse is obdurate. At this stage someone has a moral duty to take action. However, if such action is contemplated the nurse in question should be told, because it is important to be honest when dealing with colleagues as it is when dealing with patients or clients.

When making a report about a colleague there are several points to be borne in mind. A report (or reference) if it is true is not actionable, nor is it actionable if it is made in good faith and without malice to the person properly entitled to receive such a report. Privilege is lost, however, if information is passed on to a person or persons not entitled to receive it, and in the case of a district nurse this would include members of the team to whom she was not accountable. Finally, when dealing with a sick colleague it must be remembered that no approach can be made to her medical adviser without her express permission, and of course, no doctor would disclose information without the consent of his patient. In this respect it is important that district nurses understand to whom they are accountable under the Griffiths reorganisation, and whether they have a designated Nursing Officer to whom they can turn.

The records of patients

The practical considerations have been dealt with in earlier chapters but there may be ethical and legal implications. The fact that the care plan should be left in the patient's house is an indication that the plan must be factual and truthful. Other records must be kept in safe custody and should only be shown to persons entitled to see them. However, in this respect, there has recently been much disquiet about the increasing number of people who do have access to the patient's records, and with the district nurse taking a larger teaching role, this is becoming as true in the community as in the hospital. Everyone who has access to the patient's notes must be made aware of their obligation to safeguard confidentiality.

It is also important that patient's records are kept in a safe place and never lost; claims for damages may be brought at a later date, for example, a claim about the delayed effect of a drug, of which thalidomide is the prime example. For this reason, if for no other, it is important that records are accurate, legible and intelligible.

The records to be kept when administering controlled drugs are laid down by the Misuse of Drugs Acts 1985 and should be adhered to, but most authorities have their own rules to ensure that prescribing and recording habits are uniform. Although patients' records are confidential they are not the property of the practitioner and they must be disclosed to the proper authority if asked, the prospect of which is a further warning that they should never include unsubstantiated opinion. District nurses should be familiar with the UKCC's advisory paper on the administration of medicines.

Data Protection Act 1985

This Act enables people to check information held about them on computers; district nurses should be aware of its implications and the substance of the DHSS Circular 85/23.

Basically patients should be able to know what doctors and nurses have said about them, and this information should be available in all but exceptional circumstances. Many practices have computerised their records and they must now decide whether medical records should be exempt from the access requirement of the Act. Generally speaking, however, the British Medical Association and the Royal College of Nursing are in favour of patients having access to their notes except where the doctor feels such information could be a cause of distress. This Act clearly has relevance for district nurses but sharing information with the patient is in keeping with the philosophy of the nursing process.

The district nurse and the law

Confusion about accountability and professional responsibility may lead to lack of clarity about legal responsibility. When professionals were self-employed the situation was obvious; the doctor who was negligent or the architect who designed a house that fell down were clearly liable for damages. However, when professionals are employed by someone else, probably the state, the situation is less obvious, nevertheless the principle remains: professional practitioners are responsible for their own professional acts. A district nurse is a member of a primary care team and is employed by a health authority, and is personally responsible for the treatment she carries out and for the drugs she administers even though these were ordered by another professional; she is also responsible for delegating tasks to a proper person. If the patient, his property or his reputation suffer avoidable harm then the nurse in question may be liable to pay damages.

It cannot be stressed too often that each nurse is responsible for her own professional acts and for proper and safe delegation. There are no laws which lay down what a nurse should or should not do, and it is for the profession itself to determine the standards and content of nursing practice both in the basic course and in extended practice. If a nurse makes a mistake or causes harm whether acting within her role or outside it she may be held culpable. No debate about whether nursing is a profession or suggestions by other professionals can alter the realities of the law.

The duty of care—patients' rights

The nurse has a 'duty of care' for any patient with whom she deals and that patient has a right to expect that no avoidable harm will be done to him or his property, and 'harm' in this respect can include psychological factors such as anxiety caused by lack of, or even wrong, information. If the patient, or someone acting for him, feels that harm has resulted due to negligence there may be an action for damages and the action is likely to be brought against the person, persons, or corporate body against whom the claim is the most likely to succeed. However, even if the claim is initially brought against the health authority it must be remembered that the negligent person is also liable 'and indemnity may be claimed against that person'.

What constitutes negligence, and what harm, will be a matter for the law courts, and much will depend on the circumstances. If a nurse gives 1.0 mg of a well-known drug when the standard dose is 0.1 mg, even though the doctor himself misplaced the decimal point or did not make it clear, the nurse is negligent because a competent nurse should have queried the dose. The law expects a nurse to use initiative. If on the other hand, it was some esoteric drug and the wrong dose was ordered and given, the nurse could not reasonably be regarded as negligent. If harm results during the giving of treatment, a claim for damages would be unlikely to succeed if proper precautions had been taken and the treatment was given in a proper manner, and provided that the patient had given consent, understood the implications, and was the proper subject for the treatment or procedure in question. It must be remembered that 'avoidable harm' includes damage to property, and the district nurse is in a much more vulnerable position than her hospital colleagues in this respect. What about all that clutter in Mr Adam's room all too easily knocked over, or the antique table at Mr Fisher's side all too easily marked? If the nurse causes damage patients may quite rightly expect to be compensated, and if they don't it is still an embarrassment.

Finally, patients may sue not only because of physical harm but because of damage to their reputation. For this reason it is important that suspicions about cruelty, neglect or criminal activity are only made to the proper person through the correct channels. It is quite right to discuss fears that an old person is being underfed with the doctor, who would probably appreciate being informed but it may bring an action if it is discussed with the neighbours.

There are a number of points for the district nurse to remember if a claim is brought and she herself is likely to be involved. Firstly, even if the claim is against the authority she should seek advice from the professional or other organisation that manages her indemnity insurance cover. The claim may involve several members of the team who have different interests and whose evidence may conflict, and the unadvised lose out against the well-advised—there are always many versions of the same story. Secondly, the authority may settle out of court but subsequently conduct an 'unofficial' inquiry and apportion blame, or it may be concerned in defending its management role, but contending that it employed the right staff in the right place and equipment was adequate and properly maintained. On the other hand the nurse's defence might well be (and often is) that there were not enough qualified staff, or that the right equipment was not available. The managerial line of defence is not necessarily the same as that of the inidividual.

Apart from expecting that the nurse who has a duty to care will not be negligent, the patient also has the right to refuse treatment, and to touch someone without their consent is an assault. This may lead to a difficult situation with an obstinate, but ill and perhaps confused patient, who is refusing treatment or refusing to take prescribed drugs. If all persuasion by the nurse and relatives fails the patient must be left; no one can be forced to receive treatment he does not want.

The right to conscientious objection

Although the individual practitioner has 'the right to withdraw from involvement in practices that are at variance with his or her religious beliefs or to which he or she has an objection in conscience, always providing that he or she has given prior notice to the responsible authority of his or her unwillingness to participate in such practices and that as the result of his or her withdrawal, the life of a patient will not be placed in jeopardy',[4] nurses may not withdraw their services because they disagree with treatment or because they decline to nurse a certain type of patient. A test case has been the objection to ECT treatment, but more relevant has been the disinclination of some practitioners to nurse sufferers from AIDS. Nurses must take all proper precautions to protect their health but withdrawal of service is not one of them.

Although AIDS is a worrying phenomenon with maybe 30 000 people in Britain carrying the virus, with 4000 likely to die in the next few years, it must be kept in proportion; there have been scourges before. It is the duty of the district nurse to assist in the dissemination of knowledge about the transmission of the virus, but it is not for nurses to make moral judgements. All sufferers have the right to compassion and care. The doctors and nurses of the nineteenth century dealt with an alarmingly high proportion of venereal disease, which, in spite of the moral strictures of the day, they accepted as part of their duty to the sick. Syphilis has largely disappeared and there is every reason to hope that one day, in the long run, AIDS will go the same way. In the meantime sufferers have to be treated and their confidentiality respected.

The nurse's rights in relation to patients

As we have seen, the nurse may not coerce a patient; likewise the patient may not assault the nurse—unless she has forced an entrance against his wishes. If a nurse is assaulted by a patient she should withdraw as quickly as possible and a first sensible step would seem to be a discussion with the team as a whole. Maybe another member of the team would be more acceptable, or the patient may calm down, but if the patient continues to behave in a violent way to all comers then the team are quite within their rights to withdraw their services; indeed it would be folly to do otherwise. If a nurse is actually injured by a patient she should report the matter immediately and if she suffers real harm the matter should be taken up with the Criminal Injuries Board. Apart from assaults in the home district nurses have been attacked in the streets by gangs because it was thought that they were carrying drugs. Health authorities have a duty, as far as possible, to ensure the safety of vulnerable staff and in some places police protection may be advisable.

Furthermore, the nurse is entitled to expect that the premises she enters will be safe, and although the health and safety regulations do not extend to private houses, owners and occupiers are required to keep their property safe under the Occupiers' Liability Act 1957. With the obvious proviso that the nurse herself must take reasonable care, if she is injured due to faulty property, say a faulty floorboard or broken steps, she may well have a claim for compensation.

The National Insurance (Industrial Injuries) Act 1946

District nurses, who are often without trained assistance, may sustain injury to themselves when they are actually giving care; and this particularly applies to lifting patients. As far as possible nurses should avoid situations where they may either injure themselves or the patient. If the patient is injured he may have a claim against the nurse; if the nurse is injured she should report it immediately and sign the accident book, and if she is off sick she should make sure that a claim for industrial injury is lodged; this is payable no matter where the blame lies. Establishing the fact of 'industrial injury' is important, partly because injury benefit is higher than sickness benefit but, more importantly, if the disability goes on there will be a right to disablement benefit. If there is a delayed disability and the claim has not been established it is very difficult to do so retrospectively. Claims under the National Insurance Act are as of right and have nothing to do with claims for compensation.

Wills and gifts

The district nurse may become the long-standing friend of the family, but she should be wary of being drawn into too close a relationship, particularly in pecuniary matters. Nurses are sometimes asked to witness a patient's will but if so she would do him a service if she made sure all was in legal order; the two witnesses must witness the signature and sign in the presence of one another. One the whole it is better not to be involved in such transactions and some authorities have rules about this. The receiving or refusing of gifts can be a delicate matter, but any acceptance other than for the most trivial can be fraught with danger if the relatives are jealous, and large gifts, whether given or willed, may be challenged and regarded by the law as 'given under undue influence'. On the other hand, to refuse the memento from the grateful patient or relatives, or the garden produce from the proud husband, may appear churlish, and nurses must use their discretion about small gifts and be guided by good manners and common sense.

The duties and the position of the nurse

The qualified nurse is expected to be a safe practitioner within the limits of her training, but questions often arise about what are called 'grey areas'. The subject has been made unduly complicated by nurses being confused by 'certificates of authorisation' when in fact basic rules cover most problems.

The nurse should not undertake tasks outside her contract of employment. She should not, for example, agree with a doctor to do an immunisation clinic—however tempting the blandishments—unless the employing authority agrees; the doctor cannot assume responsibility for her and he does not employ her. If there is a professional accident while the nurse is doing a task outside her terms of contract, then in the eyes of the law she is doubly vulnerable, and the employing authority would certainly be under no obligation to help with her defence. However, this is not to say that nursing duties cannot or should not be extended, but if they are, there are certain precautions to be observed. The Royal College of Nursing and the British Medical Association have issued a leaflet with which all nurses should be familiar. *The Duties and Position of the Nurse*[5].

The main points—as they concern district nurses—can be summarised as follows:

1 A technique outside the scope of routine nursing should only be assigned to a nurse after consideration of the cirumstances and with the agreement of those concerned. The nurse assigned to such a task should receive proper training and supervision and be satisfied that she is competent to undertake the new duty.

2 There should be machinery for consultation between the Nursing Officers and the Family Practitioner Committees.

3 When agreement has been reached and it has been agreed that a nurse, or a group of nurses, should be deployed on duties normally considered outside the scope of routine nursing it should be reported to the employing authority and duly minuted.

4 Although Memorandum RHB 49/128 makes it clear that health authorities are expected to undertake the defence of a

nurse in proceedings against her, if the nurse has acted outside her authority such cases are to be referred to the Department of Health, but this does not absolve the nurse from personal liability for her own actions and there is no guarantee that the damages would be paid by the Department.

5   Because of the implications all nurses are urged to belong to a professional organisation *providing individual legal cover.*

6   It is important that doctors are involved in teaching programmes with reference to delegated tasks and that nursing management retains responsibility for assessing competence and ensuring that this is recorded.

If these rules are followed nurses have little to fear about extended duties, bearing in mind that they must be safe practitioners at all times and that these tasks must not be delegated to untrained persons.

However, it is not the performance of procedures 'outside the scope of routine nursing' that necessarily worries the district nurse, but the whole concept of 'prescribing care' and using initiative in planning a regime of care that is not task-orientated. Morever, the primary assessment can sometimes look perilously near 'diagnosis', but once again the same principles apply. The nurse must be a safe practitioner, inasmuch as her assessment must be based on sound knowledge and a physiological and psychological understanding of the patient's condition, and the care initiated should be that which a competent qualified nurse could be expected to prescribe. No one can expect more. Assessments are not infallible and patients may subsequently develop, or already have, an undiagnosed condition, which means that the care plan was wrong. This is not negligence. What must be borne in mind, however, is that if a wrong treatment, drug or dose is given because the nurse *herself* is out of date, for example through confusion over the metric system, this will be no excuse at law. The professional nurse has a duty to be, and to remain, a safe practitioner. Conversely, health authorities and senior nurses have a duty to see that opportunities are provided for updating and refresher courses; this is particularly important for nurses returning to district nursing after a break in service.

Stress on nurses in giving care

The UKCC code points out that registered nurses should 'have regard to the workload of and the pressures on professional colleagues and subordinates and take appropriate action if these are seen to be such as to constitute abuse of the individual practitioner and/or jeopardise safe standards of practice'. In other words, senior nurses and nurse managers have a duty to ensure that nurses do not have a workload greater than they can reasonably manage and still remain safe practitioners. That this precept is not always put into practice is clear from the report of the Professional Conduct Committee[6,7] in which it stated its concern about

> 'the ways in which, and the degree to which, second-level nurses are being placed in positions of responsibility for which their training did not prepare them and was not intended to prepare them . . .'

and

> 'The serious effects on patient safety, standards of care, and staff health and morale of manning which seemingly fails (in quantity and/or type) to match needs.'

The report goes on to say

> 'it does sometimes seem that some health authorities/boards/ employers expect practitioners to achieve the impossible. . .'

The failure to provide adequate staff to meet the reasonable needs of patients means that some practitioners either fail to provide safe practice, or due to stress, commit some misdemeanour which brings them before the Professional Conduct Committee. The same report noted with concern

> 'that there had not been a significant increase in the numbers recruited for district nurse courses. It was noted that many colleges have waiting lists and that there was no shortage of suitable applicants. . . Two difficulties were highlighted, lack of tutorial staff and restrictions on extra appointments and the increased use of unqualified staff in district nursing work with little prospect of them receiving approved training.'

Stress in district nursing is due not to lack of suitable recruits but to lack of finance. This is a political matter and district nurses must through their organisations bring these facts to light. The health needs of the community in the next decade cannot be met unless there is a political will to put more financial resource into community health care and increase the number of trained district nurses.

The district nurse and labour laws[8]

These laws, which are becoming increasingly complicated and frequently amended, apply to the district nurse as they do to any other citizen. Those most likely to affect her include:

The Contract of Employment Act 1972

This Act required that all employees, within 13 weeks of starting employment, be given a statement containing information about their rate (or scale) of remuneration, the frequency of payment, the terms and conditions of service—including the period of notice to be served—and the details of the grievance procedure. Apart from the 'contract of employment', professional workers can reasonably expect a job description and job specification, which should include the lines of accountability and the chain of command.

The Employment Protection legislation

The Employment Protection Act of 1975 extended legislation about unfair dismissal and enabled tribunals to award the reinstatement of a dismissed worker; it reduced to 26 weeks the period of completed employment necessary before the worker could complain of unfair dismissal, and was more explicit about trade union rights, time off allowed for union activities and other worker entitlements. Since then the Act has been amended several times and will be amended again. Most of the new amendments relate to union activities, reviews of closed-shop agreements, secret ballots and the like. Any nurse who feels she has been unfairly dismissed or had her contract broken in any way should get in touch with her appropriate organisation. For the purposes of industrial relations law the term 'trade union' includes those organisations who have applied successfully to the Certification Officer and have been certified as 'independent unions'. These include organisations like the Royal College of Nursing, the Royal College of Midwives and the British Medical Association.

Health and Safety at Work etc Act 1975

Although this Act does not apply to private houses, it does to clinics and old people's homes, and other public places where the nurse may work. It therefore behoves nurses to understand the main principles of the Act. These include ensuring that the working environment is safe and that equipment is in good order, that employees have adequate training and instruction, that entrances and exits are safe and there is a written-up policy on safety. The reason for the Act was that the incidence of accidents at work was unacceptably high, and the new legislation was designed to provide greater worker participation and awareness. Although there could be a danger of over-reaction, and 'safety' is not an end itself, nevertheless district nurses should set a good example and make sure that the premises in which they work are as safe as possible, lest it be said that the cobbler's children are the worst shod.

Nurses and industrial action

Whether withdrawal of labour by the caring team can be justified must be a matter for individual conscience. However, there are certain legal points to be borne in mind and a number of practical considerations.

Technically withdrawal of labour constitutes a breach of contract and can be a reason for dismissal. Although the Employment Protection Act lays down safeguards concerning such a breach in the pursuance of *bona fide* trade union activity much would depend on the particular circumstances and the attitude of the employing authority, but certainly an unofficial walk-out that left patients without cover might well be tested as a case for 'fair dismissal'. In addition, if a patient or patients suffered harm as a result of the withdrawal of labour they might well have a claim for damages. So far such a case has not arisen, but if it did there is no reason to suppose that if it were valid it would not be upheld.

Perhaps more important than the legal issues are the practical considerations. For withdrawal of labour to be effective in persuading the government to offer more money, withdrawal must be widespread and inflicting harm and hardship. But deliberately inflicted harm is something most nurses could not contemplate, nor could they visualise the 'picketing' of volunteers that would be necessary to make a strike effective. To argue that labour can be withdrawn without affecting the patients is dangerous. It implies that the absent nurses would not be missed by the patients, or that they were doing non-nursing tasks, or that they were over-staffed in the first place. Although it is possible to visualise a situation in which there is a moral duty to make a protest, the caring professions, for better or for worse, must find other means than the withdrawal of labour to put pressure on authorities. A study of wage economics reveals that public sector wages and salaries are affected by a number of factors of which industrial action has seldom been one.[9]

Although it is not always obvious, the profession's best ally is the esteem of the public. This unique esteem does not come because the district nurse is a safe practitioner who comes to the family in the time of trouble but because she 'acts always to increase trust'.

The district nurse, who is often closest to the patient, his family and other carers, has a duty to be their advocate. This was a first task of early district nurses. Miss Nightingale wrote

> 'Besides nursing the patients she shows them in their homes how they can call in official sanitary help, to make their one poor room healthy, how they can improvise appliances, how their home need not be broken up.'[10]

'Official sanitary help' may have changed and become more elaborate but it often still fails to help those in the greatest need. Miss Lees's ladies battered on the doors of sanitary officialdom; so too must we today. In 1986 it was calculated that the harsh winter caused over 100 deaths among the elderly every day because of cold-related illnesses. Help was often too little, too late and too complicated for the average citizen to understand.[11] At the same time in an affluent society there are 100 000 homeless people. District nurses may not see the really destitute sleeping rough, but they do see people whose health is impaired by living in sub-standard accommodation. They also see the results of mentally handicapped people being placed in the community without proper provision.

Sometimes help may be obtained through communication with colleagues or local agencies, but apart from that district nurses have a duty to make failures in the system known either through their own organisations or politically. 'All that is necessary for a great harm to be done is for good men to do nothing.' The Alma Ata declaration of the aim of health for all by the year 2000 AD will not be achieved unless health workers unite to strive to ensure that there is a political will to make this aim a reality.

References

1. UKCC (1984). *Code of Professional Conduct for the Nurse, Midwife and Health Visitor*, 2nd edn. London: UKCC.
2. International Council of Nurses (1974). *Code of Ethics*. Geneva.
3. Royal College of Nursing (1976). *A Code of Professional Conduct—a discussion document*. London: RCN Publications.
4. What the RCN Stands For (1976) Ethical Issues, p. 10. London: RCN Publications.
5. Royal College of Nursing (1970). *The Duties and Position of the Nurse*. London: RCN Publications.
6. Royal College of Nursing (1979). *The Extended Clinical Role of the Nurse*. London: RCN Publications.
7. Royal College of Nursing (1979). *The Extended Role of the Nurse—Legal Implications and Training Requirements*. HC27. London: RCN Publications.
8. United Kingdom Central Council (1985). *Annual Report 1984–85*. London: UKCC.
9. Baly M. E. (1980). *Nursing and Social Change* 2nd edn. London: Heinemann Medical.
10. Nightingale F. (1890). Introduction to the *'History of Nursing in the Homes of the Poor'*. London: Macmillan.
11. Age Concern (1986). *Hypothermia: the facts*. London: Age Concern.

Further reading

Baly M. E. (1984). *Professional Responsibility*, 2nd edn. Chichester: John Wiley.
Bond M. (1986). *Stress and Self-Awareness: A Guide for Nurses*. London: Heinemann Medical.
British Medical Association (1980). *Handbook of Medical Ethics*. London: BMA.
Martin A. (1978). *Watchdog for the Record*. London: RCN Publications.
Moore G. E. (1966). *Ethics*. Oxford: Oxford University Press.
Rumbold G. (1986). *Ethics in Nursing Practice*. London: Baillière Tindall.
Speller S. R. (1976). *Law Notes for Nurses*. London: RCN Publications.
Tschudin B. (1986). *Ethics in Nursing: the caring relationship*. London: Heinemann Medical.
United Kindom Central Council (1987). *Confidentiality*. UKCC Advisory Paper. London: UKCC.
Whincup N. H. (1982). *Legal Aspects of Medical and Nursing Services*. Beckenham: Ravenswood Press.

Appendices

UKCC Code of Professional Practice

Each registered nurse, midwife and health visitor shall act, at all times, in such a manner as to justify public trust and confidence, to uphold and enhance the good standing and reputation of the profession, to serve the interests of society, and above all to safeguard the interests of individual patients and clients.

Each registered nurse, midwife and health visitor is accountable for his or her practice, and, in the exercise of professional accountability shall:

1 Act always in such a way as to promote and safeguard the well being and interests of patients/clients.
2 Ensure that no action or omission on his/her part or within his/her sphere of influence is detrimental to the condition or safety of patients/clients.
3 Take every reasonable opportunity to maintain and improve professional knowledge and competence.
4 Acknowledge any limitations of competence and refuse in such cases to accept delegated functions without first having received instruction in regard to those functions and having been assessed as competent.
5 Work in a collaborative and co-operative manner with other health care professionals and recognise and respect their particular contributions within the health care team.
6 Take account of the customs, values and spiritual beliefs of patients/clients.
7 Make known to an appropriate person or authority any conscientious objection which may be relevant to professional practice.
8 Avoid any abuse of the privileged relationship which exists with patients/clients and of the privileged access allowed to their property, residence or workplace.
9 Respect confidential information obtained in the course of professional practice and refrain from disclosing such

information without the consent of the patient/client, or a person entitled to act on his/her behalf, except where disclosure is required by law or by the order of a court or is necessary in the public interest.

10   Have regard to the environment of care and its physical, psychological and social effects on patients/clients, and also to the adequacy of resources, and make known to appropriate persons or authorities any circumstances which could place patients/clients in jeopardy or which militate against safe standards of practice.

11   Have regard to the workload of and the pressures on professional colleagues and subordinates and take appropriate action if these are seen to be such as to constitute abuse of the individual practitioner and/or to jeopardise safe standards of practice.

12   In the context of the individual's own knowledge, experience, and sphere of authority, assist peers and subordinates to develop professional competence in accordance with their needs.

13   Refuse to accept any gift, favour or hospitality which might be interpreted as seeking to exert undue influence to obtain preferential consideration.

14   Avoid the use of professional qualifications in the promotion of commerical products in order not to compromise the independence of professional judgement on which patients/clients rely.

From: *Code of Professional Conduct for the Nurse, Midwife and Health Visitor*, 2nd edn (1984). London: United Kingdom Central Council for Nursing, Midwifery and Health Visiting. (With permission.)

Guide to Health and Social Services

This appendix is divided into three sections:

A Health services, provided by area health authorities (from 1982 provided by district health authorities) and by family practitioner committees.

B Personal social services provided by local authority social services departments.

C Social services provided by other agencies.

A HEALTH SERVICES

Service	Type of service provided	Notes
1 *Hospital services*	Inpatient care	Access via referral by GP
	Outpatient consultation	Referral by GP; GP can also arrange domiciliary visit by consultant
	Accident and emergency services	Self-referral to casualty departments. Some hospitals operate limited service for minor casualties only, with medical cover provided by GPs
	Maternity services—antenatal supervision, inpatient care, postnatal follow-up	Run in close conjunction with community midwifery and GP service; organisation varies greatly from district to district
2 *Hospital-based specialist services*	Diagnostic investigations	As requested by consultant or GP; for hospital inpatients and outpatients and for GP patients
	Physiotherapy	For inpatients and outpatients referred by consultants
	Occupational therapy	For inpatients and outpatients referred by consultant; limited community service provided through local authority social services

Social work	Hospital-based social workers are employed by local authority social services
Convalescence	Arranged by hospital social worker; infrequently available
Infertility and genetic counselling	Access via referral by GP or family planning clinic
Abortion	Access via referral by GP. Private clinics also available—access via referral by GP or voluntary organisation
Treatment of sexually transmitted diseases (special clinic)	Self-referral welcomed; referral by GP not necessary

3 Transport to and from hospital

Ambulance service	Sometimes run on an agency basis, e.g. London Ambulance Service. Can be ordered only by GP or hospital except: (i) for any accident (999 call) (ii) for sudden illness outside the home (999 call) (iii) maternity cases: by advance arrangement
Hospital car service	Private cars driven by volunteer owners paid a mileage allowance. Can be ordered only by hospital
Volunteer transport service	Run by many local voluntary organisations. Arrangements vary

Service	Type of service provided	Notes
	Expenses for travelling to and from hospital for visiting	Patients on low incomes or supplementary benefit may be eligible. Usually arranged by hospital social worker. See leaflet H 11 available from local social security offices or hospital social worker
4 *Community health services* (a) Health visiting	Advice about the care of young children, expectant and nursing mothers, the elderly, and others as referred or self-referred, by home visits and in clinics. Individual and group health education.	Visits *all* families following notification of birth. Access by self-referral, or referral by any health or social agency. Usually attached to general practice (see Chapter 5).
(b) District nursing	Nursing care in people's own homes and in health centres and surgeries	Access normally via referral by GP. Usually attached to general practice (see Chapter 5)
(c) Domiciliary midwifery	Home delivery now rare but antenatal and postnatal care, including health education, provided in conjunction with GP	Sometimes attached to general practice, or some other form of liaison scheme. Considerable variety of schemes for early discharge following hospital delivery
(d) Child health clinics	Health visiting advice. Developmental assessment including specific screening, e.g. vision, hearing. Immunisation (see below). Welfare foods (see below)	Held in health centres. GP surgeries, health authority clinics, and sometimes premises such as church halls hired by the health authority

(e) Immunisation	Primary immunisation for all children under 5 years against diphtheria, whooping cough, tetanus, polio, and measles. Other immunisation (e.g. TB) as necessary. Programme for older children (e.g. rubella) administered via school health service (see below)	May be given, usually by district nurse, at child health clinic or at GP's surgery. Other immunisations, i.e. for adults, come within family practitioner service (GP)
(f) Welfare foods	Vitamin drops/tablets (A, D, C) for expectant and nursing mothers and children under 5 years. Subsidised baby milks	Available at antenatal and child health clinics
(g) Family planning service	Advice on all methods of contraception including sterilisation and free contraceptive supplies. Some special clinics for phychosexual problems and for young people. Domiciliary service available in some areas	Advice also available for women patients only, through GP services
(h) Health education	Health education department acts as resource centre for advice and materials for all health service staff involved in health education. Also special programmes, and service to schools	
(i) School health service	Medical examination	Usually at school entry and at age 12 or 13. Undertaken by school nurse or health visitor at the school, with follow-up home visits if necessary
	Health surveillance, including screening for head lice, foot defects, vision and hearing. Immunisation. Specialist facilities such as speech therapy and child guidance. Dental examination and treatment.	

Service	Type of service provided	Notes
	Additional services in special schools for handicapped children	Also available through family practitioner dental service
(j) Priority dental service	Dental care for expectant and nursing mothers and children under 5 years	Usually organised in conjunction with school dental service
(k) Chiropody	Provided for elderly people in clinics or on a domiciliary basis; sometimes available for handicapped people and expectant and nursing mothers	Provided directly by health authority or by voluntary organisations such as British Red Cross Society, sometimes on an agency basis. Service very sparse in some areas
(l) Loan of equipment	Equipment necessary for nursing people at home such as commodes, hoists, incontinence pads, etc.	May be provided directly by the health authority or by voluntary organisations such as British Red Cross Society on an agency basis. Level of provision varies from area to area
5 Environmental health services	Investigation and control of outbreaks of infectious disease. Maintenance of controls on food hygiene	Run by local authority environmental health department with advice and medical staff provided by the health authority
6 Registration of nursing homes	Registration and inspection of private hospitals, nursing homes and mental nursing homes	

B PERSONAL SOCIAL SERVICES

Service	Type of service provided	Notes
1 Services for families and children		
(a) Day care	Provision of day nurseries; registration and regulation of private day nurseries and playgroups; registration and supervision of childminders	Any person who 'cares for one or more children under the age of 5, to whom they are not related, in their own home for a period of two hours or more in a day and for reward' must notify and be registered by the local authority and meet whatever conditions are required (e.g. limit on the number of children) as a condition of registration. Some authorities have training programmes for child minders
(b) Residential care	Children's homes (residential nurseries, community homes which were formerly called approved schools, hostels for teenagers)	Foster care now greatly preferred to institutional care. Foster parents are normally paid an allowance to cover cost of maintaining child; some authorities have salaried foster parents for handicapped or disturbed children
	Foster care	
	Registration and supervision of privately arranged foster care	
(c) Supervision of children in care	Residential or foster care, or supervision by social worker while child continues to live at home	Children may come 'into care' either as a result of a court order—e.g. when a child has committed a criminal offence or is 'exposed to moral danger' or 'beyond parental control', or if he is being ill-treated or neglected—or voluntarily at the request of parents

Service	Type of service provided	Notes
(d) Preventive services	Casework and counselling by social workers. Other services vary from area to area, e.g. adventure playgrounds, cash grants. Prevention of non-accidental injury to children; Area Review Committees developed jointly with health authorities	Developed since the 1963 Children and Young Persons Act Detailed procedures and guidelines vary from area to area but must conform to central guidelines laid down by DHSS
2 Services for handicapped and disabled		
(a) Social work service	Casework, counselling, and advice on obtaining services and benefits	Responsibilities laid down by 1948 National Assistance Act greatly extended by the Chronically Sick & Disabled Persons Act 1970. The local authority is required to maintain a register of disabled people
(b) Home helps	Basic housework, but often includes 'extras' such as shopping, collecting prescriptions, etc.	Charges based on means test. Persons receiving supplementary benefit usually pay nothing. Number of hours service available to each client limited by restrictions on service
(c) 'Meals on wheels'	A hot meal delivered to the home, usually two or three times per week	Usually run by a voluntary organisation (e.g. WRVS) on an agency basis. Small charge
(d) Occupational therapy	Mainly concerned with 'activities of daily living'; assesses the need for aids and adaptations to the home	

(e) Provision of aids and adaptations to the home	e.g. replacement of steps by ramps, lift, downstairs toilet	Available for privately owned and council-owned property
(f) Provision of telephone	All or part of the cost of installation and rental but not the cost of calls	Eligibility very restricted
(g) Day centres and social clubs	Premises often used as base for other services, e.g. luncheon club facilities	Service varies greatly from area to area, considerable involvement of voluntary organisations
(h) Transport facilities	Minibus or private car service, often run by voluntary organisations. Special car parking arrangements	NHS provision of 'tricycles' replaced by mobility allowance and provisions to assist in buying own cars
(i) Holidays and outings	Usually provided by voluntary organisations but paid for by local authority	Provided by several voluntary organisations, sometimes alongside other services (e.g. British Diabetic Association) sometimes as the main purpose of the organisation
(j) Residential services of various kinds	SS department may cooperate with housing department in allocation of council-owned property. Residential homes and hostels of various kinds	Severe shortage of suitable accommodation
		Also provided by voluntary organisations, e.g. Leonard Cheshire Foundation
(k) Special services for blind people	Free radio, reduced rate television licence, books and periodicals in Braille or Moon, guide dogs—these services are often administered through social services departments but not provided directly by them	Separate registration system for 'blind' and 'partially sighted' which, unlike registration as disabled, is medically assessed. Often includes elderly people whose sight is failing through age

Service	Type of service provided	Notes
3 Services for the mentally disordered All services described in previous section may also be available for the mentally disordered. In addition the NHS Act 1977 gives powers to provide additional specialist services:	Special day centres, sheltered workshops, hostels	
4 Services for the elderly Many of the services previously described are available for the elderly but in addition a DHSS circular (19/71) lists the services which the local authorities are empowered to provide specially for the elderly as follows:	(i) To provide meals and recreation in the home and elsewhere (ii) To inform the elderly of services available to them and to identify elderly people in need of services (iii) To provide facilities or assistance in travelling to and from their homes for the purpose of participating in services provided (iv) To assist in finding suitable households for boarding elderly persons (v) To provide visiting and advisory services and social work support (vi) To provide practical assistance in the home including assistance in carrying out adaptations or providing additional facilities to secure greater safety, comfort or convenience	

	(vii) To contribute to the cost of employing a warden or welfare function in warden-assisted housing schemes	
	(viii) To provide warden services for occupiers of private housing	
Residential accommodation	Old people's homes	Originally provided under Part III of the 1948 National Assistance Act hence often referred to as 'Part III accommodation'. Charges on a means tested basis. Privately owned residential and rest homes for elderly people are registered as residential homes by the local authority. Homes which provide nursing care must be registered as nursing homes by the district health authority. Homes which provide both forms of care must be registered with both authorities
	Sheltered (warden assisted) accommodation usually flats or bed-sitting rooms	Provided in association with local authority housing department
5 *Services for other groups*		
e.g. vagrants, alcoholics, battered women	Residential services—hostels of various kinds, with or without social workers' support	Services vary greatly from area to area. Special schemes in city areas funded by the Urban Aid Programme
	Day services—clubs and day centres of various kinds	

Service	Type of service provided	Notes
6 Family practitioner services (a) Medical (general practitioner)	Primary medical care as defined in Chapter 5. GP is contracted to provide services 24 hours a day and 7 days a week and is responsible for arrangements to cover his absence Some GPs provide special services, e.g. obstetrics, family planning Emergency treatment is available to anyone	See Chapter 5 Individuals register with GP of their choice; GP also has the right to accept or not accept a particular patient A patient who cannot find a GP willing to accept him/her will be allocated to a GP by the FPC. List of local GPs is available from Post Office or Family Practitioner Committee
(b) Dental services	Dental examination. Dental treatment. Supply of dentures. Preventive measures (e.g. fluoride treatment) not usually available as NHS but may be available privately	Lists of local dentists are available from Family Practitioner Committee. Patients do not register with a dentist as with a GP. Some dentists give only limited NHS services. Examinations free of charge but charges up to specified maximum payable for treatment except for: (i) children under 16 years, (ii) children over 16 years attending full-time school (iii) expectant and nursing mothers (i.e. within 1 year of delivery) (iv) persons in receipt of FIS or SB, (v) other persons with low income. See leaflet NHS 4

(c) Ophthalmic services

Ophthalmic opticians can examine and test eyes, prescribe spectacles and supply them. Dispensing opticians can only supply spectacles prescribed elsewhere. Ophthalmic medical practitioners can examine and test eyes and prescribe glasses but do not supply them. More complicated eye disorders are treated by the hospital services.

Initial eye test no longer depends on referral by GP.

Examination and eye tests are free, but there is a charge for spectacles except for under-fives, schoolchildren and people with low incomes (see leaflet F1 available from opticians). This exemption covers only the cheapest NHS frames; more expensive NHS frames and privately manufactured frames have to be paid for and if chosen frames do not fit NHS lenses the lenses have to be paid for as well

(d) Pharmaceutical services

Supply of drugs, dressings and appliances prescribed by GP, by hospital outpatient department, or by a dentist

Each item is charged for, except for patients in the following groups:

(i) children under 16 years

(ii) men over 65 years and women over 60 years

(iii) expectant and nursing mothers (i.e. within one year of birth)

(iv) people suffering from certain specified conditions

(v) people receiving SB or FIS

(vi) war pensioners for treatment of their accepted war disabilities

(vii) people with low incomes

Non-exempt persons who need frequent prescriptions can buy a 'season ticket'. See leaflet M11

C SOCIAL SERVICES PROVIDED BY OTHER AGENCIES

Service	Agency	Type of service provided
(a) Housing	Local authority housing department (non-metropolitan district councils)	(1) Demolition of old housing, building new housing, improvement, management and repair of existing local authority housing (2) Assistance to private house owners—improvement schemes and mortages (3) Responsibility for dealing with homelessness transferred from social services departments under the Housing (Homeless Persons) Act 1977
	Housing associations	Specialise in providing accommodation to meet the special needs of elderly, mentally handicapped, physically disabled or mentally ill people
(b) Education	Local authority education department	(1) Preschool education—nursery schools (2) Primary and secondary education (3) Further and higher education—polytechnics and colleges of further and higher education administered by local authorities, universities by University Grants Committee In addition to the schools and colleges themselves, the following services are also provided:

(i) school health service (provided by the NHS, see page 000)
(ii) special schools for handicapped children
(iii) social work (education welfare service)
(iv) school meals
(v) financial grants for fares, maintenance and clothing
(vi) careers advice
(vii) youth and community service (youth clubs)
(viii) grants and awards for further and higher education

(c) Employment services — Manpower Services Commission

Job centres
Rehabilitation and resettlement service for disabled people (disabled resettlement officer) Training Opportunities Scheme (TOPs), Youth Opportunities Programme, Careers Service

(d) Legal services — Legal Aid scheme

Free legal advice from solicitors who choose to participate in the scheme; subject to means test
Further information available from citizens advice bureau

(e) Probation and aftercare — Home office

Supervision of people placed 'on probation' by the courts
Prison welfare—social work support for prisoners' families
After care of ex-prisoners

Appendix 3

Guide to Voluntary Organisations

There are thousands of voluntary organisations and this appendix lists only a few of those most relevant to district nursing. Directories which give more information include:

> Darnbrough A., Kinrade D. (1985). *Directory for Disabled People.* London: Woodhead-Faulkner Ltd.
> Family Welfare Association (published annually). *Guide to the Social Services.* London: Family Welfare Association.
> Family Welfare Association (published annually). *Charities Digest.* London: Family Welfare Association.
> National Council for Voluntary Organisations (1985). *Voluntary Organisations: A NCVO Directory.* London: National Council for Voluntary Organisations.

It is important for nurses working in the community to find out at local level w' ich organisations operate in their area and what services they provide. Information about local services can be obtained from the following sources: public library; town hall or council offices; citizens advice bureau; community health council.

The main types of voluntary organisations are:

1 *Large nationally organised societies* which provide a wide range of services, sometimes acting as the agent of the local authority or the health authority to provide services such as 'meals on wheels', or transport services which the statutory authorities have a duty or the power to provide, e.g. British Red Cross Society, Citizens Advice Bureau, Salvation Army, St John's Ambulance Brigade, Women's Royal Voluntary Service. These organisations have local branches whose address and telephone number will be found in the local telephone directory.

2 *Charities which provide financial help* for certain groups in need, or for research, e.g. National Society for Cancer Relief, Lady Hoare Trust for Physically Disabled Children.

3 *Education and pressure groups* set up to promote understanding and stimulate government action to deal with a particular problem, e.g. National Association for Improvements in the Maternity Services.

4 *Self-help groups* made up of people who suffer from a particular disability, and their relatives. Some of these groups have local branches as well as national offices. The range of services provided varies from area to area, but at national level most of these organisations provide useful information services and act as pressure groups like those in group (3), e.g. Alcoholics Anonymous, Mastectomy Association.

5 *Local 'good neighbour' schemes* run by local churches, local women's organisations etc., which meet particular local needs such as home visiting, transport services, night-sitting, etc. Information about these organisations must be sought at local level from the sources listed above.

The organisations listed below are grouped, somewhat arbitrarily, under nine headings defined by 'client group'. This list is by no means comprehensive but the main organisations in each group can usually provide information about other organisations concerned with the same client group.

The blind

Royal National Institute for the Blind, 224 Great Portland St, London W1N 6AA

There are many organisations which provide specialist services for the blind and many 'special interest' groups covering a variety of recreational activities. Several are listed in directories mentioned above.

Carers

Association of Carers, 21–23 New Road, Chatham, Kent ME4 4JQ

Association of Crossroads Care Attendant Schemes Limited, 94 Coton Road, Rugby, Warwickshire, CV21 4LN

National Council for Carers and their Elderly Dependents, 29 Chilworth Mews, London W2 3RG

The deaf

Royal National Institute for the Deaf, 105 Gower St, London WC1E 6AH

British Association for the Hard of Hearing, 16 Park St, Windsor, Berks. SL4 1LU

Both of these organisations provide specialist advice and information about other organisations, and there are many 'special interest' organisations for deaf people.

Mental handicap, mental illness, behavioural problems

Mental handicap

MENCAP (Royal Society for Mentally Handicapped Children and Adults), 123 Golden Lane, London EC1Y 0RT

This organisation has over 450 local branches and 12 regional offices to provide help and advice for mentally handicapped people.

Mental illness

MIND (National Association of Mental Health), 22 Harley Street, London W1N 2ED

This organisation provides a wide range of services itself, especially through its local branches, and also acts as a coordinator and information centre for many other voluntary organisations concerned with mental illness and mental health.

Specialist organisations of particular relevance to district nurses include:

Al-Anon Family Groups, 61 Great Dover St, London SE1 4YE

Alcoholics Anonymous, PO Box 514, 11 Redcliffe Gardens, London SW10 9BG (for local branches see local telephone directory)

Depressives Associated, 19 Merleys Way, Wimborne Minster, Dorset BH21 1QN

Open Door Association, c/o 447 Pensby Rd, Heswall, Merseyside L61 9PQ (agoraphobia sufferers)

Phobics Society, 4 Cheltenham Rd, Charlton-cum-Hardy, Manchester M21 1QN

Samaritans, 17 Uxbridge Road, Slough, Bucks (over 100 local branches—see local telephone directory)

Physically disabled and handicapped (general)

Association of Disabled Professionals, The Stables, 73 Pound Rd, Banstead, Surrey SM7 2HU

Disabled Living Foundation, 380–384 Harrow Road, London W9 2HU

Disablement Income Group, Attlee House, Toynbee Hall, 28 Commercial St, London E1 6LR

Disability Alliance, 25 Denmark St, London WC2 8NJ

Motability, Boundary House, 91–93 Chaterhouse St, London EC1M 6BT

PHAB (Physically Handicapped and Able Bodied), 42 Devonshire St, London W1N 1LN

Royal Association for Disability and Rehabilitation (RADAR), 25 Mortimer St, London W1N 8AB (Formerly Central Council for the Disabled)

SPOD (Committee on Sexual Problems of the Disabled), 40 Victoria St, London SW1

Wheelchair Action, 2 Merthyr Terrace, Barnes, London SW13

Specific disorders

Association for Spina Bifida and Hydrocephalus (ASBAH), 22 Upper Woburn Place, London WC1H 0EP

Back Pain Association, Grundy House, Teddington, Middx TE11 8TD

British Association of Cancer United Patients and their families and friends (BACUP), 121/123 Charterhouse Street, London EC1M 6AA

British Diabetic Association, 10 Queen Anne St, London W1M 0BD

British Epilepsy Association, Crowthorne House, Bigshotte, New Wokingham Road, Wokingham, Berks. RG11 3AY

British Migraine Association, Evergreen, Ottermead Lane, Ottershaw, Chertsey, Surrey KT16 0HJ

British Rheumatism and Arthritis Association, 6 Grosvenor Crescent, London SW1X 7ER

Cancer Aftercare and Rehabilitation Society (CARE), Lodge Cottage, Church Lane, Timsbury, Bath BA3 1LF

Chest, Heart and Stroke Association, Tavistock House North, Tavistock Square, London WC1 9JE

Coeliac Society, PO Box 181, London NW2 2QY

Colostomy Welfare Group, 38–9 Eccleston Square, London SW1V 1PB

CRACK (the young arm of the Multiple Sclerosis Society), 286 Munster Road, Fulham, London SW6 6BE

Cystic Fibrosis Research Trust, 5 Blyth Road, Bromley, Kent BR1 3RS

Haemophilia Society, PO Box 9, 16 Trinity St, London SE1

Ileostomy Association, 1st floor, 23 Winchester Road, Basingstoke, Hants.

Invalids At Home Trust, 23 Farm Avenue, London NW2

Leukaemia Society, 45 Craigmoor Avenue, Queens Park, Bournemouth

Marie Curie Memorial Foundation, 124 Sloane St, London SW1X 9BP

Mastectomy Association, 1 Colworth Road, Croydon, Surrey CR0 7AD

Multiple Sclerosis Society, 286 Munster Rd, London SW6 6BE

Muscular Dystrophy Group, Nattrass House, 35 Macaulay Rd, London SW4 0QP

National Ankylosing Spondylitis Society, 4 Beaconsfield Rd, Clifton, Bristol BS8 2TS

National Society for Cancer Relief, 30 Dorset Square, London NW1 6QL

Parkinsons Disease Society, 36 Portland Place, London W1N 3DG

Renal Society, Oak Cottage, Wises Lane, Borden, Sitting-bourne, Kent

Sickle Cell Society, Green Lodge, Barretts Green Rd, London NW10 7AP

Spastics Society, 12 Park Crescent, London W1N 4EQ

Spinal Injuries Association, 5 Crowndale Rd, London NW1 1TU

Urinary Conduit Association, 36 York Rd, Denton, Manchester

Children

BREAK (Davison Morley Trust), 20 Hooks Hill Rd, Shering-ham, Norfolk NR26 8NL (holidays and short-stay emergency care)

Invalid Children's Aid Association, 126 Buckingham Palace Rd, London SW1 9SB

National Association for the Welfare of Children in Hospital, 7 Exton Street, London SE1

National Society for the Prevention of Cruelty to Children, 1 Riding House St, London W1

Voluntary Council for Handicapped Children, 8 Wakley St, London EC1V 7QE

(*Note*: all the societies dealing with specific disorders provide information, advice, and support for parents)

Marriage and family problems

Brook Advisory Centres, 233 Tottenham Court Rd, London W1A 9AE

Family Planning Association, Margaret Pyke House, 27–35 Mortimer St, London W1N 7RJ

Gingerbread (The Association for One-Parent Families), 35 Wellington St, London WC2

National Council for the Divorced and Separated, 13 High St, Little Shelford, Cambridge CB2 5ES

National Marriage Guidance Council, Harbert Gray College, Little Church St, Rugby, Warwicks (*Note*: there are specialist organisations for Jews and for Catholics with marital problems)

National Women's Aid Federation, 374 Grays Inn Rd, London WC1

National Council for One-Parent Families, 225 Kentish Town Rd, London NW5 2LX

Pregnancy Advisory Service, 40 Margaret St, London W1N 7FB

Elderly People

Age Concern England, Bernard Sunley House, 60 Pitcairn Rd, Mitcham, Surrey CR4 3LL (formerly National Old People's Welfare Council)

Counsel and Care for the Elderly, 131 Middlesex St, London E1 7JF

Help the Aged, 16–18 St. James's Walk, London EC1R 0VE

There are also many locally based voluntary organisations which provide a variety of benefits and services for elderly people; information can be obtained from the local branch of Age Concern, whose address and telephone number will be found in the local telephone directory.

Bereavement

Compassionate Friends, 5 Lower Clifton Hill, Clifton, Bristol. (Bereaved parents)

Cruse: National Organisation for Widows and their Children, Cruse House, 126 Sheen Rd, Richmond, Surrey (for widows, widowers and their children)

Guide to Social Security and Other Financial Benefits

The system of financial support provided by the state to individuals in need is highly complex. The government department which is responsible for the main benefits, i.e. social security benefits, is the Department of Health and Social Security, operating through local DHSS offices. Some financial benefits are administered through other departments, e.g. tax allowances through the Inland Revenue Department.

Leaflets about DHSS benefits, including details of who is eligible and how to apply, can be obtained from local DHSS offices, or from the DHSS Information Division, Leaflets Unit, Block 4, Government Buildings, Honeypot Lane, Stanmore, Middlesex HA7 1AY. Leaflet FB2 gives basic information on the social security system of benefits and contains an order form. The level of benefit is adjusted each year.

It is now possible to obtain general advice about contributions and benefits by telephone; dial 100 and ask for Freephone DHSS. A good summary of the system of cash benefits, including the amounts payable, is included in *Guide to the Social Services*, published annually by the Family Welfare Association.

Appendix 5

A Synoptic History of District Nursing

1850–1900

Health services and related legislation	Related nursing events	District nursing	Contemporary events
Population: 18 million	1854 Miss Nightingale takes a party of nurses to Scutari	1854 Mrs Fry's Institute	1854 Cholera epidemic (Dr Snow and the Broad St pump)
1855 John Simon at the Board of Health	1860 Foundation of the Nightingale Nursing School	1859 Mr Rathbone employs a 'district nurse'	1854–56 The Crimean War
1858 Regstration of Doctors Board of Health dissolved	1862 Manchester & Salford Ladies Health Society	1864 District Nursing Ass. in Liverpool, Manchester and Salford	1864 The Geneva Convention
1866 Sanitary Act	1865 Ladies Medical College—gives instruction in midwifery	1868 Mrs Ranyard founds the Bible Women and Nurses Mission	1867 2nd Reform Act (male franchise extended)
1867 Metropolitan Poor Act (Poor Law able to build hospitals)	1887 British Nursing Ass. founded	1874 Metropolitan Nursing Ass. for District Nurse Training set up	1870 Franco–Prussian War (Red Cross used)
1870 Education Act (Foster)	1890 First Preliminary Training School	1887 Queen Victoria Jubilee Institute for Nurses founded (Rosalind Paget the first Superintendent)	1876 Royal Sanitary Inst. founded by Chadwick
1872 Public Health Acts	1894 Training course for health visitors in Buckinghamshire	1888 Rural Nursing Ass. set up	1882 Koch discovers the tubercle bacillus
1875 (urban and rural sanitary authorities)	1892 The first School Nurse (Amy Hughes)	1889 The Jubilee Institute receives a Royal Charter	1890 Diphtheria antitoxin used
1886 Idiots Act	1899 The International Council of Nurses founded		1892 Booth's report Life and Labour in London
1888 Local Government Act (creates county and county borough authorities)			1898 The Boer War (Queen Alexandra Military Nursing Service used)
1890 Lunacy Act (lays down regulations about 'certification')			

1900–1950

Health services and related legislation

- 1901 *Population 33 million*
- 1902 Education Act (Balfour—schools under LEAs)
- 1907 School Medical Inspections
- 1907 Notification of Births Act (permissive)
- 1908 Old Age Pensions Act
- 1908 Children's Act (Child Life Protection)
- 1911 National Insurance Act (Lloyd George)
- 1918 Maternity & Child Welfare Act
- 1918 Education Act (Fisher) (school health service extended)
- 1919 Ministry of Health formed
- 1920 Dawson Report on the Health Services
- 1929 Local Government Act
- 1944 Education Act (Butler)
- 1945 Family Allnces. Act
- 1946 National Health Service Act
- 1948 National Assistance Act

Related nursing events

- 1902 Midwives Act
- 1904 Committee on Nursing Registration
- 1916 College of Nursing Founded
- 1919 Nurses Registration Act (General Nursing Council)
- 1925 Regulations for health visitor training—first examinations with the RSI
- 1925 Student Nurses Ass.
- 1932 The Lancet Commission on Nursing
- 1937 Interdepartmental Com. on Nursing (Athlone)
- 1943 Rushcliffe Committee on pay
- 1943 Nurses Act (Assistant Nurse)
- 1942–45 Horder Committee
- 1947 Working Party on Recruitment & Training

District nursing

- 1902 Village nurse midwifery training in East London
- 1912 Highlands & Islands medical service
- 1918 Maternity & Child Welfare Act Requires home nurses for infectious cases
- 1925 Queen Victoria's Jubilee Inst. becomes Queen's Inst. of District Nursing
- 1928 Supplementary Charter issued to the Queen's Inst.
- 1946 National Health Service Act—district nurses now part of the local authority health services
- 1947 Queen's Inst. offers training to male nurses

Contemporary events

- 1901 *Edward VII*
- 1904 Report of the Interdepartmental Committee on Physical Deterioration
- 1904–9 Royal Commission on the Poor Law
- 1910 *George V*
- 1914–18 *First World War*
- 1918 Representation of the People Act (votes for women)
- 1926 The General Strike
- 1931 Gold Standard suspended
- 1933 Unemployment 22%
- 1933 Nazi revolution in Germany
- 1935 Italy invades Ethiopia
- 1936 *George VI*
- 1938 Nazis seize Austria. Munich Agreement
- 1939 Florey prepares stable penicillin
- 1939–45 *Second World War*
- 1942 Beveridge Report
- 1945 Labour Government (Attlee)

1950–1986

1951 *Population 44 million*
1951 Min. of Health becomes Min. of Housing & Local Gov.
1956 Guillebaud Report on NHS costs
1959 The Mental Health Act
1962 The Hospital Plan
1970 The Peel report on midwifery services
1970 Social Services Act
1971 Industrial Relations Act
1972 White Paper on a Reorganised health service
1974 Reorganisation of the health services
1974 Reorganisation of Local Government Act
1974 Health and Safety at Work Act
1975 Employment Protection Act
1979 Report of the Royal Commission on the NHS
1979 Consultative document on NHS reorganisation
1980 The Health Services Act
1982 NHS reorganisation
1985 NHS management inquiry (Griffiths)
1986 Green Paper—primary health care

1951 Midwives Act
1956 Inquiry into Health Visiting (Jameson)
1962 Health Visitors & Social Workers Training Council
1964 Reform of Nursing Education (Platt)
1966 Committee on Senior Nursing Structure (Salmon)
1969 Joint Board of Clinical Nursing Studies
1972 Committee on Nursing
1974 Halsbury Report
1979 EEC Regulations on Nursing
1979 Nurses, Midwives and Health Visitors Act
1980 New UK Central Council for Nurses, Midwives and Health Visitors set up with National Boards
1983 UKCC and National Boards take over functions
1983 Pay Review Body established
1985 RCN Judge Report
1986 UKCC *Project 2000* (interim report)
1986 Cumberlege Report

1955 Working Party on the Training of District Nurses Panel of Assessors—National Cert. of District Nursing
1959 Revision of GNC syllabus student nurses to have experience in the community
1963 Future Scope of General Practice (Gillie report recommends 'attachment')
1969 Mayston Report; nursing officer grade introduced
1970 Arrangements for extending district nurse training to enrolled nurses Circular 8/70
1972 Revised syllabus
1974 Panel of Assessors issue handbook for training and education centres
1976 Working Party Report of the Panel of Assessors. Proposed that new curriculum replace the old syllabus
1981 New curriculum mandatory
1983 District Nursing Joint Committee established

1952 Conservative victory
1953 *Elizabeth II*
1956 Suez crisis
1957 The Treaty of Rome
1957 Macmillan administration
1964 Labour administration (Wilson)
1970 Conservative administration (Heath)
1973 *Yom Kippur War*—oil and sterling crisis
1973 Britain joins the EEC
1974 The 'three day week'
1974 Labour administration (Wilson)
1975 The 'social contract'
1979 Conservative administration (Thatcher)
1980 Unemployment 2 million
1980 *The Gulf War*
1981 Cuts in public services
1982 *The Falklands War*
1982 Health service cuts (Fowler)
1983 Conservative government re-elected (Thatcher)
1986 Unemployment 3 million

Curriculum in District Nursing

For Registered General Nurses

Produced by the former Panel of Assessors for District Nurse Training. Issued by the National Boards for Nursing, Midwifery and Health Visiting in England, Northern Ireland, Scotland and Wales.

Aim of the course in district nursing

The aim of the course is to prepare a district nurse who is competent to undertake nursing duties in the community and able to accept individual responsibility for the professional standards of her own performance. To satisfy this aim the curriculum has been designed to emphasise the use of a problem-solving approach to district nursing and reference is made throughout to the 'nursing process'.

Course objectives

Four main objectives are incorporated in the outline curriculum and elaborated in the detailed guide. It is intended that the principles are applied throughout the course of study and not limited to specific units of learning.

Objective 1 To assess and meet the nursing needs of patients in the community.

Objective 2 To apply skills and knowledge and to impart them effectively to patients, relatives, other carers and the general public.

Objective 3 To be skilled in communications, establishing and maintaining good relationships and able to coordinate appropriate services for the patient, his family and others involved with delivery of care.

Objective 4 To have an understanding of management and organisation principles within the multidisciplinary team and a positive approach to future developments to meet health care needs.

Entry requirements

The curriculum will make considerable demands upon students and candidates should preferably be in possesion of 5 'O' levels of the General Certificate of Education. To ensure, however, that people with the right qualities for district nursing are not excluded solely on the grounds of lack of academic qualifications, a form of assessment should be devised to select candidates who have the competence and ability to undertake the course. Candidates should be those whose names appear on Part 1 of the professional register of the United Kingdom Central Council for Nursing, Midwifery and Health Visiting, i.e. RGNs or those formerly designated SRN or RGN (Scotland). Further nursing experience since registration is desirable.

Length of course

Course must be of at least 26 weeks duration exclusive of annual leave, planned on the basis of two-thirds theory to one-third practice. This must be followed by a period of supervised practice, the recommended length of which is 12 weeks.

Plan of course

Correlation of theory and practice

Theory and practice should be correlated throughout the course.

Theory

There should be flexibility in planning the timetable to include study blocks or days but some concentration of study at the beginning and end of the course would be expected.

Practical experience

One-third of the course should be allocated to practical experience. The student should be placed with a practical work teacher who would assume responsibility for planning the student's practical work programme, allocating a controlled caseload, and teaching the skills of district nursing within a primary health care team.

Supervised practice

The student should be placed in a setting where she will continue to work as a district nurse and be a member of a primary health care team. The student should be supervised throughout the period by a named person who has attended a course for supervisors of supervised practice.

Associated training

It is desirable that training should take place in association with health visitors and social work students. There are also obvious advantages to district nurse students if practical work teachers can be based in practices which are used for general medical practice vocational training and such practices should be utilised wherever possible.

Examination procedure

Examination for the Certificate in District Nursing will be based upon:

(a) Principles and practice of district nursing

A written examination in the principles and practice of district nursing and related subjects is taken at the end of the course. This paper will be a minimum of three hours. Training institutions have discretion in the way this is planned.

(b) Assessment of course work

During the course the student will be required to undertake four assignments; it will be for the training institution to determine the type of assignment, e.g. extended essays, case studies, project work. These should be marked internally but external assessors should be appointed to check the assessment procedure and to examine some of the work produced by the students.

(c) Assessment of taught practice

The practical work teacher will be required to make a continuous assessment of the student's progress throughout the 6 months of the course and report upon the student having reached a level of competence to proceed to supervised practice.

(d) Assessment of supervised practice

The supervisor will be required to make a continuous assessment of the student's progress throughout the period of supervised practice.

Award of the Board's certificate leading to the qualification District Nurse will be dependent upon the student achieving a pass in (a), (b), (c) and (d).

Approval of centres and courses

A formal application must be made to the Boards by any training institution wishing to conduct a course in district nursing. Guidance on approval procedures is issued separately.

OUTLINE CURRICULUM COURSE CONTENT

Skills	Knowledge	Attitudes
	Principles and practice of district nursing techniques. Development of social policy	
1 Information gathering	Interviewing methods. Principles and problems of confidentiality	Awareness of the need to preserve confidentiality
2 Observation	Effect of the environment on the individual. Sociological concepts and their significance in health and disease	Respect for the values held by all persons with whom she comes into contact
3 Assessment of physical, social and emotional needs	Criteria for assessment of total needs of individual and groups of patients. Normal and disordered body functions. Psychological concepts and their significance in health and disease. Needs of crisis groups	Demonstration of an enquiring mind
4 Planning of care	Problem solving techniques. Programmes of care to meet assessed needs. Referral techniques	Respect for the patients' and carers' perception of their needs

5 Implementing care	Organisation of the nursing environment. Dietetics. Drugs and other therapeutic measures for conditions commonly met in the community. Rehabilitation	Respect for patient's property
6 Evaluation	Methods of evaluating care. Prevention of further ill health. Promotion of health	Awareness of the need for continual reassessment of care provided and willingness to modify previously made plans
7 Supportive care	Determinants of stress in the family situation	Acceptance of professional responsibility for the welfare of people other than patients
8 Imparting skill and knowledge	Introduction to principles of learning and teaching. Skills analysis. Demonstration and teaching techniques. Self analysis. Assessment of performance of others. Programmes of nurse education and training	Understanding of the importance of teaching and willingness to accept this responsibility

Appreciation of the value of health education in its widest sense and and need to develop an individual approach as necessary

Willingness to learn and relearn |

Skills	Knowledge	Attitudes
9 Communication	The basic principles of written and verbal communication. Record keeping. Report writing.	Awareness of communication as an important part of total patient care
10 Establishment and maintenance of effective relationships	The dynamics of individual and group relationships. The psychological and social needs of families. The role and function of the primary care team. The management structure of the National Health Service. An outline of central and local government	Acceptance of her responsibility as clinical nursing expert within the primary care team
11 Coordination of services	The policies, structure and contribution of other health, social and voluntary services	Appreciation of, and respect for, the skilled contribution of others concerned with patient care
12 Organisation and supervision of the nursing team	The principles of management as adapted to the needs of community care. Basic understanding of the principles of motivation.	Appreciation of the importance of teamwork. Willingness to accept managerial responsibility
13 Appreciation of methods of critical investigation	Development of new procedures and techniques. Information retrieval and use of resources. Ethical, legal, professional implications of research	Awareness of the value of research and its contribution to better patient care
		Respect for human dignity

Selected Relevant Official Reports, Related Legislation

1842 *Report on the Sanitary Conditions of the Labouring Population* (Edwin Chadwick). Edinburgh University Press.

1892 *Report of Life and Labour in London* (Charles Booth). London: Macmillan.

1904 *Report of the Interdepartmental Committee on Physical Deterioration.* Gave rise to much of the social legislation 1905–1913, including the School Health Service.

1909 *Report of the Poor Law Commission*, including the Minority Report by Beatrice Webb.
Minority report recommended a 'comprehensive health service based on local government'—blueprint for subsequent reports.

1911 *The National Insurance Act.*
Established the 'insurance principle' as a means of providing a limited health service.

1919 *The Nurses Registration Act.*
General Nursing Councils set up.

1920 *Report on the Future Provision of Medical and Allied Services* (Dawson).

1937 *Report of the Interdepartmental Committee on Nursing* (Athlone).
Recommended the Assistant Nurse.

1942 *Report on Social Insurance and Allied Services* (Beveridge).
The basis of most postwar social legislation.

1946 *The National Health Service Act.*
NHS came into being 1 July 1948.

1955 *Report of the Working Party on the Training of District Nurses.*
Recommended the National Certificate of District Nursing.

1956 *Report of the Inquiry into Health Visiting* (Jameson).

1962 Health Visitors and Social Workers Training Council set up.

1963 *Report on the Future Scope of General Practice* (Gillie).
Encouraged attachement of nursing staff to general practice.

1966 *Report of the Committee on Senior Nursing Staff Structure* (Salmon).
Recommended a new simplified structure of nurse managers to match the National Health Service structure.

1968 *Report of Local Authority and Allied Social Services* (Seebohm)
Recommended setting up social services departments.

1969 *Report on the Management Structure in the Local Authority Nursing Service* (Mayston). London: DHSS.

1971 *Report of the Committee on the Organisation of Group Practice* (Havard Davis).

1972 *Report of the Committee on Nursing* (Briggs).

1974 *The Reorganisation of the Health Services Act.*

1974 *Report of the Committee of Inquiry into Pay and Related Conditions for Nurses* (Halsbury).

1976 *Report of the Working Party of the Panel of Assessors on the Education and Training of the District Nurse* (Carr). London: DHSS.

1976 *Report on the Future of Child Health Services. 'Fit for the Future'* (Court).

1979 EEC Directives for Nurses comes into force.

1979 *The Nurses Midwives and Health Visitors Act.*
Established UKCC and National Boards.

1979 *Report of the Staffing of Mental Handicap Residential Care* (Jay).

1980 The new curriculum for district nurse training issued; came into force 1981. London: DHSS.

1980 *Report on the education and training in district nursing for the enrolled nurse.*

1980 *Health Services Act.*

1981 *Patients First* report (basis for 1982 reorganisation).

1981/82 Arrangements for restructuring the National Health Service into district health authorities under the provisions of the Health Services Act (1980).

1983 *NHS Management Inquiry* (Griffiths).

1985 *The Education of Nurses: A New Dispensation* (Judge).

1986 *Review of Community Nursing Services in England* (Cumberlege).

1986 *Primary Health Care: An Agenda for Discussion* (Green Paper).

1986 UKCC. *Project 2000.* London: UKCC.

(Unless otherwise specified, these reports are published by Her Majesty's Stationery Office, London.)

Index

Abortion, 375
Accident/emergency services, 374
Acquired immune deficiency
    syndrome (AIDS), 25, 350,
    351, 358–9
Acute illness, patient with, 218–21
    assessment care, 220
    implementation/evaluation, 220–1
    planning care, 220
Adaptations in the home, 381
Adolescence, 50–1
Adulthood, 51
Aftercare of ex-prisoners, 387
Ager, J. W., 181
Age Concern, England, 394
Aggleton, P., 105
Aids to daily living, 159, 381
Al-Anon Family Groups, 390
Alcoholics Anonymous, 390
Alcoholism, 23, 211
    services, 383
Allen, I., 229
*All our Tomorrows: Growing Old in
    Britain* (BMA, 1986), 229–30
Ambulance service, 375
Amendment Act (1834), 333
Anderson, W. F., 232
Antecedents, 39
Anticipatory grief, 250
Anxiety, 41–3
Approaches to care, 97–9
Aristotle, (348–322 BC), 347
Aseptic technique, 157–9
Assessment man, 116, 117 (Fig.)
Assessment of need, 112–32
    assessment of carers, 125
    assessment of environment, 123–4
    assessment of patient, 124–5
    barriers to communication, 121

gathering information, 116–29
    before first visit, 118–19
    first visit, 119
    interviewing, 119–21
    information required, 112–13
    measurement, 121–3
    needs, 114–16
    nursing history, 113–16
    nursing history chart, 126–7
    where to keep, 128–9
Assistant nurse, 319
Association of Carers, 240, 389
Association of Crossroads Care
    Attendent Schemes, 389
Association of Disabled Professionals,
    391
Association of Spina Bifida and
    Hydrocephalus (ASBAH), 391
Association of Sports Medicine, 199
Atmospheric pollution, 28
Attention, 39
Attitudes, 39–40

Back Pain Association, 391
Backrest, 160
Balint, M., 44
Ball, J. A., 182
Barber, J. H., 223
Battered woman, services for, 383
Bed cradle, 160
Behaviour
    goal-orientated, 39
    individual, 37–41, 47–53
    reflex, 38
Behaviourist school of psychology,
    36–7
Bereavement, 69
Bereavement visiting, 152
Bevan, Aneurin, 274

Beveridge report (1942), 262–3
Birth rate, 11–12
Black report (*Inequalities in Health*, 1980), 65, 269, 277
Blind people, services for, 381
BMA working party on primary health care, 82–3
Board of Control, 273, 317
Body image disturbance, 45
Body types, 36
Booth, Charles, 300
Booth, William Bramwell (General), 307
Boroch, R. M., 166
Bowel cancer, 23
Bowlby, J., 190, 222
Brain tumour, 211–12
BREAK (Davison Morley Trust), 393
Briggs report (Committee on Nursing, 1972), 298
British Association of Cancer United Patients (BACUP), 252, 391
British Association for the Hard of Hearing, 390
British Council for Rehabilitation of the Disabled, 205
British Diabetic Association, 392
British Epilepsy Association, 392
British Migraine Association, 392
British Rheumatism and Arthritis Association, 392
British Sports Association for the Disabled, 205
Brocklehurst, J. C., 235
Bronchitis, chronic, 24, 25–6
Brook Advisory Centres, 393
Broome, W. E., 158
Brown, G. W., 69
Bruce, N., 92, 93, 219
Buttimore, A., 219

Caird, F. I., 232
Cancer Aftercare Rehabilitation Society (CARE), 392
Caplan, G., 151
Car accidents, 28, 29

Care in the Balance (L. Hockey, 1968), 276, 277
Carers
    burn-out, 173, 226
    evaluation of, 173
    looking-glass self, 173
    of elderly people, 240–1
    role fatigue/disillusionment, 223
Carr, C., 250
Case conference, 92, 174–5
Castledine, G., 105, 108
Central Council for the Disabled, 205
Central Midwives Board, 318
Central nervous system, 38
Central sterile services department (CSSD), 158
Cerebral accident, 211
Certificate of Higher Education, 320
Certificate of Industrial Nursing, 318
Certificate of Social Service, 298
Cervical cancer, 24
Chadwick, Edwin, 16, 269, 277
Changing patterns of health and disease, 15–18
Chalmers, H., 105
Changing plan of care, 172–3
Chapman, C., 44 (Fig.)
Charity Organisation Society, 307
Chemical toilet, 159
Chest, Heart and Stroke Association, 392
Child abuse (non-accidental injury), 221, 295–6, 349
Child health clinics, 376
Childhood, 50
Children
    in care, 379
    problem, 214–15
    sick, 189–96
        assessments, 191–2
        evaluation of care, 195
        implementation of care, 194
        planning care, 192–4
        reasons for keeping at home, 190–1
Children Act (1975), 295
Children and Young Persons Act (1963), 295

Chiropody, 378
Cholera, 16–17
Chronically Sick and Disabled
    Persons Act (1970), 197, 200,
    296
Chronic illness, patient with, 221–6
    assessment for care, 223–4
    evaluation, 226
    intervention, 226
    planning care, 224–6
    retraining, 224
    role reversal, 224
Cirrhosis of liver, social class
    differences, 65
Citizens Advice Bureau, 205
Clark, J., 106
Clark, M., 222
Clements, I. M., 106, 116
Clinic-based services, 79
Clinic nurse, 87
Code of Professional Conduct for the Nurse,
    Midwife and Health Visitor
    (1984), 170
Coeliac Society, 392
Collaboration, 156–7
College of Midwives, 317–18
College of Nursing, 315–16
Collier, M. M., 182
Colostomy Welfare Group, 392
Commission on Housing (1885), 291
Committee on Future Scope of
    General Practice, 277
Committee on Nursing (Briggs
    report, 1972), 298, 320
Committee on Physical Deterioration
    (1904), 302
Committee on Residential Care for
    the Mentally Handicapped
    (Jay committee), 298
Committee on Senior Nursing
    Structure (Salmon committee,
    1966), 312, 324–5
Committee on Sexual Problems for
    the Disabled (SPOD), 391
Commode, 159
Communication, 156–7
Community, 71–5

rural, 73
urban, 73–4
Community care, role-reversal, 77–8
Community Health Council, 205
Community hospital, 78–9
Community mental handicap nurse,
    87
Community nursing, 19th century,
    333–6
Community psychiatric nurse, 87, 88,
    214, 297
Community Psychiatric Nurses
    Association, 214, 297
Community services
    child health clinics, 376
    chiropody, 378
    dental, priority, 378
    district nursing, 376
    health education, 377
    health visiting, 376
    immunisation, 377
    loan of equipment, 378
    school health service, 302–3, 377
    welfare foods, 377
Compassionate Friends, 252, 394
Compensation, 42
Computers, 129
Conditioning, 40–1
Confidentiality, 349–50
Contract of Employment Act (1972),
    364
Convalescence, 375
Conversion hysteria, 42
Coordination, 156–7
Copperman, H., 251
Coronary heart disease, 23, 24
Council for the Education and
    Training of Health Visitors,
    89, 318
Counsel and Care for the Elderly, 394
Counselling, 154–6
Counselling, Help and Advice
    Together (CHAT), 300
Court report (*Fit for the Future; Report*
    of the Committee on Child Health
    Services, 1976), 194, 200, 304
CRACK, 392

Criminal activities, suspicions of, 352
Cruse: National Organisation for Widows and their Children, 252, 394
Cultural differences, 57–9
Culture, 57
Cumberlege report *see Neighbourhood Nursing: a focus for care*
Curriculum in District Nursing for State Registered Nurses and Registered General Nurses (1978), 98
Curtis report, 294
Cystic Fibrosis Research Trust, 392

Dahrendorf, R., 309
Data Protection Act (1985), 355–6
Davison, V., 157
Day care, 379
Day centre, 381
Day surgery, 219–20
Death rate, 12
Declaration of Alma Ata (WHO, 1978), 81
Demographic changes, 11–14
Dental caries, 23, 29
Dental services, 384
  priority, 378
Depression, 212–13
Depressives Associated, 391
Diagnostic investigations, 374
Diet, faulty, 23
Diploma in Nursing, 318
Director of nursing services, 286
Disability
  assessment, 200–3
  definition, 97
  implementation/evaluation, 207–8
  physical, 199–200
  planning care, 203–6
  sexual problems, 206
Disabled allowance, 205, 391
Disabled Living Foundation, 224–5, 391
Disabled Persons (Employment) Act, 296
Disablement resettlement officer, 205
Discharge from care, 175–7

Discharge from hospital, 219
Diseases, self-inflicted, 22–5
  alcoholism, 23
  drug addiction, 23
  smoking associated, 24
  venereal, 24
Disengagement, 53
Disposal of dirty dressings/used instruments, 159
District enrolled nurse (DEN), 84–5
District nurse, 79, 84
  attachment to general practice, 79
  definition, 174
  duties/position, 361–2
  increase in workload, 270–1
  industrial action, 365–7
  labour laws, 364–7
  number, 270
  role and function, 107–10
  prescription of medications, 327
  role as rehabilitation progresses, 104 (Fig.)
  safe practitioner, 342–4
  social conditions affecting role, 32
  stress on, 363
  working day (1893), 8–11
District nursing
  as profession, 339–42
  curriculum for Registered General Nurses, 400–6
  development, 333–45
  nature of, 101–11
  settings, 78–80
  synoptic history, 396–9
  work load, 141
District Nursing Joint Committee, 321
Diverticular disease, 23
Divorce, 30
Dobbs, J., 151, 183, 218, 230
Dorothy House (Bath), 249
Dressing packs, Hampshire, 158
Drive, 39
Drug addiction, 23
Drug administration, 162–4
  controlled drugs, 164–5
Dunnell, K., 151, 183, 218, 230

Duties and Position of the Nurse, The
  (Royal College of Nursing),
  361

Education, 386
Education Act (1902), 291, 301
Education (Administrative
  Provisions) Act (1907), 302
Education Act (1944), 296, 301–2
Education Act (1975), 298
Education Act (1981), 197, 302, 303,
  304
Education service, 301–2
Ego integrity, 53
Elderly people, 228–53
  carers, 240–1
    elderly children, 14
  diseases/disabilities, 22
  drugs/drug-containers, 233
  hypothermia associated, 232
  falls, 234
  health education, 230–1
  hypothermia, 231–3
  incidence, 228
  living in own homes, 229–30
  NHS nursing homes, 229
  residential care, 228–9, 383
    short-stay, 229
  services for, 298, 382–3
  sex, 237
  use of health services, 13, 14 (Fig.)
  see also Psychogeriatric care
Eliopoulous, C., 252
Employment Protection Act (1975),
  364
Employment protection legislation,
  364–5
Employment Resettlement Centre,
  205
Employment services, 307, 387
Enrolled nurses, 319
Environment
  control and personal freedom, 28
  new hazards, 28
  physical, 25–8
  services, 27
  social, 29–31

Environmental health services, 378
Equipment
  loan, 378
  use, 159–61
Erikson, E., 51, 53
Erikson, R., 116
Ethics, 346–56
  communication about colleagues,
    353–4
European Community regulations,
  327–8
Evaluation, 170–86
  carers, 173–4
  district nurse's responsibility, 174
  changing plan of care, 172–3
  definition, 170
  goals of care, 171–7
  nursing performance, 178–82
    assessment, 179
    evaluation, 180
    implementation, 179–80
    planning, 179
    recording, 177–8
    superior/subordinate, 181–2
    system of care, 182–4
Experience, individual, 36–7
Extravert, 36

Families in Stress (S. Harrison), 191
Family, 66–71
  definition, 30
  extended, 67
  illness and, 69, 70–1
  nuclear, 67
  of origin, 67
  of marriage, 67
  role in care, 71
Family Planning Association, 393
Family planning nurse, 87
Family planning service, 377
Family practitioner committee, 286–7
Family practitioner services, 384
Feedback, 150
Feeling the Pulse (L. Hockey, 1966),
  276
Fenwick, Bedford, 314
Fever nursing, 313

Financial benefits, 395
*Fit for the Future: Report of the Committee
on Child Health Services* (Court
report, 1976), 194, 200, 304
Fletcher, R., 67
Fluoride, 29
Frail elderly patients, 153
Fry, Elizabeth, 333

General Nursing Councils, 316
Disciplinary and Penal Committee,
341
General practitioners, 81
group practice, 81
Genetic counselling, 375
Gifts, 360
Gilmore, M., 92, 93, 219
Gingerbread (Association for One-
Parent Families), 393
Goldberg, K., 253
Goldstone, L. A., 182, 183
Goldthorpe, J. H., 64 (Table)
Good neighbour services, 89
Group(s), 56–76
attitudes, 57
primary, 56
values, 57
Group teaching, 153
Guide to the Social Services (Family
Welfare Association), 395
Guillebrand Committee (1953), 263

Haemophilia Society, 392
Hall, C., 218
Hamby, R. C., 233
Hand washing, 158
Handicap
definition, 197
mental *see* Mental handicap
Handicapped/disabled, service for
aids/adaptations in home, 381
holidays/outings, 381
meals on wheels, 380
occupational therapy, 380
residential services, 381
social clubs, 381
social work service, 381

telephone, 381
transport facilities, 381
*Handicapped and Impaired in Great
Britain* (Harris report, 1971),
197
Happier Old Age, A—a discussion document
(DHSS, 1978), 299
Hardie, J., 240
Harris report (*Handicapped and
Impaired in Great Britain* (1971),
197
Harrison, S., 191
Hawthorn, P. J., 190
Health, WHO definition, 103
Health at School (W. Nash, M.
Thruston, M. Baly, 1985), 296
Health care expenditure
international companions, 260–1
per capita, 261 (Table)
Health centres, 81
treatment room, 79
*Health Divide, The: Inequalities in Health
Care in the 1980s* (Health
Education Council, 1987), 269
Health education, 151, 377
primary prevention, 151
secondary prevention, 152
tertiary prevention, 152–3
Health education officer, 153
Health and Safety at Work etc. Act
(1975), 365
Health services
internationl comparison, 260–1
nineteenth century, 292 (Fig.)
Health Services Supervisory Board,
284
Health of Towns Commission (1845),
313
Health visitor, 83–4, 318
training, 314, 318
Heartbreak death, 213
Hector, W., 251
Help the Aged, 394
Henderson, V., 101, 106, 107, 114–15,
165
Hibiscol, 158
Hibiscrub, 158

Hibitane-impregnated tissue, 158
Himsworth, Sir Harold, 340
HIV virus, 24
Hockey, L., 84, 85, 183, 201, 219
  Care in the Balance (1968), 276, 277
  Feeling the Pulse (1966), 276
  Home from Hospital (M. Skeet), 139,
    276, 277
Home helps, 380
Horder report (Report of the Nursing
    Reconstruction Committee), 319
Hospice, 246
Hospital-based specialist services
  abortion, 375
  convalescence, 375
  diagnostic investigations, 374
  infertility and genetic counselling,
    375
  occupational therapy, 374
  physiotherapy, 374
  sexually transmitted diseases, 375
  social work, 375
Hospital car service, 375
Hospital services
  accident/emergency, 374–5
  inpatient care, 374
  maternity services, 374
  outpatient consultation, 374
Household, definition, 30
Housing, 27–8, 386
Housing Acts (1885, 1890), 305
Housing services, 305–7
  rights of tenants, 306–7
Hunt, J. M., 147
Hunt, M., 92, 93, 219
Hyperactivity, 42
Hypothermia, 231–3

Identification, 42
Identification of problems, 129–31
Ileostomy Association, 392
Illness
  definitions, 43–4
  emotional responses, 45
  individual responses, 44–5
  perceptions, 44
  religious attitudes, 59

Illness behaviour, 44
Immigrants, 57–8
  integration, 58
Immunisation, 377
Impairment, definition, 197
Implementation of plan, 146–69
  teaching patient, 147–53
  teaching personnel, 153–4
Individual
  human uniqueness, 34–5
  people as, 34–5
Individual care, nursing process and,
    106–7
Inequalities in Health (Black report,
    1980), 65, 269, 277
Infant mortality rate, 261
Infancy, 49–50
Infertility, 375
Inpatient care, 374
International Year of Disabled People
    (1980), 197
Introvert, 36
Invalid Children's Aid Association,
    393
Invalids At Home Trust, 392

James, D., 42
Jay Committee (Committee on
    Residential Care for the
    Mentally Handicapped), 298
Jellinik, E. M., 211
Jenkins, S. M., 193
Jones, C., 106

Kant, Immanuel (1724–1804), 348
Kastenbaum, R., 237
Kennedy, R. D., 232
King's College Hospital, School of
    Midwives, 317
Körner, E., 185
Kratz, C. R., 135, 221, 222, 223
Kron, T., 170, 180
Kubler-Ross, E., 244, 247
Kutscher, A., 253

Lady Superintendents, 339
Laing, R. D., 37, 69

Law, 356–62
  conscientious objection, 358–9
  duty of care, 356–8
  nurse's rights, 359
Learning, 40–1
  by patient, 147–50
  see also Health education
Lees, Florence, 335
Legal services, 387
Leisure activities, 25
Leukaemia Society, 392
Liaison between hospital and
      community, 139–40
Liaison nurse, 88–9
Lifting, 161–2
Liverpool Infirmary, 334
Local Authority Social Services Act
      (1970), 278, 294
Local Government Act (1888), 291
Local Government Act (1972), 279,
      294
Lockwood, D., 64 (Table)
Logan, W., 115
Lückes, Miss, 317
Lunacy Commission, 273, 317
Lung cancer, 24

McCathy, M., 221–2
McCarthy, N. C., 133
McClymont, M., 223
MacDonald, J. B., 233
MacDonald, E. T., 233
McFarlane, J. K., 105, 108
McIntosh, J., 141, 231
McKeown, T., 15, 16
Macmillan nurses, 246
Mahler, Halfden, 289
Male nurses, 85
Manic-depressive illness, 212
Marie Curie Memorial Foundation,
      249, 392
Marital breakdown, 216
Marriage guidance counsellor, 216
Maslow, A. H., 115, 136
Mastectomy Association, 392
Maternal mortality, 17–18, 19 (Fig.)
Maternity services, 374

Mathieson, A., 233
Matrons' Council, 315
Maurer, I. M., 157
Maxwell, R., 261
Mayston report, 325
Meals on wheels, 380
Mechanic, D., 44
Medical Act (1858), 314
Medical officer of health, 291
Memory, 40
Mental defence mechanisms, 42–3, 45
Mental handicap, 198–9
  services, 297–8, 382
Mental illness, 209–17
  assessing need for care, 210–13
  drug-induced, 211
  evaluating plan, 216–17
  implementing plan, 215–16
  infection-induced, 211
  planning care, 214–15
  services, 297–8, 382
Mental nursing, 317
Metropolitan Asylums Board, 313
Metropolitan Nursing Association,
      335–6
Metropolitan Poor Act (1867), 313
Middle age, 51–2
Middle-class perceptions, 64 (Table)
Midwifery, domiciliary, 376
Midwives, 87, 317–18
Midwives Act (1902), 318, 337
Midwives Act (1936), 337
Millard, P., 221–2
Milne, A., 92
MIMS (Monthly Index of Medical
      Specialities), 165
Ministry of Health, 316
Ministry of Town and Country
      Planning, 305
Misinterpretation, 39
Misuse of Drugs Act (1971), 164–5,
      355
  modifications (1985), 164–5
Mitchell, P. H., 165
Monitor system, 182
Mood, 36
Morbidity, 21–2

Mortality today, 19
  deaths in age groups, 20 (Fig.)
Motability, 391
Motivation, 39
Muller, H. J., 35
Multiple Sclerosis Society, 392
Munley, A., 247
Muscular Dystrophy Group, 392

National Ankylosing Spondylitis
  Society, 392
National Association of Mental
  Health (MIND), 390
National Association for the Welfare
  of Children in Hospital, 190,
  393
National certificates, 318
National Council for Carers and their
  Elderly Dependents, 390
National Council for the Divorced
  and Separated, 393
National Council of Nurses, 315
National Council for One-Parent
  Families, 394
National Health Service, 259–90
  criticism of, 276–7
  development, 273–90
  distribution, geographically/
    branches of service, 269–71
  financing, 259–72
    allocation, 266
    alternative ways, 267–8
    comparison of price indices, 264
      (Fig.)
    international comparisons, 260
      (Fig.)
    per capita expenditure, 261 (Fig.)
    source of money, 265–6
    total budget, 264–5
  future, 271–2
  reform, 278–9
  reorganisation, 279–81
    criticism of, 281–2
    reorganising, 283–6
  structure, 273–4
    1948, 274, 275 (Fig.)
    1974, 280 (Fig.)

  1984, 285 (Fig.)
  use of, by elderly, 13, 14 (Fig.)
National Health Service Act (1946),
  274, 338, 407
National Insurance Act (1911), 262,
  337, 407
National Insurance (Industrial
  Injuries) Act (1946), 360
National Marriage Guidance
  Council, 393
National Society for Cancer Relief,
  392
National Society for the Prevention of
  Cruelty to Children, 295, 307,
  393
National Women's Aid Federation,
  394
Needs
  Henderson, 114–15
  Maslow, 115, 136
  Roper, 115
Neighbourhood Nursing: a focus for care
  (Cumberlege Report, 1986),
  83, 86, 88, 90, 91
  community nurse management,
    326
  model agreement, 93–4
  nurse practitioner, 218, 323
  training proposals, 323
New towns, 75
Night sitter, 89
Nightingale, Florence, 101
  district nursing, 272
  elements of nursing, 105
  home nursing, 255, 334
  nurse as sanitary missioner, 339
  reforms, 311–14
  school of midwives, 317
  *Suggestions for Improving the Nursing
    Service for the Sick Poor*, 335
  vow not to found a religious order,
    334
Nightingale Fund, 311–12
Noise, 28
Non-accidental injury to children
  (child abuse), 221, 295–6, 349
Normalisation, 198

Norms of behaviour, 57
Norton pressure sore rating scale,
     122–3
Notification of Births Act (1907,
     1915), 303, 337
Nurse, G., 155
Nurse management, 324–5
Nurse practitioner, 218, 323–4, 326–7
Nurse research officers, 344
Nurses Act (1943), 319
Nurses Registration Act (1919), 407
Nurses, Midwives and Health
     Visitors Act (1979), 320
Nurses Working in the Community (K.
     Dunnel & J. Dobbs, 1982),
     151, 183
Nursing
   definitions, 101–3
   problem-solving approach, 107
   process, individual care and, 106–7
Nursing bag, 159
Nursing care plan, 133–45
   abilities of patient/family, 138
   desired outcome of care, 134–5
   group of patients, 141–4
   liaison between hospital and
        community, 139–40
   nursing action, 136–7
   patient's role, 137–8
   people giving care, 138–40
   priority setting, 135–6
   referral to other agencies, 139
   where to keep, 140–1
Nursing education, 319–24
Nursing home registration, 378
Nursing model, 105–6
Nursing organisations, 315–17
Nursing in Primary Health Care (DHSS,
     1977), 108
Nursing schools, 304
Nursing techniques, adapted, 157–62
   aseptic technique, 157–9
   drug administration, 162–4
      controlled drugs, 164–5
   lifting, 161–2
   use of equipment, 159–61
Nutrition, 26–7

O'Brien, J., 198
Observational visits, 177
Occupation, 27
Occupational health nurse, 87
Occupational therapy, 374, 380
Occupier's Liability Act (1957), 359
Oliver, J., 240–1
Old age, 52–3: *see also* Elderly people;
     Psychogeriatric care
Old Age Pension Act (1908), 262
One-parent families, 30
Open Door Association, 391
Ophthalmic services, 385
Order of St. John of Jerusalem, 335
Orem, D. E., 101, 106, 116
Outpatient consultation, 374

Panel of Assessors for District Nurse
     Training, 338, 339
Parasuicide, 213
Parkinson's Disease Society, 392
Parsons, T., 46
Patient(s)
   as people, 3–7
   saving them from themselves,
        351–2
Patient assessment form, 122 (Fig.)
Patients First, 283
Pearson, A., 181
Perception, 38
Peretz, D., 253
Perinatal mortality, 24, 261
Personal social services
   day care, 379
   preventive services, 380
   residental care, 379
   supervision of children in care, 379
Personality, 35–6
   stable/unstable, 212
   traits, 36
   type, 36
Phaneuf, M. C., 182
Pharmaceutical services, 385
Phillipson, C., 230
Phobics Society, 391
Physically Handicapped and Able
     Bodied (PHAB), 391

Physiotherapy, 374
Planning nurse, 87
Plato (427–348 BC), 347
Platt report (*A Reform of Nursing Education*), 319
Policies for care, 255–7
Policies for nursing, 311–29
  developing new roles, 326–7
  interwar years, 317–18
  since establishment of NHS, 318–27
Poor Law, 262, 273
Population, age structure, 11–13
Practice nurse, 86
Pregnancy Advisory Service, 394
Premenstrual syndrome, 213
Prevention and Health (DHSS, 1977) 151
Preventive medicine, 151
Primary health care, 81–2
Primary health care team, 80, 82–9, 277, 287–8
  administrative staff, 86
  members, 83–6
  nucleus team, 83
  nursing staff, 138
  wider team, 87–9
Primary Health Care Teams (Harding report, 1981), 90
Primary medical care, 80–1
Prisoners of war, 212
Probation, 387
Profession
  district nursing as, 339
  hallmarks, 340–1
  is nursing a profession?, 341–2
  nursing as research-based profession, 344–5
Professional Ethic, The (N. Mackenzie), 340
Progress notes, 167
Projection, 42
Psychiatric illness, social class differences, women, 65
Psychiatric social worker, 297
Psychogeriatric care, 234–41
  assessment, 235
  evaluation, 239–41
  implementation, 239
  planning, 237–8
Psychological concepts and nursing, 43
Psychosocial development, 48 (Fig.)
Psychosomatic illness, 42

Qualpacs, 181–2
Queen's Institute of District Nursing, 273, 318, 334
Queen Victoria's Jubilee Institute for Nurses, 336–9
Quirm, S., 70

Rathbone, William, 334–5, 336
Rationalisation, 42
Records
  confidentiality, 354–5
  keeping, 184–5
Redman, B. K., 148
Reedy, B., 86
Referral to other agencies, 139
Reflex behaviour, 38
Reform of Nursing Education, A (Platt report), 319
Refuse disposal, 27
Regression, 42
Rehabilitation, 165–7
Reilly, D. E., 171, 179
Reinforcement, 41
Relieving officer, 293
Religion, 59
Renal Society, 393
Report of Committee on Education of Handicapped Children and Young People (Warnock report, 1978), 200, 302
Report on Confidential Enquiries into Maternal Deaths, 18
Report of Nursing Reconstruction Committee (Horder report), 319
Report of Royal Commission on the NHS (1979), 29
Report on Sanitary Conditions of the Labouring Population of Great Britain (Chadwick, 1842), 16–17, 407

Report on Working Party on the Recruitment and Training of Nurses (Wood report), 319
Reports, official, 407–8
Repression, 40, 42
Research, 344–5
  ethics, 353
Residential care, 379
Resource Allocation Working Party, 269
Respiratory diseases, social class differences, 65
Retirement areas, 74–5
Richardson, I. M., 141, 241
Roberts, F. B., 106, 116
Robertson, J., 190
Robinson, Kenneth, 277
Robinson, Mrs., 334
Robottom, B. M., 193
Rogers, M. R., 102
Rogerson, B., 241
Roper, N., 115
Role reversal, 224
Roy, C., 106
Royal Association for Disability and Rehabilitation (RADAR), 391
Royal British Nurses' Association, 314, 315, 316
Royal College of General Practitioners, 218
Royal College of Nursing, 318
  Research Society, 344
Royal Commission on Health Service (1979), 267, 268
Royal Commission on Local Government (1969), 278, 279
Royal National Institute for the Blind, 389
Royal National Institute for the Deaf, 390
Royal Sanitary Institute, 318
Royal Society for Mentally Handicapped Children and Adults (MENCAP), 390
Rural District Nursing Association, 336
Russell, Bertrand, 348

St. Thomas's Hospital, 312
Salford Ladies Health Society, 313
Salmon Committee (Committee on Senior Nursing Structure, 1966), 312, 324–5
Samaritans, 391
Sartre, Jean Paul, 37, 228
Saunders, C., 246, 247
Schizophrenia, 209
Schmeidman, E. S., 250
Schoenberg, B., 250
School board attendance officer, 293
School health service, 302–3, 377
School meals/milk, 302
School nurse, 87, 214, 303
Schwartz, D., 232
Scottish Home and Health Department, report on district nurse, 108–9
Seat belts, 29
Seebohm, Sir Frederick, 278, 294
Sewage, 27
Sexual behaviour, 24, 206
Sexuality, loss of, 223
Sexual Problems of the Disabled (SPOD), 205
Sexually transmitted disease, 375
Shetland, M. L., 102, 110, 118
Short-term care, 219
Sickle Cell Society, 393
Skeet, M., 139, 152, 201, 219, 220
Smoking, 24
Snow, John, 17
Social class, 60–3
  health/health care, 63–6
Social club, 381
Social conditions, role of nurse, 32
Social interaction, 56
Socialisation, 57
Social network, 60, 61 (Fig.)
Social position, 59–60
Social role, 59–60
Social services, 291–310
  children, 294–6
  elderly *see* Elderly people
  financing, 259–72
  mentally handicapped, 297–8

mentally ill, 297–8
personal, 293–4
physically handicapped, 296–7
poverty, 300–1
reform, 277–8
Social Services Act (1970), 297
Social system, 56
Social worker, 86, 375
Society, 56
Society of Primary Health Care
  Nursing, 87–8
Sociology for Nurses (C. Chapman,
  1977), 44 (Fig.)
Socrates (469–399 BC), 347
Spastics Society, 393
Special schools, 304
Specialist nurses, 87–9
Spinal Injuries Association, 393
Sports injuries, 25
State registration, campaign for,
  314–15
Stevenson, T. H. C., 61
Stigma, 197
Stockwell, F., 222
Stoma therapist, 87
Strang, P., 230
Strehlow, M. S., 153
Stress, 41–3
Student nurse, community
  experience, 153
Sublimation, 42
Suburban housing estates, 74
Suicide, 213
Syphilis, mental illness due to, 209

Teaching, 150
Team
  case conference, 92
  common purposes/goals, 90–1
  communication, 94
  concept, 89–95
  dynamics of teamwork, 90
  management, 92–3
  pooling knowledge and skills, 92
  understanding different roles, 91–2
Technology, effects of, 31–2
Teenage pregnancies, 303

Temperament, 36
Terminal care, 243–52
  assessment for, 245
  evaluation, 251–2
  implementation, 251
  patient's wishes, 352–3
  planning, 352–3
Termination of care, 175–6
Tierney, A., 115
Tinkham, C. W., 133
Titmuss, R., 291
Trade union, independent, 365
Transport to/from hospital
  ambulance service, 375
  expenses for visiting, 376
  hospital car service, 375
  volunteer transport service, 375
Treatment room nurse, 85–6
Treatment room service, 79
Triple-duty nurse, 85
Tuberculosis, death rate, 10, 16
Tudor Hart, J., 65
Turton, P., 231

Unemployment, 31, 293
United Kingdom Central Council for
  Nurses, Midwives and Health
  Visitors (UKCC), 320–1, 338
  Annual Report (1984–5), 286
  Code of Professional Practice, 371–2
  District Nursing Joint Committee,
    321–3
  Professional Conduct Committee,
    363
  Project 2000, 322–3
Unpopular patient, 222
Urinary Conduit Association, 393
Utilitarianism, 348

Vagrants, services for, 383
Values, 39–40
Voluntary Council for Handicapped
  Children, 393
Voluntary organisations, 307–9,
  388–94
Volunteer transport service, 375
Voorhies, E. F., 133

Wandelt, M. A., 181
Ward Sisters' Certificate, 318
Wardroper, Mrs., 312
Warnock report (*Report of the
    Committee on the Education of
    Handicapped Children and Young
    People*, 1978), 200, 302
Water supply, 27
Welfare of Children in Hospital (Platt
    report, 1959), 190
Welfare foods, 377
Welfare officer (housing department),
    293

Welfare state, 293
Werner Beland, J. A., 221
Wheelchair Action, 391
Whitfield, S., 251
Will making, 250, 360
Withdrawal, 42
Wolff, H., 116
Working-class perspectives, 64
    (Table)
World Health Organisation
    definition of health, 103
    health for all by year 2000, 288–9
Worrall, J., 186